SEVENTH EDITION

Handbook of
Patient Care in
Cardiac Surgery

SEVENTH EDITION

Handbook of
Patient Care in
Cardiac Surgery

John H. Lemmer, Jr., MD

The Oregon Clinic
Legacy Good Samaritan Hospital
Clinical Assistant Professor, Department of Surgery
Oregon Health and Science University
Portland, Oregon

Gus J. Vlahakes, MD

Professor of Surgery
Harvard Medical School
Massachusetts General Hospital
Boston, Massachusetts

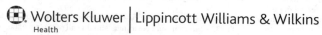

Philadelphia · Baltimore · New York · London
Buenos Aires · Hong Kong · Sydney · Tokyo

Acquisitions Editor: Brian Brown
Senior Product Manager: Erika Kors
Manufacturing Manager: Benjamin Rivera
Marketing Manager: Lisa Lawrence
Design Coordinator: Terry Mallon
Production Services: Aptara, Inc.

7th Edition
© 2010 by Lippincott Williams & Wilkins, a Wolters Kluwer business
530 Walnut Street
Philadelphia, PA 19106
LWW.com

Printed in China

Library of Congress Cataloging-in-Publication Data

Handbook of patient care in cardiac surgery. — 7th ed. / edited by John H. Lemmer Jr., Gus J. Vlahakes.
  p. ; cm.
  Rev. ed. of: Handbook of patient care in cardiac surgery. 6th ed. / John H. Lemmer Jr., Wayne E. Richenbacher, Gus J. Vlahakes. c2003.
  Includes bibliographical references and index.
  ISBN 978-0-7817-7385-0 (alk. paper)
  1. Heart—Surgery. 2. Postoperative care. 3. Therapeutics, Surgical.
I. Lemmer, John H. II. Vlahakes, Gus J.
  [DNLM: 1. Cardiac Surgical Procedures—methods. 2. Perioperative Care—methods. 3. Patient Care Planning. 4. Postoperative Complications—prevention & control. WG 169 H236 2010]
  RD598.B39 2010
  617.4′12—dc22
                                                              2009037994

The publishers have made every effort to trace copyright holders for borrowed material. If they have inadvertently overlooked any, they will be pleased to make the necessary arrangements at the first opportunity.

To purchase additional copies of this book, call our customer service department at (800) 638-3030 or fax orders to (301) 223-2320. International customers should call (301) 223-2300.

Visit Lippincott Williams & Wilkins on the Internet at LWW.com. Lippincott Williams & Wilkins customer service representatives are available from 8:30 am to 6 pm, EST.

10 9 8 7 6 5 4 3 2 1

We dedicate this book to its creators and
our surgical mentors, Drs. Douglas M. Behrendt and
W. Gerald Austen, who coauthored the first four editions and
co-authored with us the fifth edition.
Their teachings, both in person and in print, have greatly
benefited countless surgeons, students, residents, nurses,
and most important, the patients for whom they care.

CONTRIBUTORS

Chapter 7: Management of Infants and Children

Jeff L. Myers, MD, PhD
Lecturer in Surgery, Harvard Medical School
Chief, Pediatric Heart Surgery
Massachusetts General Hospital
Boston, Massachusetts

Chapter 8: Mechanical Cardiac Support and Transplantation

Marco E. Larobina, MB.BS (Hons), FRCAS
Consultant Cardiothoracic Surgeon
The C. J. Officer-Brown Cardiothoracic Unit
The Alfred
Melbourne, Australia

Bruce R. Rosengard, MD, FRCS
Associate Professor of Surgery, Harvard Medical School
Surgical Director, Cardiac Transplantation
Massachusetts General Hospital
Boston, Massachusetts

Begun as a typewritten manual for house officers at Massachusetts General Hospital nearly 40 years ago, *Handbook of Patient Care in Cardiac Surgery* has evolved into its seventh edition. Drs. Douglas M. Behrendt and W. Gerald Austen wrote the first four editions and the subsequent three editions have been produced by Drs. John H. Lemmer, Jr., and Gus J. Vlahakes. Dr. Wayne E. Richenbacher contributed to the sixth edition. Initially, the *Handbook* reflected patient care practices at Massachusetts General Hospital but, over the years, has absorbed influences from the University of Michigan, The University of Iowa, and Legacy Good Samaritan Hospital in Portland, Oregon. In this edition, we are pleased to add the expertise of guest authors Dr. Jeff Myers (Chapter 7; Management of Infants and Children) and Drs. Marco Larobina and Bruce Rosengard (Chapter 8; Mechanical Cardiac Support and Transplantation). Their expertise in these specialized areas of cardiac surgery is a valuable addition to this edition of the *Handbook*.

This handbook is simply a book small enough to fit the hand or the pocket of a white coat. There are larger, more detailed, and multivolume textbooks on the subject of cardiac surgery, particularly with regard to the surgical technical issues. There are also other small comprehensive books on the subject of thoracic surgery, which are in more of an outline form. The *Handbook* falls in between these two ends of the spectrum, with the goal of providing concise, useful information on the essentials of cardiac surgery patient care in a readable fashion. It is centered on the care of the patient before and after heart surgery. Operative management is reviewed with an emphasis on issues that affect the overall perioperative care of the patient, not on how to perform heart surgery.

In the preface to the sixth edition, Drs. Austen and Behrendt wrote: "Just as the sailor who claims never to have run aground probably has not sailed much, the surgeon who claims never to have experienced complications either is not operating much or is not to be believed." The goals of cardiac surgery are to improve the patient's cardiac status and to avoid complications in the process. It is not unusual to achieve the first goal (for example, by replacing a severely stenotic aortic valve) but then to have the end result be marred by a complication (for example, a stroke). It has long been observed that the heart is often more resilient than other organs, and it is often noncardiac complications that lead to a poor operative result. Thus, the *Handbook* places considerable emphasis on the prevention and management of the perioperative complications that will inevitably occur in a busy, contemporary cardiac surgery practice.

In many ways, this is a "how we do it" manual that is a compilation of patient care practices used by us at our hospitals. We do, however, fully realize that there are many ways to achieve excellent results and do not propose that these management suggestions are the only road to success. Our goal is to provide evidence-based recommendations with extensive contemporary literature references that will lead the reader to more detailed information.

While a technically perfect operation can be ruined by poor perioperative care, appropriate management of perioperative problems can often save a less-than-perfect technical result. That is the importance of providing high-quality care to patients undergoing heart surgery. The *Handbook of Patient Care in Cardiac Surgery* has been, and continues to be, a sincere effort to provide guidance in this complex, but rewarding, endeavor. Over time, surgical procedures will evolve, newer agents will replace currently used drugs, and management recommendations will change. But, quoting Austen and Behrendt once again, it will remain true that "the secret of successful patient care is caring for the patient."

John H. Lemmer, Jr., MD

Gus J. Vlahakes, MD

CONTENTS

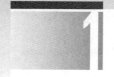

Preoperative Evaluation and Management

Patient care in cardiac surgery begins with a thorough evaluation of the pathophysiology, anatomy, and abnormal hemodynamics associated with the patient's heart disease. Although the referring cardiologist has often performed the necessary diagnostic studies, the surgeon should be certain that the evaluation is complete and that all surgically relevant information needed to plan and perform the proposed operation is obtained. In addition to developing an operative plan, the surgeon must identify the patient's coexisting diseases to estimate the surgical risk and to optimize the surgical outcome. Over the years, there has been a shift to outpatient preoperative management of elective cardiac surgery patients that can complicate the preoperative preparation process. Because the elective surgery patient is most often admitted to the hospital on the day of the operation, it is important to develop a system that ensures that all preoperative issues are addressed prior to admission. This includes the medical history evaluation, physical examination, laboratory and diagnostic tests, anesthesia evaluation, risk assessment, consultations if needed, and patient education regarding the planned operation.

MEDICAL HISTORY

Obtaining a medical history begins with signs and symptoms referable to the patient's heart disease. For patients with coronary artery disease, the presence and severity of angina should be documented and characterized according to the Canadian Cardiovascular Society Angina Classification System (Table 1.1) (1). The patient's need for nitroglycerin tablets provides insight as to the severity of the angina. Severity of the angina, a reflection of the ischemic threshold, helps to determine the urgency of the subsequent evaluation and surgical plan. If the patient suffers from chronic stable angina, the work-up can be performed on an outpatient basis. If, however, the patient presents with accelerating angina, urgent evaluation and treatment are warranted (2). If the patient suffered a previous myocardial infarction, he or she is evaluated for signs or symptoms of congestive heart failure and questioned with regard to palpitations or dizzy spells potentially indicative of ventricular arrhythmias. The history of a recent anterior wall myocardial infarction may indicate the need for preoperative echocardiography to rule out wall motion abnormality and the presence of

TABLE 1.1   Canadian Cardiovascular Society Functional Classification of Angina Pectoris

Class I	Angina resulting from strenuous exertion. Normal activity does not cause angina.
Class II	Slight limitation of normal activity. Walking more than two blocks on the level or more than one flight of stairs at a normal pace causes angina.
Class III	Marked limitation of normal activity. Walking one or two blocks on the level or climbing one flight of stairs at a normal pace causes angina.
Class IV	Angina occurs with any physical activity. Angina may be present at rest.

Adapted from Campeau L. Grading of angina pectoris. *Circulation* 1976;54:522–523.

left ventricular mural thrombus. If clot is identified, this finding may impact the surgical technique and timing of the operation to reduce the chance of clot embolization.

Patients with valvular heart disease may have a history of rheumatic fever or a known cardiac murmur. Such patients may have symptoms of congestive heart failure such as easy fatigability, dyspnea on exertion, orthopnea, paroxysmal nocturnal dyspnea, and ankle swelling. The degree of functional disability present in heart failure may be classified using the New York Heart Association Functional Classification system (Table 1.2) (3). A newer classification system (stages A through D) has been proposed that emphasizes the development and progression of heart failure and treatment options (4). For some patients, the change in activity level over time may have been gradual as the patient often accommodates to the limitations caused by a progressive valvular abnormality. As a result, the decline in functional capability can be insidious. Asking the patient to compare his or her activity level 1 year ago with the current status is useful. The presence of syncopal episodes or angina (both potentially associated with aortic stenosis) and arrhythmias should be noted.

Previous cardiac interventions such as coronary angioplasty or stent placement should be documented. The history of previous cardiac surgery has a major impact on a repeat surgery. For repeat ("redo") procedures, the previous surgeon's dictated operative note should be carefully reviewed. Knowledge concerning previous cannulation sites, the appearance and quality of the native coronary arteries, the location of old bypass grafts, and whether or not the pericardium was closed at the time of the first operation facilitates reoperative heart surgery.

The complete relevant medical history includes family history (including age and cause of death of parents and siblings) and heart disease risk factors. Although the preoperative evaluation is not geared toward immediate risk factor modification, identification of

TABLE 1.2	New York Heart Association Functional Classification for Heart Failure
Class 1	No symptoms with ordinary physical activity
Class 2	Symptoms with ordinary activity. Slight limitation of activity.
Class 3	Symptoms with less than ordinary activity. Marked limitation of activity.
Class 4	Symptoms with any physical activity or even at rest.

Adapted from Criteria Committee of the New York Heart Association. *Diseases of the heart and blood vessels: nomenclature and criteria for diagnosis of the heart and great vessels*, 6th ed. New York: New York Heart Association/Little Brown, 1964.

risk factors will allow targeted education during the patient's convalescence. The commonly recognized risk factors for coronary artery disease are shown in Table 1.3. These factors may be used in an age-weighted scoring system to predict a patient's risk of coronary heart disease (5,6).

The purpose of the medical history and review of systems evaluation is to identify disease processes that impact the conduct and results of the cardiac operation. For example, patients with diabetes have increased rates of postoperative complications including renal insufficiency, stroke, infections, and, in some series, death (7–9). The presence of diabetes may be a contraindication to the use of bilateral internal mammary artery grafts as conduit for coronary bypass grafting (10–12). Patients with diabetes who are insulin dependent may also be at risk for an allergic response to protamine administration (13). These patients benefit from aggressive serum glucose management during the perioperative period (14). Preoperative identification of the patient with diabetes and determination of the degree of glycemic control in the patient with known diabetes are aided by measurement of the patient's serum glycosylated hemoglobin level (hemoglobin A_{1c}). Further discussion regarding serum glucose management is provided in Chapter 3.

Patients with hypothyroidism should receive their thyroid hormone supplementation preoperatively (15). In particular, women with hypothyroidism undergoing coronary artery bypass surgery may be at increased risk for mortality and thus identification and treatment of these patients are warranted (16). Routine preoperative testing of the patients' thyroid-stimulating hormone levels will help to identify the patients with subclinical hypothyroidism.

Patients with a history of excessive bleeding (such as easy bruisability or long-lasting bleeding following a previous operation) or excessive clotting (such as the history of thrombophlebitis) may be more likely to experience postoperative hemorrhagic or thrombotic complications (17). Therefore, inquiry regarding these and related topics should be made and appropriate additional testing should be performed.

TABLE 1.3   Risk Factors for Coronary Heart Disease

Major Independent Risk Factors
  Male gender
  Cigarette smoking
  Hypertension
  Elevated serum total (and low-density lipoprotein) cholesterol
  Low serum high-density lipoprotein cholesterol
  Diabetes mellitus
  Advancing age

Predisposing Risk Factors
  Obesity
  Abdominal obesity
  Physical inactivity
  Family history of premature coronary heart disease
  Psychosocial factors

Conditional Risk Factors
  Elevated serum triglycerides
  Small low-density lipoprotein particles
  Elevated serum homocysteine
  Elevated serum lipoproteins
  Prothrombotic factors (e.g., fibrinogen)
  Inflammatory markers (e.g., C-reactive protein)

From Grundy SM, Pasternak R, Greenland P, et al. Assessment of cardiovascular risk by use of multiple-risk-factor assessment equations: a statement for healthcare professionals from the American Heart Association and the American College of Cardiology. *J Am Coll Cardiol* 1999;34:1348–1359, with permission.

Patients with transient ischemic attacks or a previous stroke are at risk for neurologic complications and should undergo preoperative carotid duplex study (18,19). Carotid ultrasound imaging may be indicated for patients with one or more of the following: carotid bruit, age above 65 years, left main coronary artery stenosis, peripheral arterial disease, and/or a history of smoking (20,21). Patients with aortic stenosis often have a murmur that radiates to the neck that may interfere with the detection of a carotid bruit, and carotid imaging is needed to rule out stenosis. If the carotid duplex identifies a severe internal carotid artery stenosis (>80%), carotid endarterectomy at the time of the cardiac procedure may be indicated depending on the patient's anatomy and symptoms. The recommendation for a combined approach to this problem should, however, be individualized and is dependent on the patient's anatomy and symptoms. Although patients who undergo combined procedures do have increased complication rates, the increase appears to be due to their greater inherent risk and not due to the addition of the carotid procedure to the coronary bypass operation (22–24).

Patients who provide a history of leg claudication or have nonhealing foot ulcers likely suffer from arterial insufficiency. The ankle–brachial index (the ratio of the upper to lower extremity systolic blood pressure) documents the severity of the problem. Patients with lower extremity vascular disease are at increased risk for wound-healing complications following saphenous vein removal. Patients with saphenous vein varicosities, or who have undergone previous vein stripping or sclerosis, may have insufficient venous conduit for use in a coronary bypass operation. For these patients, alternative conduit choices such as bilateral internal mammary arteries and/or radial artery grafts may need to be considered.

The history of cancers that are of particular interest to the cardiac surgeon includes mediastinal tumors and breast carcinoma (25). Both may be associated with previous chest wall or mediastinal surgery and/or posttreatment radiotherapy. In such patients, the mammary arteries should be studied by angiography at the time of cardiac catheterization to rule out radiation-induced stenoses if their use in coronary revascularization is planned. Patients with extensive preoperative radiation therapy have an increased incidence of radiation heart disease, perioperative complications, and reduced survival. Although previous mediastinal radiotherapy is not necessarily a contraindication to sternotomy, it may be associated with sternal radiation-induced necrosis, constrictive pericarditis, and significant intrapericardial adhesions (26,27).

MEDICATIONS

The patient's current medications are carefully reviewed, because these can impact the conduct of an open heart surgery. Patients undergoing coronary artery bypass graft (CABG) surgery are often receiving oral *nitrate* therapy and this is continued up to the time of surgery to avoid precipitating an ischemic event. Likewise, *β-adrenergic blocking agents* are administered preoperatively (and continued after surgery) to reduce perioperative arrhythmias (in particular, atrial fibrillation) and ischemia. Preoperative β-blockers may be associated with reduced operative mortality (28–31). The importance of perioperative β-blocker therapy in patients without contraindications has been well established. In fact, the incidence of β-blocker administration to CABG patients has become a measurable quality indicator for heart surgery programs. It is our practice to continue these drugs in all patients up until the time of surgery, including a dose with a sip of water on the morning of surgery. Patients undergoing CABG surgery who are not taking a β-blocker are started on therapy, most often metoprolol at low dose (12.5 to 25 mg twice daily). Contraindications include hypotension (systolic pressure < 90 mm Hg) and bradycardia (heart rate < 60 beats per minute).

The use of coenzyme A reductase inhibitors, known as *statins*, has become widespread in patients with coronary artery disease. These drugs appear to be of benefit in reducing postoperative morbidity and/or mortality in patients undergoing both cardiac and noncardiac surgery (32–34). They are, therefore, continued up until surgery. For patients undergoing surgery who have dyslipidemia and who are not receiving statin therapy preoperatively, it is begun before operation and continued afterward as indicated. Patients taking these drugs do, however, require follow-up to monitor for potential hepatic toxicity. Arrangements for this should be made at the time of the patient's discharge from the hospital.

Amiodarone is commonly used to treat cardiac surgery patients with rhythm disturbances. Because it has an extended half-life, discontinuation of this medication preoperatively will usually have no impact upon serum levels at the time of the operation and may, in fact, exacerbate the patient's underlying rhythm disorder. Preoperative prophylactic amiodarone administration has a protective effect against postoperative atrial fibrillation (see Chapter 4) (35). It should be recognized that chronic amiodarone administration may be associated with a number of side effects, including corneal microdeposits, optic neuritis, bluish skin discoloration, photosensitivity, hypothyroidism, hyperthyroidism, pulmonary toxicity, peripheral neuropathy, and liver toxicity (36).

Calcium channel blocking agents are generally continued until surgery because withdrawal may increase the risk of coronary artery spasm or acceleration of the ventricular response in patients with chronic atrial fibrillation. Generally, antihypertensive drugs, including *angiotensin-converting enzyme inhibitors* (such as *captopril* and *lisinopril*), *angiotensin II receptor antagonists* (such as *losartan* and *valsartan*), and *diuretics*, are held on the morning of surgery to avoid intraoperative hypotension (37). *Clonidine*, however, is continued until surgery, because abrupt discontinuation of this medication may result in rebound hypertension. *Digitalis* preparations that are being administered for rate control in patients with atrial tachyarrhythmias are usually administered on the day of surgery.

Patients with *insulin*-dependent diabetes receive half their usual dose of insulin on the morning of surgery. This is combined with the administration of a glucose-containing parenteral fluid. Oral glucose-lowering agents (such as *glyburide, glipizide, miglitol, nateglinide*, and *tolazamide*) are not administered on the morning of surgery. The oral hypoglycemic agent *metformin* has been associated with perioperative lactic acidosis and is held for several days before surgery, although this is somewhat controversial (38,39). For the patient who takes steroids (usually *prednisone*) on a chronic basis, a supraphysiologic dose of hydrocortisone [100 mg intravenous (IV)] is given preoperatively.

Patients with unstable angina are frequently maintained on IV *heparin* until surgery, and this generally presents no problem as the heparin is usually reversed intraoperatively by the administration of protamine. For these patients, we usually stop the heparin infusion 2 to 4 hours prior to arrival in the operating room unless they are very unstable or have very critical coronary anatomy. In contrast to unfractionated heparin, *low-molecular-weight heparin* is not effectively neutralized by protamine, and preoperative treatment (within 12 to 24 hours) is associated with increased bleeding and transfusions in CABG patients (40,41). We, therefore, recommend that the patient be switched from low-molecular-weight heparin to unfractionated heparin at least 24 hours prior to surgery. Patients who have received preoperative heparin (especially unfractionated) are, however, more likely to experience a reduced response to heparin administered during surgery, so-called heparin resistance, which is most likely the result of reduced antithrombin III activity (see Chapter 2) (42).

Patients who have recently been treated with heparin are at risk for the development of *heparin-induced thrombocytopenia (HIT)*. This serious immune-mediated reaction is characterized by significant thrombocytopenia and the development of thromboembolic complications (both venous and arterial). Re-exposure to heparin may precipitate thrombotic complications leading to stroke, myocardial infarction, limb ischemia, and death. The diagnosis may be made on the basis of thrombocytopenia and serologic antibody assay, although these criteria are not foolproof. If HIT is present and anticoagulation of the patient is absolutely required [for cardiopulmonary bypass (CPB), for example], an alternative anticoagulant regimen other than heparin as sole therapy is used (43,44). If possible, it may be prudent to defer surgery with the patient being treated with warfarin, until the patient's antibody titer is reduced.

Patients with coronary disease are treated with platelet inhibitors, most commonly *aspirin* (45,46). In the past, it was common practice to discontinue aspirin for several days prior to surgery, but this is no longer the case. Although preoperative aspirin treatment may increase postoperative bleeding, transfusion requirements, and the need for postoperative re-exploration for bleeding, reports in this regard are not consistent (47,48). In fact, published results indicate that preoperative aspirin treatment is associated with improved outcomes, including lower mortality, in CABG patients (49–51). Thus, for CABG patients, preoperative aspirin treatment is generally continued up until surgery except for those who are at increased risk for bleeding problems or who refuse blood product transfusion. Using a lower dose, 81 mg daily, may confer the benefits of mild platelet inhibition with a reduced risk of bleeding complications (52).

Patients suffering acute coronary syndromes or who are undergoing percutaneous coronary interventions (such as stent placement) are often treated with other platelet inhibitors in addition to aspirin (2). The adenosine diphosphate receptor inhibitor *clopidogrel* irreversibly inhibits platelet function and has the duration of action of several days (the life of the platelet). Unless it is absolutely necessary, clopidogrel should be discontinued for 5 days prior to surgery, as preoperative treatment is associated with increased bleeding, transfusions, and the need to be returned to the operating room for excessive bleeding (48,53–56). The platelet IIb/IIIa glycoprotein receptor inhibitors include *abciximab, tirofiban,* and *eptifibatide*. Because abciximab has a longer duration of action, it is preferable to discontinue the drug 12 to 24 hours prior to surgery, if the patient's clinical status and coronary anatomy allow. If emergency surgery is required for the abciximab-treated patient, however, it can be successfully accomplished and indicated surgery should not be denied (57,58). Tirofiban and eptifibatide have short durations of action and may be continued up until the time of surgery. See Chapter 3 for further discussion of these drugs.

Warfarin is used to treat patients who have prosthetic valves, atrial fibrillation, cardiomyopathy with severe left ventricular dysfunction, venous thromboembolism, or other conditions. When these patients require elective surgery, the drug is usually discontinued approximately 4 to 6 days prior to the operation (59). If the patient is at high risk for thromboembolism (e.g., with a mechanical valve in place), he or she is admitted to the hospital about 2 days prior to surgery and treated with IV heparin while the effect of warfarin wears off. Alternatively, low-molecular-weight heparin has been used to "bridge" patients on anticoagulation treatment from warfarin to surgery, although clear-cut guidelines in this regard are lacking (59,60). Sometimes patients taking warfarin require urgent or emergency surgery, not an uncommon occurrence in prospective heart transplant recipient patients. In these cases, the prolonged prothrombin time may be corrected with fresh frozen plasma and/or vitamin K administration. Complete reversal of warfarin may not, however, be required and preoperative warfarin treatment may, in fact, be associated with less postoperative bleeding and fewer transfusions (perhaps due to less thrombin generation during CPB) (61). In general, vitamin K should not be given to patients who have an implanted mechanical valve, because rapid correction of the prothrombin time may precipitate valve thrombosis. Gradual reversal with fresh frozen plasma, however, is safe in patients with very elevated prothrombin times who must be operated on urgently. If vitamin K is used, only a small dose is indicated (1.0 to 2.5 mg) and the oral route is

TABLE 1.4	Commonly Used Herbal Supplements

Echinacea
Ephedra
Feverfew[a]
Garlic[a]
Ginger[a]
Ginkgo biloba[a]
Ginseng[a]
Kava
Saw palmetto[a]
St. John's wort
Valerian
Vitamin E[a]

[a]Reported to increase the risk of bleeding.

preferred (62). Excessive preoperative treatment with vitamin K will result in warfarin resistance postoperatively, possibly prolonging the patient's hospitalization.

Recently, nonprescription herbal supplements have gained increasing popularity (Table 1.4) (63–65). These medications have not been the subject of animal studies, controlled clinical trials, or postmarket surveillance, and their efficacy and safety are not well studied. Garlic, ginseng, and ginkgo (the three "G's"), in particular, have been associated with excessive bleeding. We request that patients discontinue all herbal supplements for at least 1 week prior to elective surgery.

Medication allergies, either documented or suspected, should be recorded and nonmedication allergies should be investigated. A latex-free operating room environment is used for the patient with a latex allergy (66). Patients with an allergy to iodine are prepped with a topical agent other than povidone–iodine (67).

PHYSICAL EXAMINATION

A thorough physical examination is warranted in all presurgical patients. Particular attention should be directed to findings that impact the proposed open heart surgery. The patient's height and weight are determined and used to calculate the body surface area (BSA) and body mass index (BMI) using readily available hand-held computer freeware programs such as those found at MedCalc (68). Patients with extreme obesity (BMI > 45) undergoing cardiac surgery have higher morbidity and mortality rates as compared with smaller patients (69). The BSA is used in the calculations of the arterial perfusion flow rate during CPB and the thermodilution cardiac index using the pulmonary artery catheter and for guiding the size of valve prostheses that are to be implanted. The patient's preoperative weight is used for comparison with the weight after surgery. The use of CPB during surgery is associated with capillary leakage, increases in interstitial fluid, and weight gain. Postoperatively the patient is treated with diuretics to reduce his or her weight to the baseline value; thus, an accurate preoperative weight determination is important.

Examination determines the patient's heart rate and rhythm. Cardiac auscultation will identify a cardiac murmur and suggest its etiology. Patients should be evaluated for congestive heart failure. Signs of congestive heart failure include a laterally displaced cardiac apex (not to be confused with the point of maximum impulse), an S_3 gallop, pulmonary rales that do not clear with coughing, peripheral edema, and jugulovenous distention. Patients with end-stage right heart failure may have a prominent, or even pulsatile, liver margin and ascites. Arterial desaturation, whether cardiac or pulmonary in origin, is demonstrated by cyanosis of the nail beds and mucous membranes.

Because atherosclerosis is a systemic disease, the patient should be carefully examined for peripheral vascular disease. The carotid arteries are auscultated. If there is a bruit or the history of cerebrovascular occlusive disease, a carotid duplex study is performed. Pulses in the upper extremities are palpated and blood pressures determined in both of the patient's arms. A difference in blood pressure between the two arms suggests a stenosis of the subclavian artery. This might preclude the use of the ipsilateral internal mammary artery as an *in situ* bypass conduit or suggest the need for preoperative stenting of the subclavian artery on that side (70). This finding is also a marker for the presence of increased carotid and proximal atherosclerotic aortic disease (71). Similarly, a patient who has a reduction in palmar perfusion or a decrease in the pulsation from the palmar arch by Doppler examination during compression of the radial artery may not be a candidate for use of the radial artery as a bypass graft. In anticipation of the use of the radial artery as conduit, the patient's nondominant hand should be identified and an Allen's test and digital pulse oximetry performed. These tests will help to ensure that the ulnar artery and palmar arch are intact and that the patient's hand perfusion will not be jeopardized following removal of the radial artery (72,73). Femoral, posterior tibial, and dorsalis pedis pulses are palpated. If the pulses are diminished, this may prompt further investigation with determination of ankle–brachial indices. If a patient has an ankle–brachial index of <0.6, some surgeons recommend not harvesting the saphenous vein from that leg because of concerns about wound healing following saphenous venectomy (74). Others will restrict the vein removal to the thigh portion only in legs with severe vascular insufficiency. If the femoral pulse is markedly decreased, it may not be possible to insert an intra-aortic balloon pump (IABP) through that vessel.

For patients undergoing CABG surgery, evaluation of the lower extremities includes inspection of the greater and lesser saphenous veins. With the patient standing, the greater saphenous vein is located on the medial aspect of the ankle, anterior to the medial malleolus. The patient is examined for the presence of venous varicosities and for brawny edema or skin changes suggestive of chronic venous insufficiency. If the greater saphenous vein is surgically absent, or of poor quality, the lesser saphenous vein (located on the posterolateral aspect of the calf) is inspected. Preoperative venous duplex mapping is helpful in CABG patients to determine the location and diameter of the greater and lesser saphenous veins (75,76). The skin overlying the located veins is marked with an indelible marker to facilitate intraoperative vein removal. This is particularly helpful in patients who are obese.

The patient's skin is inspected for the presence of infections or a localized rash. The presence of acne in the presternal area or groin fungal infection increases the risk of a wound infection. If indicated, elective patients are treated with antistaphylococcal or antifungal therapy prior to surgery. If the patient is to undergo valve replacement or implantation of prosthetic material, the patient's dentition is carefully inspected. Elective valve surgery patients undergo complete evaluation by their dentist to rule out occult infections. Any necessary dental work should be completed prior to surgery (with appropriate endocarditis prophylaxis) to avoid postoperative endocarditis.

LABORATORY TESTING

A variety of laboratory and noninvasive diagnostic studies are performed as screening tools (Table 1.5). The complete blood cell count identifies the patient with undiagnosed anemia, an unsuspected elevation in white blood cell count, and unsuspected thrombocytopenia. Preoperative anemia is associated with increased postoperative complications although it is not clear that preoperative transfusion will reverse this association (77,78). Leukocytosis should initiate a further evaluation to determine the source. The presence of a subnormal platelet count may reflect drug-induced thrombocytopenia or, if the patient has been exposed to heparin, the presence of HIT. HIT is a serious immune-mediated prothrombotic disorder that is important to recognize prior to surgery (43,79). If present, a nonheparin form of anticoagulation for CPB may be required (44,80).

Serum electrolyte measurements assess the adequacy of potassium repletion in the patient on diuretic therapy, whereas the serum

TABLE 1.5	Preoperative Testing

Blood studies
   Complete blood cell count with platelet count
   Serum electrolytes, with creatinine and BUN
   Serum glucose and glycosylated hemoglobin level
   Liver function tests and albumin
   Thyroid-stimulating hormone
   Hemoglobin A_{1c}
   Fasting lipid panel

Urinalysis

Chest x-ray

Electrocardiogram

BUN, blood urea nitrogen.

sodium level provides an estimate of the patient's hydration status. Although the serum creatinine level is a gross measure of kidney function, the preoperative calculation of the creatinine clearance (CrCl) is a more reliable indicator of operative risk for complications including mortality and prolonged hospital stay. This is especially true for small older women who may have a normal serum creatinine level but "occult" renal insufficiency based on the CrCl (81). An estimate of the patient's CrCl may be calculated using the Cockroft-Gault equation (82).

$$CrCl = \frac{(140 - age) \times weight}{serum\ Cr \times 72}$$

Units are weight (kg), age (years), serum Cr (mg/dL). For women, the calculated CrCl is multiplied by 0.85 to correct for their proportionally lower muscle mass. Patients with preoperative renal dysfunction will benefit from adequate hydration prior to cardiac catheterization to minimize the toxic effect of the contrast medium. If the abnormal renal function is new or worsened by the contrast agent load associated with cardiac catheterization, it is prudent to wait until the creatinine returns to baseline levels prior to proceeding with surgery. Surgery within 5 days of the catheterization procedure is associated with an increased risk of postoperative renal failure (83). Moderate renal dysfunction (creatinine level >2.5 mg/dL) is associated with an increased operative morbidity, need for postoperative dialysis, and mortality (84,85).

An elevated blood glucose level may identify the previously unsuspected diabetic patient; determination of the patient's hemoglobin A_{1c} level may aid in the diagnosis of diabetes mellitus. This reliable measure of long-term glucose control is also a useful predictor of postoperative complications such as mortality, renal failure, and sternal wound infection in patients undergoing CABG surgery (86).

Extensive coagulation studies are not required for patients who have no history of bleeding or excessive bruising although platelet function testing may be of value in patients who have been receiving platelet inhibitor therapy, in particular clopidogrel. For most patients, measurement of the platelet count, activated partial thromboplastin time, and prothrombin time is sufficient (87). The patient with liver dysfunction, as may occur with significant right ventricular dysfunction and systemic hypertension, may have an elevated prothrombin time that may predict an increased possibility of postoperative coagulopathy.

The serum *B-type natriuretic peptide* (*BNP*) level is a useful tool for the diagnosis and quantification of congestive heart failure. BNP is released from the heart in response to pressure and volume overload and high serum levels are highly suggestive of underlying myocardial disease although the underlying cause cannot be based simply on the abnormal test result (88).

A preoperative chest x-ray is performed. Signs of congestive heart failure include an enlarged cardiac silhouette, pulmonary interstitial edema, and pleural effusions. Although the enlarged cardiac silhouette usually suggests left ventricular enlargement secondary to volume overload as a result of congestive heart failure, the enlarged cardiac silhouette may also be seen with left ventricular hypertrophy or a large pericardial effusion. A densely calcified ascending aorta can also be identified on the chest x-ray and suggests an increased risk of atherosclerotic embolism during surgery (89). The presence of a very severely calcified or "porcelain" aorta may necessitate a change in operative plan (avoidance of ascending aorta cannulation, all arterial conduit rather than aortocoronary bypass in the revascularization patient), or preclude operative intervention altogether. The lateral chest x-ray is of particular value in reoperative patients as it shows the proximity of the cardiac structures and internal mammary artery pedicle clips to the posterior table of the sternum (90). As discussed in the section on Diagnostic Studies, the chest computed tomography (CT) scan is also useful for this situation.

The preoperative electrocardiogram (ECG) demonstrates the cardiac rate and rhythm, evidence of an old myocardial infarction, and/or ongoing myocardial ischemia. It also is the reference for comparison for postoperative ECGs.

The urinalysis will identify an occult urinary tract infection (surprisingly common in the elderly), microscopic hematuria, or poor blood glucose control. Usually, CABG patients found to have a urinary tract infection are treated immediately with an appropriate antibiotic (typically trimethoprim/sulfa or levofloxacin) and the surgery is performed as scheduled. If, however, the patient is scheduled to undergo elective placement of foreign material (e.g., valve replacement or prosthetic patch placement), the procedure is postponed until the urinary tract infection is definitively treated and the follow-up urinalysis is negative for infection.

For the stable patient who is being evaluated as an outpatient, some of these studies (such as the chest x-ray and ECG) need only be performed within 30 days of surgery. If new symptoms develop (such as a new cough or chest pain), then it is wise to repeat any studies that may have potentially changed. Likewise, patients with a chronic condition (such as renal insufficiency or mild anemia) should have follow-up studies performed near to the day of surgery to be sure that the condition has not worsened.

DIAGNOSTIC STUDIES

Patients who present with chronic stable angina often undergo noninvasive assessment of myocardial ischemia by the referring cardiologist prior to a cardiac catheterization. The *exercise stress test* evaluates the patient's heart rate and blood pressure responses to exercise while walking on a treadmill according to a graded protocol. Development of symptoms, electrocardiographic changes (>2 mm ST-segment depression), or a reduced or blunted blood pressure response is indicative of ischemia (91).

A more quantitative means of documenting myocardial perfusion can be accomplished with *myocardial perfusion imaging* (92). During peak exercise, thallium-201 or technetium-99m is injected. These tracers are taken up by viable myocardium, whereas irreversibly infarcted myocardium demonstrates no tracer uptake. Delayed images document the redistribution of tracer into ischemic myocardium. If the patient is unable to exercise, drugs, such as adenosine, dipyridamole, or dobutamine, may be administered to mimic the effect of exercise on the distribution of blood flow (93). The adenosine, dipyridamole, or dobutamine myocardial perfusion scan provides results comparable to exercise-induced ischemia.

Stress echocardiography is also used to identify patients with myocardial ischemia (94). This imaging modality is based upon the principle that exercise-induced ischemia caused by occlusive coronary artery disease results in regional wall motion abnormalities. If the patient cannot exercise, dobutamine may be used to increase myocardial oxygen demand. If the increase in myocardial oxygen demand cannot be met by an increase in blood flow, a regional wall motion abnormality results and is observed on the echocardiogram.

Cardiac catheterization with coronary angiography remains the gold standard in the preoperative evaluation of most types of cardiac disease although it may be contraindicated in patients with an acute aortic dissection or those with aortic valve endocarditis vegetations. Even if the preoperative patient does not have a history or symptoms of coronary insufficiency, coronary angiography is generally performed in patients older than 40 years, and in younger patients who have hyperlipidemia, diabetes, a history of tobacco abuse, or a strong family history of coronary artery disease. The complete cardiac catheterization study usually includes a left ventriculogram to identify wall motion abnormalities and the presence of a ventricular aneurysm and to provide a gross estimate of mitral regurgitation severity. The ventriculogram catheter measures pressures within the left ventricle and provides a pullback gradient determination when it is withdrawn into the aortic root. This allows calculation of the aortic valve area (95). The aortic root injection demonstrates aortic valve insufficiency and reveals the size and length of an ascending aortic aneurysm, if present. Coronary and bypass graft angiography defines the anatomy as well as the presence, location, and severity of obstructions. Visualization of the native internal mammary arteries is useful for the patient being considered for repeat CABG surgery to confirm the suitability of these vessels for use as bypass conduits.

A right heart catheterization study is performed in patients who present with signs or symptoms of congestive heart failure, patients with low ejection fractions, and those with valvular heart disease. The purpose is to determine the patient's preoperative cardiac output and pulmonary artery pressures. The pulmonary capillary wedge pressure provides an estimate of left ventricular preload and the reversibility of pulmonary hypertension, if present, can be assessed. Significant V waves in the pulmonary capillary wedge pressure tracing are indicative, but not diagnostic, of mitral regurgitation. Parameters derived from the right heart catheterization allow an accurate assessment of heart failure and intrinsic pulmonary hypertension and can facilitate targeted therapeutic intervention.

Echocardiography provides details about intracardiac anatomy, left ventricular function, and valve function and anatomy (96). Transthoracic echocardiography is noninvasive but can provide a less than ideal view of the heart in a patient who is obese, or in a patient who has undergone recent chest surgery. Transesophageal echocardiography (TEE) provides highly detailed anatomic information about the mitral valve (imperative when planning a mitral valve repair) and usually provides better views of the ascending aorta (important for diagnosing an ascending aortic dissection). TEE is, however, invasive in that it requires placement of an esophageal probe under IV sedation. Echocardiography is valuable in evaluating the patient with a suspected malfunction of a prosthetic heart valve, because it demonstrates paravalvular leaks and abnormal leaflet motion and identifies failed bioprosthetic valves (97,98). Echocardiography effectively defines the presence and location of vegetations on valve leaflets associated with endocarditis (99). Thrombus within the atrial appendage associated with atrial fibrillation and intraventricular thrombus associated with a transmural myocardial infarction are readily seen by echocardiography. Echocardiography can be used to estimate valve areas and pulmonary artery pressures. Echocardiography is readily performed, is associated with little risk, and can provide highly detailed information regarding cardiac anatomy and physiology, but the utility of the study is dependent upon the quality of the equipment and the knowledge and experience of the echocardiographer.

Preoperative *myocardial viability imaging* is of great value in evaluating the patient with depressed left ventricular function who is being considered for CABG surgery. Viability imaging can identify "hibernating myocardium" that may recover function following revascularization (100). Thallium scintigraphy, as described previously, documents the presence and location of ischemic myocardium. Further confirmation of the presence of viable myocardium in ischemic segments can be obtained from positron emission tomography (PET) scan (101). A PET scan identifies metabolically active myocardium. If present in the ischemic wall segment supplied by a stenotic coronary artery, the assumption is that the patient would benefit from coronary revascularization in spite of a depressed ejection fraction.

CT is used for the diagnosis of aortic aneurysms and acute aortic dissections and has largely replaced the more invasive procedure, aortography. CT is also helpful in evaluating the thickness of the pericardium in patients with constrictive pericarditis. For patients with suspected calcific atherosclerosis of the ascending aorta, noncontract CT helps to delineate the location and severity of calcified plaques that may interfere with aortic cannulation and placement of the crossclamping and put the patient at increased risk of embolic intraoperative stroke. *CT angiography* has become an increasingly important imaging technique for patients undergoing evaluation for cardiac surgery. It does require pharmacologic slowing of the heart rate (by β-blocker infusion) and practitioners who are experienced in interpreting the images. These scans can provide very valuable information regarding the location and patency of native coronary arteries and previously placed bypass grafts, the proximity of the aorta and/or right ventricle to the sternum (useful for patients undergoing repeat sternotomy), and the size and condition of the aortic root and the thoracic aorta (102,103). *Aortography* was the diagnostic gold standard for patients with traumatic tears of the proximal descending thoracic aorta, but CT has become increasingly useful for making the diagnosis (104). *Magnetic resonance imaging (MRI)* provides information regarding cardiac ventricular volumes, function, myocardial mass, and intracardiac tumors (105). MRI provides a quantitative evaluation of ventricular function, an accurate assessment of chamber volume and ventricular mass, and an assessment of pericardial disease. These modalities have also been used to evaluate coronary artery anatomy and myocardial perfusion. *Magnetic resonance angiography* provides excellent imaging of the aorta and its branches and intrathoracic venous structures. These modalities have also been used to evaluate coronary artery anatomy and myocardial perfusion. MRI is not as useful as CT for delineating vascular calcifications. MRI procedures are contraindicated in patients with ferromagnetic implants such as currently available pacemakers.

Pulmonary function testing is not routinely performed on the cardiac surgery patient but is of value if the patient has a history of extensive tobacco use, chronic obstructive pulmonary disease, asthma, or unexplained exertional dyspnea. In these patients, preoperative testing provides an assessment of the patient's pulmonary reserve and risk for surgery (106). The patient's response to bronchodilators can be determined and this information is used to guide postoperative therapy. Likewise, preoperative measurement of the patient's room air arterial blood gas will identify patients suffering chronic hypoxia or hypercarbia. This information facilitates weaning the patient from mechanical ventilation following surgery.

PRESURGERY VISIT

Most elective adult cardiac surgery patients are admitted to the hospital on the day of surgery. Thus, they are seen as outpatients within a few days prior to surgery for completion of their workup and preoperative preparation. Elimination of the preoperative hospital stay has reduced costs and has improved patient satisfaction, as most patients are more comfortable in an out-of-hospital environment the night prior to surgery. However, the associated reduction in patient contact places greater emphasis upon the final clinic visit prior to surgery. It is important to ensure that all preoperative issues are addressed and that final preparations are completed at this time.

The final preoperative visit includes an interval history and physical examination and laboratory studies as needed (including a sample for blood bank purposes). The chest x-ray and ECG need only be checked within 30 days of surgery. However, if there has been an intervening event or an increase in shortness of breath or angina, these studies are repeated at this time.

Preoperative teaching is performed as an outpatient. Interactive teaching modules and videotapes facilitate patient education. These may review basic cardiac anatomy, touch on operative detail (but in no way replace an operative discussion with the surgeon), and place emphasis on the postoperative issues such as tubes, catheters, pacing wires, invasive hemodynamic monitoring lines, and pulmonary care. The patients and their families are introduced to the intensive care unit environment as well as monitoring equipment and nursing routines. These teaching tools include interviews with dieticians and cardiac rehabilitation personnel to ensure that the patient has adequate home-going education. Emphasis is placed upon appropriate level of postoperative activity and cardiac rehabilitation as well as dietary management. The patients are informed of likely postoperative medications. The patients are instructed and then asked to perform the routine for exiting a bed or chair. They are taught how to support a sternotomy incision to ensure adequate coughing and deep breathing postoperatively and how to use the incentive spirometer.

The patient has a brief, final visit with the operating surgeon to ensure that all questions and concerns are addressed. A thorough discussion of the operative plan and potential complications is conducted and documented. Complications to be discussed include, but are not limited to, bleeding, infection, myocardial infarction, stroke, the risks of blood transfusion, and death. For procedures involving the tissue adjacent to the cardiac conduction system (such as in valve replacement), the potential for heart block requiring a permanent cardiac pacemaker is also mentioned. The potential adverse events are not belabored, but they are outlined and listed on the informed consent form, which is signed and witnessed.

The preoperative anesthesia evaluation focuses on airway management and previous anesthetic experiences. Obesity and a history of gastroesophageal reflux increase the potential for aspiration. The anesthesiologist reviews the patient's cardiac evaluation to determine how intensively the patient needs to be monitored during surgery. In general, if the patient has a history of congestive heart failure, a low ejection fraction, or recent myocardial infarction, a pulmonary arterial (Swan–Ganz) catheter is employed. If the patient is stable with well-preserved ventricular function and is undergoing a relatively uncomplicated procedure, the use of a pulmonary arterial catheter is optional. The neck and upper extremities are inspected by the anesthesiologist to ensure that appropriate monitoring lines can be placed. If a radial artery is to be employed as a bypass conduit, that arm (usually nondominant) is not used for IV catheters or blood pressure monitoring (either with a blood pressure cuff or with an arterial line). The presence, absence, and condition of the patient's teeth are documented. The anesthesiologist inquires with regard to a history of esophageal disease, especially if TEE is planned.

Postoperative discharge planning begins with the preoperative visit. If the patient lives alone or has an inadequate social support network, a social worker may see the patient before surgery to facilitate arrangements for postoperative placement.

PREOPERATIVE PREDICTION OF POSTOPERATIVE COMPLICATIONS

An important aspect of the preoperative evaluation of the cardiac surgery is an assessment of the patient's operative risk. This has become increasingly important as the population of adult cardiac surgery patients becomes older, with more coexisting diseases and greater degrees of cardiac impairment (107). The development of large clinical practice databases has provided for evaluation of surgical results (including complication and mortality rates) for commonly performed procedures such as CABG surgery and valve replacement. This allows surgeons and institutions to compare their results with those of the database and thus serves as a method of quality assessment and as a basis for quality improvement. In addition, these large databases provide the necessary data from which predictive formulas for risk estimation may be derived. These formulas can provide, for the individual patient, a prediction of expected operative mortality based on easily assessed preoperative risk factors. A number of different risk classification indexes are available, most of which have been developed using multiple regression analysis or Bayes theorem techniques. These risk-adjusted outcome predictive tools may utilize computer software or paper-and-pencil technique (108–113). By entering a number of preoperative clinical variables into the computer program (Table 1.6) or into a worksheet, a relatively reliable estimate of the patient's predicted chance of death is derived. It is also possible to predict the probability of specific postoperative complications such as stroke, renal failure, wound infection, atrial fibrillation, and prolonged mechanical ventilation using similar methods (114–117). A particularly useful outcomes predictor tool (the "Risk Calculator") is available at the Society of Thoracic Surgeons' Web site (www.sts.org). A very simple mortality risk prediction score, based only on age, creatinine, and ejection fraction has recently been described (118). The information obtained by preoperative estimation of postoperative complications provides a basis for a risk-versus-benefit discussion with the patient and his or her family. Such a discussion is an integral part of the decision-making process regarding the proposed cardiac surgical procedure.

SPECIAL PREOPERATIVE PROBLEMS

Depressed Left Ventricular Function

Because of advances that have been made in cardiac surgery, patients previously judged to be "inoperable" due to poor left ventricular function

TABLE 1.6	Preoperative Variables Commonly Used to Assess Surgical Risk

Patient age
Left ventricular function (ejection fraction)
Nature of procedure
Gender
Previous cardiac procedure
Timing of surgery (elective, urgent, emergency)
Previous myocardial infarction
Presence of congestive heart failure
Need for preoperative IABP
Diabetes mellitus
Dialysis dependency
Chronic obstructive pulmonary disease, severe
Elevated pulmonary artery pressure (systolic > 60 mm Hg)
Morbid obesity (BMI > 34)
Cerebrovascular disease
Hypertension

BMI, body mass index [weight (kg)/height (m^2)]; IABP, intra-aortic balloon pump.
See references 99 to 103.

are now considered for operation. Likewise, patients with advanced coronary artery disease who have intractable rest pain or life-threatening coronary artery anatomy face a dismal prognosis without revascularization, and CABG surgery is often recommended. Although it is attractive to consider coronary angioplasty and stent placement as a good alternative for the high-risk surgical candidate, these patients often have severe, diffuse, multivessel coronary disease that often precludes percutaneous interventions. Thus, cardiac surgeons are frequently called on to manage these challenging patients. To the extent possible, congestive heart failure should be controlled medically before surgery in these high-risk patients.

In situations where left ventricular function is very poor (e.g., ejection fraction < 25%), when revascularization may not be complete, and where operative ischemic time is likely to be long, it is useful to initiate preoperative IABP counterpulsation (119–121). This is in recognition of the higher-than-usual need for IABP support after surgery for these patients. In some patients, the IABP may be inserted 1 day prior to surgery for a short term of preoperative support prior to undergoing surgery. Typically this is performed, with fluoroscopic guidance, in the catheterization laboratory. The balloon pump catheter is inserted over a guidewire using percutaneous techniques, usually on the side opposite from that where saphenous vein harvesting is anticipated. Alternatively, patients are taken to the catheterization laboratory during transfer to the operating room for IABP insertion. IABP placement in the catheterization laboratory may be particularly useful in patients who have peripheral vascular disease for whom fluoroscopic guidance is helpful. Under other circumstances, the IABP insertion can be performed in the operating room before the induction of anesthesia. In our experience, and that of others, prophylactic preoperative use of the IABP in CABG patients with poor left ventricular function and other risk factors for mortality is associated with significantly improved surgical results (122). Further discussion regarding IABP management is included in Chapter 3.

Left Main Coronary Artery Disease

Patients with significant obstruction of the left main coronary artery will frequently present with unstable angina and are at risk for sudden death. These patients can develop arrhythmias or instability during coronary arteriography, during the induction of anesthesia, and even during the handling of the heart before CPB. Maintenance of medical therapy including the use of nitrates, aspirin, β-blockers, and heparin is useful to maintain the patient's stability while awaiting surgery. Other antiplatelet drugs, in particular, one of the short-acting glycoprotein IIb/IIIa inhibitors, tirofiban or eptifibatide, may also be indicated. Should evidence of ischemia develop on such a regimen, immediate surgery is indicated, at times with preoperative IABP support.

Recent Acute Myocardial Infarction

The optimal timing for CABG procedure for patients who have suffered an acute myocardial infarction has been unclear. For the stable patient, not requiring emergency revascularization, delaying the procedure for 3 or more days after admission to the hospital for the infarction is associated with reduced mortality (123).

Critical Aortic Valve Stenosis

Patients with severe aortic valve stenosis may become suddenly unstable or die unexpectedly. Unlike patients with coronary artery disease, there are no options for support with IABP and really there is no effective medical therapy that alters the pathophysiology of this lesion (124). Because of the imbalance between myocardial oxygen supply and demand, the maintenance of adequate systemic blood pressure is crucial, because hypotension will further compromise coronary flow and may be disastrous. Excessive treatment with diuretics should be avoided, even though the patient may be in heart failure, because they produce volume depletion and hypotension that could reduce coronary perfusion further and result in severe instability. Likewise, vasodilator therapy is to be avoided. IABP counterpulsation does little to stabilize these patients, and in instances where aortic stenosis is accompanied by regurgitation, it may actually worsen the hemodynamic state. Thus, patients with critical aortic stenosis should undergo surgery as soon as reasonable. If increasing heart failure is noted, the procedure should be performed on an emergency basis. Occasionally concurrent medical issues, such as pneumonia, may preclude an urgent aortic valve replacement. In these circumstances, surgery can be delayed for a short period of time by percutaneous aortic valvuloplasty. This provides short-term reduction of the critical aortic valve gradient. This technique may also be used in patients with poorly controlled congestive heart failure and prohibitively reduced left ventricular function. Temporary reduction in the aortic valve gradient by balloon valvuloplasty may result in improved left ventricular function, stabilization of the patient, and a reduction in the patient's subsequent operative risk.

Acute Valve Regurgitation and Malfunctioning Prosthetic Valves

Patients presenting with severe, acute, mitral valve regurgitation have usually experienced a ruptured papillary muscle because of a myocardial infarction. If the lesion is severe enough to produce cardiogenic shock, these patients may be stabilized temporarily with an IABP and then undergo surgery on an emergency basis.

Patients with aortic or mitral valve regurgitation due to endocarditis usually do not exhibit cardiogenic shock. These patients may often be stabilized with antibiotic therapy, diuresis, and inotropic or afterload medications. Ideally, they should have a period of appropriate antibiotic therapy before valve replacement to sterilize the native valve or at least clear the bacteremia. Indications for early valve replacement include uncontrollable heart failure, valvular obstruction, septal perforation, fistula formation, recurrent emboli, and new-onset conduction disturbance (125). Persistent bacteremia may also be an indication for early valve surgery.

Patients with acute aortic valve regurgitation usually have this lesion as a complication of aortic dissection or endocarditis. It results in wide pulse pressure with a low diastolic pressure. A natural cardiac reflex to minimize the effects of aortic regurgitation is tachycardia, which decreases the amount of time that the heart spends in diastole, during which time the regurgitation occurs. Thus, when these patients develop tachycardia, drugs such as β-blockers are contraindicated. Mechanical support with an IABP is not an option for acute aortic regurgitation, as it requires a competent aortic valve. Surgical replacement or repair of the acutely and severely regurgitant aortic valve should generally be undertaken as soon as possible.

Acutely malfunctioning prosthetic valves produce relative surgical emergencies. One situation is thrombosis of a mechanical prosthesis because of inadequate systemic anticoagulation, most commonly in the mitral position. This usually creates a clinical picture of mitral valve stenosis (± regurgitation) and severe heart failure. Preoperative management includes immediate systemic heparinization and echocardiographic evaluation. Thrombolytic therapy has been used with some success, especially in critically ill patients with a very high operative risk. There is, however, a significant risk of arterial embolization with this treatment, up to 19% (126–128). Generally, emergency valve replacement is indicated for patients who are relatively stable, patients with large thrombi visible on echocardiography, and those with thrombosed mitral prostheses (because the results of thrombolysis are not as good as for thrombosed aortic prosthetic valves). Thrombosis of aortic valve prosthesis is much less common because of the higher rate of blood flow past the prosthetic orifice. Thrombolytic therapy of mechanical tricuspid or pulmonary valves is generally preferable as the consequences of emboli are less severe. Acute prosthetic regurgitation may occur with older-model bioprosthetic tissue valves although much more commonly the leakage develops over time as the valve gradually deteriorates. Rarely, a mechanical valve may experience strut or disc fracture or disc occluder escape resulting in acute regurgitation.

The Patient with Chronic Kidney Disease

End-stage renal disease patients on dialysis may require heart surgery for coronary heart or valvular disease. In the past, these patients were at increased risk for operative mortality and complications, but the results of surgery have improved and the number of patients referred for surgery is increasing (129–131). It is not uncommon to perform CABG surgery in the dialysis-dependent patient in preparation for subsequent kidney transplantation. Close collaboration with the patient's nephrologists is essential to successful perioperative management. Usually, dialysis is performed the day prior to surgery and then on the first postoperative day unless required sooner after surgery for indications such as hypervolemia or hyperkalemia. Use of the internal mammary artery on the same side as the patient's upper extremity arteriovenous dialysis fistula may be contraindicated. If the ipsilateral internal mammary artery is used, flow steal and resultant myocardial ischemia during dialysis may occur (132).

Patients with lesser degrees of chronic kidney disease (CrCl < 30 mL per minute) who are not dialysis dependent may also benefit from preoperative dialysis treatment in terms of reduced complications and length of hospital stay (133).

Pregnancy

Pregnancy imposes a substantial stress on the cardiovascular system (134). Cardiac output progressively rises during pregnancy reaching a peak nearly 1.5 times baseline during the 25th to 27th weeks. Although cardiac operations during pregnancy are rare, the usual circumstance involves a woman with underlying (most often valvular) heart disease and limited cardiovascular reserve who develops worsening congestive heart failure. Cardiac surgery, including open procedures on CPB, may be performed on pregnant women although risk to the parturient is increased and fetal mortality may be high (135–137). With respect to timing, the risk of surgery to the mother is lowest in the early stages of pregnancy but this is also the period of critical fetal development. In preoperative consultation, the potential for fetal malformation or death and relative risks to the mother are discussed if the mother does not accept therapeutic abortion and cardiac surgery cannot be avoided. The management of long-term anticoagulation for pregnant patients requires special considerations because warfarin may cause fetal bleeding and teratogenicity (138).

SKIN PREPARATION AND ANTIBIOTIC PROPHYLAXIS

The patient showers with chlorhexidine the night before surgery and is asked to not eat or drink anything beginning 12 hours prior to surgery. The preoperative outpatient returns to the hospital several hours in advance of the anticipated operative time. On arrival, the patient's body hair is clipped, including the anterior chest, abdomen, and, for coronary revascularization patients, the entire legs. The clip stops at the knees for patients undergoing valve replacement or another cardiac operation. An IV catheter is placed and the preoperative antibiotic administered. A dose of prophylactic antibiotic is administered within 60 minutes prior to the incision. The preferred antibiotic for adult cardiac surgery is usually cefazolin (2 g IV) (139). In addition to the preoperative dose, an intraoperative cephalosporin dose is also recommended. Vancomycin is administered, in addition to cefazolin, for patients at institutions that have a high rate of infections caused by methicillin-resistant *Staphylococcus aureus* and *Staphylococcus epidermidis*. For patients with penicillin or cephalosporin allergy, vancomycin plus an aminoglycoside or fluoroquinolone (to provide Gram-negative coverage) is given. When administered, vancomycin must be infused slowly to avoid hypotension, which can be severe. The patient's name and identification number and operative plan are confirmed and the patient is transported to the operating room at the appropriate time.

References

1. Gibbons RJ, Abrams J, Chatterjee K, et al. ACC/AHA 2002 guideline update for the management of patients with chronic stable angina: a report of the American College of Cardiology/American Heart Association Task Force on Practice Guidelines (Committee to Update the 1999 Guidelines for the Management of Patients with Chronic Stable Angina). *Circulation* 2003;107:149–158.
2. Anderson JL, Adams CD, Antman EM, et al. ACC/AHA 2007 guidelines for the management of patients with unstable angina/non–ST-elevation myocardial infarction: a report of the American College of Cardiology/American Heart Association Task Force on Practice Guidelines (Writing Committee to Revise the 2002 Guidelines for the Management of Patients with Unstable Angina/Non–ST-Elevation Myocardial Infarction): developed in collaboration with the American College of Emergency Physicians, American College of Physicians, Society for Academic Emergency Medicine, Society for Cardiovascular Angiography and Interventions, and Society of Thoracic Surgeons. *J Am Coll Cardiol* 2007;50:1–157.
3. Criteria Committee of the New York Heart Association. *Diseases of the heart and blood vessels: nomenclature and criteria for diagnosis of the heart and great vessels*, 6th ed. New York: New York Heart Association/Little Brown, 1964.
4. Bonow RO, Carabello BA, Chatterjee K, et al. ACC/AHA 2006 guidelines for the management of patients with valvular heart disease: a report of the American College of Cardiology/American Heart Association Task Force on Practice Guidelines (Writing Committee to Develop Guidelines for the Management of Patients with Valvular Heart Disease). *J Am Coll Cardiol* 2005;46:1116–1143.
5. Grundy SM, Pasternak R, Greenland P, et al. Assessment of cardiovascular risk by use of multiple-risk-factor assessment equations: a statement for healthcare professionals from the American Heart Association and the American College of Cardiology. *J Am Coll Cardiol* 1999;34:1348–1359.
6. Smith SC, Allen J, Blair SN, et al. AHA/ACC guidelines for secondary prevention for patients with coronary and other atherosclerotic vascular disease: 2006 update. *J Am Coll Cardiol* 2006;47:2130–2139.
7. Rajakaruna C, Rogers CA, Surinamala C, et al. The effect of diabetes mellitus on patients undergoing coronary surgery: a risk-adjusted analysis. *J Thorac Cardiovasc Surg* 2006;132:802–810.
8. Estrada CA, Young JA, Nifong LW, et al. Outcomes and perioperative hyperglycemia in patients undergoing coronary artery bypass grafting. *Ann Thorac Surg* 2002;75:1392–1399.
9. Woods SE, Smith JM, Sohail S, et al. The influence of type 2 diabetes mellitus in patients undergoing coronary artery bypass graft surgery. *Chest* 2004;126:1789–1795.
10. The Parisian Mediastinitis Study Group. Risk factors for deep sternal wound infection after sternotomy: a prospective, multicenter study. *J Thorac Cardiovasc Surg* 1996;111:1200–1207.

11. Lu JC, Grayson AD, Jha P, et al. Risk factors for sternal wound infection and mid-term survival following coronary artery bypass surgery. *Eur J Cardiothorac Surg* 2003;23:943–949.

12. Nakano J, Okabayashi H, Hanyu M, et al. Risk factors for wound infection after off-pump coronary artery bypass grafting: should bilateral internal arteries be harvested in patients with diabetes mellitus? *J Thorac Cardiovasc Surg* 2008;135:540–545.

13. Porsche R, Brenner ZR. Allergy to protamine sulfate. *Heart Lung* 1999;28: 418–428.

14. Lazar HL, Chipkin SR, Fitzgerald CA, et al. Tight glycemic control in diabetic coronary artery bypass graft patients improves perioperative outcomes and decreases recurrent ischemic events. *Circulation* 2004;109:1497–1502.

15. Gomberg-Maitland M, Frishman WH. Thyroid hormone and cardiovascular disease. *Am Heart J* 1998;135:187–196.

16. Edward FH, Ferraris VA, Shahian DM, et al. Gender-specific practice guidelines for coronary artery bypass surgery: perioperative management. *Ann Thorac Surg* 2005;79:2189–2194.

17. Klopfenstein CE. Preoperative clinical assessment of hemostatic function in patients scheduled for a cardiac operation. *Ann Thorac Surg* 1996;62: 1918–1920.

18. Puskas JD, Winston AD, Wright CE, et al. Stroke after coronary artery operation: incidence, correlates, outcome, and cost. *Ann Thorac Surg* 2000;69: 1053–1056.

19. Bucerius J, Gummert JF, Borger MA, et al. Stroke after cardiac surgery: a risk analysis of 16,184 consecutive adult patients. *Ann Thorac Surg* 2003;75: 472–478.

20. Eagle KA, Guyton RA, Davidoff R, et al. ACC/AHA 2004 guideline update for coronary artery bypass graft surgery: summary article. A report of the American College of Cardiology/American Heart Association Task Force on Practice Guidelines (Committee to Update the 1999 Guidelines for Coronary Artery Bypass Graft Surgery). *J Am CollCardiol* 2004;44:1146–1154.

21. Sheiman RG, Janne d'Othee B. Screening carotid sonography before elective coronary artery bypass graft surgery: who needs it. *Am J Roentgenol* 2007;188:W475–W479.

22. Borger MA, Fremes SE. Management of patients with concomitant coronary and carotid vascular disease. *Semin Thorac Cardiovasc Surg* 2001;13:192–198.

23. Chiappini B, Amore AD, Di Marco L, et al. Simultaneous carotid and coronary arteries disease: staged or combined surgical approach. *J Card Surg* 2005;20:234–240.

24. Ricotta JJ, Wall LP, Blackstone E. The influence of concurrent carotid endarterectomy on coronary bypass: a case controlled study. *J Vasc Surg* 2005;41:397–402.

25. Erez E, Eldar S, Sharoni E, et al. Coronary artery operation in patients after breast cancer therapy. *Ann Thorac Surg* 1998;66:1312–1317.

26. Chang AS, Smedira NG, Chang CL, et al. Cardiac surgery after mediastinal radiation: extent of exposure influences outcome. *J Thorac Cardiovasc Surg* 2007;133:404–413.

27. Handa N, McGregor CGA, Danielson GK, et al. Valvular heart operation in patients with previous mediastinal radiation therapy. *Ann Thorac Surg* 2001;71:1880–1884.

28. Geraci SAZ, Haan CK. Effect of beta blockers after coronary artery bypass in postinfarct patients: what can we learn from available literature? *Ann Thorac Surg* 2002;74:1727–1732.

29. Ferguson TB Jr, Coombs LP, Peterson ED. Preoperative β-blocker use and mortality and morbidity following CABG surgery in North America. *JAMA* 2002;287:2221–2227.

30. Rahme E, Eisenberg MJ. Perioperative use of cardiac medical therapy among patients undergoing coronary artery bypass graft surgery: a systematic review. *Am Heart J* 2007;154:407–414.

31. Weisbauer F, Schlager O, Domanovits H, et al. Perioperative beta-blockers for preventing surgery-related mortality and morbidity: a systematic review and meta-analysis. *Anesth Analg* 2007;104:27–41.

32. Collard CD, Body SC, Shernan SK, et al. Preoperative statin therapy is associated with reduced cardiac mortality after coronary artery bypass graft surgery. *J Thorac Cardiovasc Surg* 2006;132:392–400.

33. Tabata M, Khalpey Z, Cohn LH, et al. Effect of statins in patients without coronary artery disease who undergo cardiac surgery. *J Thorac Cardiovasc Surg* 2008;136:1510–1513.

34. Katznelson R, Djaiani GN, Borger MA, et al. Preoperative use of statins is associated with reduced early delirium rates after cardiac surgery. *Anesthesiology* 2009;110:67–73.

35. Barnes BJ, Kirkland EA, Howard PA, et al. Risk-stratified evaluation of amiodarone to prevent atrial fibrillation after cardiac surgery. *Ann Thorac Surg* 2006;82:1332–1337.

36. Vassalo P, Trohman RG. Prescribing amiodarone: an evidence-based review of clinical indication. *JAMA* 2007;298:1312–1322.

37. Brabant SM, Bertrand M, Eyraud D, et al. The hemodynamic effects of anesthetic induction in vascular surgical patients chronically treated with angiotensin II receptor antagonists. *Anesth Analg* 1999;88:1388–1392.

38. Chan NN, Brain HPS, Feher MD. Metformin-associated lactic acidosis: a rare or very rare clinical entity? *Diabetic Med* 1999;16:273–281.

39. Duncan AI, Koch CG, Xu M, et al. Recent metformin ingestion does not increase in-hospital morbidity or mortality after cardiac surgery. *Ann Analg* 2007;104:42–50.

40. Clark SC, Vitale N, Zacharias J, et al. Effect of low molecular weight heparin (Fragmin) on bleeding after cardiac surgery. *Ann Thorac Surg* 2000;69:762–765.

41. Jones HU, Muhlestein JB, Jones KW, et al. Preoperative use of enoxaparin compared with unfractionated heparin increases the incidence of re-exploration for postoperative bleeding after open-heart surgery in patients who present with an acute coronary syndrome. *Circulation* 2002;106(suppl I):I-19–I-22.

42. Lemmer JH, Despotis GJ. Antithrombin III concentrate to treat heparin resistance in patients undergoing cardiac surgery. *J Thorac Cardiovasc Surg* 2002;123:213–217.

43. Levy JH, Tanaka KA, Hursting MJ. Reducing thrombotic complications in the perioperative setting: an update on heparin-induced thrombocytopenia. *Anesth Analg* 2007;105:570–582.

44. Koster A, Dyke CM, Aldea G, et al. Bivalirudin during cardiopulmonary bypass in patients with previous or acute heparin-induced thrombocytopenia and heparin antibodies: results of the CHOOSE-ON trial. *Ann Thorac Surg* 2007;83:572–577.

45. Woo YJ. Cardiac surgery in patients on antiplatelet and antithrombotic agents. *Semin Thorac Cardiovasc Surg* 2005;17:66–72.
46. Meadows T, Bhatt DL. Clinical aspects of platelet inhibitors and thrombus formation. *Circ Res* 2007;100:1261–1275.
47. Ferraris VA, Ferraris VP, Joseph O, et al. Aspirin and postoperative bleeding after coronary artery bypass grafting. *Ann Surg* 2002;235:820–827.
48. Ferraris VA, Ferraris SP, Saha SP, et al. Perioperative blood transfusion and blood conservation in cardiac surgery: the Society of Thoracic Surgeons and The Society of Cardiovascular Anesthesiologists clinical practice guideline. *Ann Thorac Surg* 2007;83: S27–S86.
49. Mangano DT; Multicenter Study of Perioperative Ischemia Research Group. Aspirin and mortality after coronary bypass surgery. *N Engl J Med* 2002;347: 1309–1317.
50. Dacey LJ, Munozzz JJ, Johnson EZR, et al. Effect of preoperative aspirin use on mortality in coronary artery bypass patients. *Ann Thorac Surg* 2000;70: 1986–1990.
51. Bybee KA, Powell BD, Valeti U, et al. Preoperative aspirin therapy is associated with improved postoperative outcomes in patients undergoing coronary artery bypass grafting. *Circulation* 2005;112(suppl I):I-286–I-292.
52. Campbell CL, Smyth S, Montalescot G, et al. Aspirin dose for the prevention of cardiovascular disease. *JAMA* 2007;297:2018–2024.
53. Filsoufi F, Rahmanian PB, Castillo JG, et al. Clopidogrel treatment before coronary artery bypass graft surgery increases postoperative morbidity and blood product requirements. *J Cardiothorac Vasc Anesth* 2008;22:60–66.
54. Purkayastha S, Athanasiou T, Malinovski V, et al. Does clopidogrel affect outcome after coronary artery bypass grafting? A meta-analysis. *Heart* 2006;92: 531–532.
55. Reichert MG, Robinson AH, Travis JA, et al. Effects of a waiting period after clopidogrel treatment before performing coronary artery bypass grafting. *Pharmacotherapy* 2008; 28:151–155.
56. Berger JS, Frye CB, Harshaw Q, et al. Impact of clopidogrel in patients with acute coronary syndromes requiring coronary artery bypass surgery: a multicenter analysis. *J Am Coll Cardiol* 2008;52:1693–1701.
57. Lemmer JH Jr. Clinical experience in coronary bypass surgery for abciximab-treated patients. *Ann Thorac Surg* 2000;70:S33–S37.
58. De Carlo M, Maselli D, Cortese B, et al. Emergency coronary artery bypass grafting in patients with acute myocardial infarction treated with glycoprotein IIb/IIIa receptor inhibitors. *Int J Cardiol* 2008;123:229–233.
59. Whitlock RP, Crowther MA, Warkentin TE, et al. Warfarin cessation before cardiopulmonary bypass: lessons learned from a randomized controlled trial of oral vitamin K. *Ann Thorac Surg* 2007;84:103–109.
60. Spyropoulos AC, Bauersachs RM, Omran H, et al. Periprocedural bridging therapy in patients receiving chronic oral anticoagulation therapy. *Curr Med Res Opin* 2006;22: 1109–1122.
61. Dietrich W, Spannagl M, Schramm W, et al. The influence of preoperative anticoagulation on heparin response during cardiopulmonary bypass. *J Thorac Cardiovasc Surg* 1991;102:505–514.
62. Ansell J, Hirsh J, Dalen J, et al. Managing oral anticoagulant therapy. *Chest* 2001;119: 22S–38S.
63. Ang-Lee MK, Moss J, Yuan C-S. Herbal medicines and perioperative care. *JAMA* 2001;286: 208–216.

64. Norred CL, Finlayson CA. Hemorrhage after the preoperative use of complementary and alternative medicines. *AANA J* 2000;68:217–220.
65. Valli G, Giardina EG. Benefits, adverse effects and drug interactions of herbal therapies with cardiovascular effects. *J Am Coll Cardiol* 2002;39:1083–1095.
66. Poley GE Jr, Slater JE. Latex allergy. *J Allergy Clin Immunol* 2000;105:1054–1062.
67. Erdmann S, Hertl M, Merk HF. Allergic contact dermatitis from povidone-iodine. *Contact Dermatitis* 1999;40:331–332.
68. Hu C, Kneusel R, Barnas G. MedCalc: body surface area, body mass index (BMI). http://www.medcalc.com/body.html.
69. Tyson GH, Rodriguez E, Elci OC, et al. Cardiac procedures in patients with body mass index exceeding 45: outcomes and long-term results. *Ann Thorac Surg* 2007;84:3–9.
70. Rogers JH, Calhoun RF. Diagnosis and management of subclavian artery stenosis prior to coronary artery bypass grafting in the current era. *J Cardiac Surg* 2007;22:20–25.
71. Baribeau YM, Westbrook BW, Charlesworth DC, et al. Brachial gradient in cardiac surgical patients. *Circulation* 2002;106(suppl I):I-11–I-13.
72. Greene MA, Malias MA. Arm complications after radial artery procurement for coronary bypass operation. *Ann Thorac Surg* 2001;72:126–128.
73. Asif M, Sarkar PK. Three-digit Allen's test. *Ann Thorac Surg* 2007;84:686–687.
74. Avrahami R, Haddad M, Koren A, et al. Saphenous vein harvesting for coronary artery bypass grafting. Retrospective analysis of possible causes of major wound complications in patients with peripheral arterial disease. *Eur J Vasc Endovasc Surg* 2001;21:423–426.
75. Head HD, Brown MF. Preoperative vein mapping for coronary artery bypass operations. *Ann Thorac Surg* 1995;59:144–148.
76. Lemmer JH Jr, Meng RL, Corson JD, et al. Preoperative saphenous vein mapping for coronary artery bypass. *J Card Surg* 1988;3:237–240.
77. Karkouti K, Wijeysundera DN, Beattie WS. Reducing Bleeding in Cardiac Surgery (RBC) Investigators. Risk associated with preoperative anemia in cardiac surgery. *Circulation* 2008;117:478–484.
78. Bell ML, Grunwald GK, Baltz JH, et al. Does preoperative hemoglobin independently predict short-term outcomes after coronary artery bypass surgery? *Ann Thorac Surg* 2008;86:1415–1423.
79. Baldwin ZK, Spitzer AL, Ng VL, et al. Contemporary standards for the diagnosis and treatment of heparin-induced thrombocytopenia (HIT). *Surgery* 2008;143:305–312.
80. Riess F-C. Anticoagulation management and cardiac surgery in patients with heparin-induced thrombocytopenia. *Semin Thorac Cardiovasc Surg* 2005;17:85–96.
81. Najafi M, Goodararzynejad H, Karimi A, et al. Is preoperative serum creatinine a reliable indicator of outcome in patients undergoing coronary artery bypass surgery? *J Thorac Cardiovasc Surg* 2009;137:304–308.
82. Robertshaw M, Lai KN, Swaminathan R. Prediction of creatinine clearance from plasma creatinine: comparison of five formulae. *Br J Pharmacol* 1989;28:275–280.
83. Del Duca D, Iqbal S, Rahme E, et al. Renal failure after cardiac surgery: timing of cardiac catheterization and other perioperative risk factors. *Ann Thorac Surg* 2007;84:1264–1271.
84. Durmaz I, Büket S, Atay Y, et al. Cardiac surgery with cardiopulmonary bypass in patients with chronic renal failure. *J Thorac Cardiovasc Surg* 1999;118:306–315.

85. Penta de Peppo A, Nardi P, De Paulis R, et al. Cardiac surgery in moderate to end-stage renal failure: analysis of risk factors. *Ann Thorac Surg* 2002;74: 378–383.

86. Halkos ME, Puskas JD, Lattouf OM, et al. Elevated preoperative hemoglobin A1c level is predictive of adverse events after coronary artery bypass surgery. *Ann Thorac Surg* 2008;136:631–640.

87. De Moerloose P. Laboratory evaluation of hemostasis before cardiac operations. *Ann Thorac Surg* 1996;62:1921–1925.

88. Tang WHW. B-type natriuretic peptide: a critical review. *Congest Heart Fail* 2007;13:48–52.

89. Mills NL, Everson CT. Atherosclerosis of the ascending aorta and coronary artery bypass. Pathology, clinical correlates, and operative management. *J Thorac Cardiovasc Surg* 1991;102:546–553.

90. Gillinov AM, Casselman FP, Lytle BW, et al. Injury to a patent left internal thoracic artery graft at coronary reoperation. *Ann Thorac Surg* 1999;67:382–386.

91. Gibbons RJ, Balady GJ, Bricker JT, et al. ACC/AHA 2002 guideline update for exercise testing: summary article. A report of the American College of Cardiology/American Heart Association Task Force on Practice Guidelines (Committee to Update the 1997 Exercise Testing Guidelines). *J Am Coll Cardiol* 2002;40:1531–1540.

92. Klocke FJ, Baird MG, Lorell BH, et al. ACC/AHA/ASNC guidelines for the clinical use of cardiac radionuclide imaging—executive summary: a report of the American College of Cardiology/American Heart Association Task Force on Practice Guidelines (ACC/AHA/ASNC Committee to Revise the 1995 Guidelines for the Clinical Use of Cardiac Radionuclide Imaging). *J Am Coll Cardiol* 2003;42:1318–1333.

93. Geleijnse ML, Elhendy A, Fioretti PM, et al. Dobutamine stress myocardial perfusion imaging. *J Am Coll Cardiol* 2000;36:2017–2027.

94. Lewis JF. Current status of stress echocardiography. *Clin Cardiol* 2000;23: 242–246.

95. Gorlin R, Gorlin SG. Hydraulic formula for calculation of the area of the stenotic mitral valve, other cardiac valves, and central circulatory shunts. *Am Heart J* 1951;41:1–29.

96. Douglas PS, Khandheria B, Stainback RF, et al. ACCF/ASE/ACEP/ASNC/SCAI/SCCT/SCMR 2007 appropriateness criteria for transthoracic and transesophageal echocardiography. *J Am Coll Cardiol* 2007;50:187–204.

97. Daniel WG, Mügge A, Grote J, et al. Comparison of transthoracic and transesophageal echocardiography for detection of abnormalities of prosthetic and bioprosthetic valves in the mitral and aortic positions. *Am J Cardiol* 1993;71:210–215.

98. Bach DS. Transesophageal echocardiographic (TEE) evaluation of prosthetic valves. *Cardiol Clin* 2000;18:751–771.

99. Ryan EW, Bolger AF. Transesophageal echocardiography (TEE) in the evaluation of infective endocarditis. *Cardiol Clin* 2000;18:773–787.

100. Perrone-Filardi P, Chiariello M. The identification of myocardial hibernation in patients with ischemic heart failure by echocardiography and radionuclide studies. *Prog Cardiovasc Dis* 2001;43:419–432.

101. Maddahi J, Schelbert H, Brunken R, et al. Role of thallium-201 and PET imaging in evaluation of myocardial viability and management of patients with coronary artery disease and left ventricular dysfunction. *J Nucl Med* 1994;35: 707–715.

102. Hartnell GG. Imaging of aortic aneurysms and dissection: CT and MRI. *J Thorac Imaging* 2001;16:35–46.
103. Rybicki FJM, Seth T, Chen FY. Cardiac surgical imaging. In: Cohn LH, Edmunds LH Jr, eds. *Cardiac surgery in the adult*. New York: McGraw-Hill, 2003:179–198.
104. Brinkman WT, Szeto WY, Bavaria JE. Overview of great vessel trauma. *Thorac Surg Clin* 2007;17:95–108.
105. Hendel RC, Patel MR, Kramer CM, et al. ACCF/ACR/SCCT/SCMR/ASNC/ NASCI/SCAI/SIR 2006 appropriateness criteria for cardiac computed tomography and cardiac magnetic resonance imaging: a report of the American College of Cardiology Foundation/American College of Radiology, Society of Cardiovascular Computed Tomography, Society for Cardiovascular Magnetic Resonance, American Society of Nuclear Cardiology, North American Society for Cardiac Imaging, Society for Cardiovascular Angiography and Interventions, and Society of Interventional Radiology. *J Am Coll Cardiol* 2006;48: 1475–1497.
106. Durand M, Combes P, Eisele JH, et al. Pulmonary function tests predict outcome after cardiac surgery. *Acta Anaesthesiol Belg* 1993;44:17–23.
107. Ngaage DL, Griffin S, Guvendik L, et al. Changing operative characteristics of patients undergoing operations for coronary artery disease: impact on early outcomes. *Ann Thorac Surg* 2008;86:1424–1430.
108. Ferguson TB, Dziuban SW, Edwards FH, et al. The STS National Database: current changes and challenges for the new millennium. *Ann Thorac Surg* 2000;69:680–691.
109. Bernstein AD, Parsonnett V. Bedside estimation of risk as an aid for decision-making in cardiac surgery. *Ann Thorac Surg* 2000;69:823–828.
110. Dupuis J-Y, Wang F, Nathan H, et al. The cardiac anesthesia risk evaluation score: a clinically useful predictor of mortality and morbidity after cardiac surgery. *Anesthesiology* 2001;94:194–204.
111. Nashef SA, Roques F, Hammill BG, et al. Validation of European System for Cardiac Operative Risk Evaluation (EuroSCORE) in North American cardiac surgery. *Eur J Cardiothorac Surg* 2002;22:101–105.
112. Ambler G, Omar RZ, Royston P, et al. Generic, simple risk stratification model for heart valve surgery. *Circulation* 2005;112:224–231.
113. Singh M, Gersh BJ, Li S, et al. Mayo Clinic Risk Score for percutaneous coronary intervention predicts in-hospital mortality in patients undergoing coronary artery bypass graft surgery. *Circulation* 2008;117:356–362.
114. Charlesworth DC, Likosky DS, Marrin CAS, et al. Development and validation of a prediction model for strokes after coronary bypass grafting. *Ann Thorac Surg* 2003;76:436–443.
115. Fowler VG Jr, O'Brien SM, Muhlbaier LH, et al. Clinical predictors of major infections after cardiac surgery. *Circulation* 2005;112 (suppl):I358–I365.
116. Magee MJ, Herbert MA, Dewey TM, et al. Atrial fibrillation after coronary artery bypass grafting surgery: development of a predictive risk algorithm. *Ann Thorac Surg* 2007;83:1707–1712.
117. Reddy SLC, Grayson AD, Griffiths EM, et al. Logistical risk model for prolonged ventilation after adult cardiac surgery. *Ann Thorac Surg* 2007; 84:528–536.
118. Ranucci M, Castelvecchio S, Menicanti L, et al. Risk of assessing mortality risk in elective cardiac operations. *Circulation* 2009;119:3053–3061.
119. Dyub Am, Whitlock RP, Abouzahr LL, et al. Preoperative intra-aortic balloon pump in patients undergoing coronary bypass surgery: a systematic review and meta-analysis. *J Card Surg* 2008;23:79–86.

120. Dietl CA, Berkheimer MD, Woods EL, et al. Efficacy and cost-effectiveness of preoperative IABP in patients with ejection fraction of 0.25 or less. *Ann Thorac Surg* 1996;62:401–409.
121. Christenson JT, Simonet F, Badel P, et al. Optimal timing of preoperative intraaortic balloon pump support in high-risk coronary patients. *Ann Thorac Surg* 1999;68:934–939.
122. Dyub AM, Whitlock RP, Abouzahr LL, et al. Preoperative intra-aortic balloon pump in patients undergoing coronary bypass surgery: a systematic review and meta-analysis. *J Card Surg* 2008;23:79–86.
123. Weiass ES, Chang DD, Joyce DL, et al. Optimal timing of coronary artery bypass after acute myocardial infarction: a review of California discharge data. *J Thorac Cardiovasc Surg* 2008;135:503–511.
124. Carabello BA, Paulus WJ. Aortic stenosis. *Lancet* 2009;373:956–966.
125. Oloaison L, Pettersson G. Current best practices and guidelines: indications for surgical intervention in infective endocarditis. *Cardiol Clin* 2003;21:235–251.
126. Manteiga R, Souto JC, Altès A, et al. Short-course thrombolysis as the first line of therapy for cardiac valve thrombosis. *J Thorac Cardiovasc Surg* 1998;115:780–784.
127. Lengyel M, Fuster V, Keltai M, et al. Guidelines for management of left-sided prosthetic valve thrombosis: a role for thrombolytic therapy. *J Am Coll Cardiol* 1997;30:1521–1526.
128. Vongpatanasin W, Hillis LD, Lange RA. Prosthetic heart valves. *N Engl J Med* 1996;355: 407–416.
129. Horst M, Melhorn U, Heoerstrup SP, et al. Cardiac surgery in patients with end-stage renal disease: a 10-year experience. *Ann Thorac Surg* 2000;69:96–101.
130. Bechtel JFM, Detter C, Fischlein T, et al. Cardiac surgery in patients on dialysis: decreased 30-day mortality, unchanged overall survival. *Ann Thorac Surg* 2008;85: 147–153.
131. Rahmanian PB, Adams DH, Castillo JG, et al. Early and late outcome of cardiac surgery in dialysis-dependent patients: single-center experience with 245 consecutive patients. *J Thorac Cardiovasc Surg* 2008;135:915–922.
132. Gaudino M, Serricchio M, Luciani N, et al. Risks of using internal thoracic artery grafts in patients in chronic hemodialysis via upper extremity arteriovenous fistula. *Circulation* 2003;107:2653–2655.
133. Khan JH, Davis EA, Dean LS, et al. The role of elective perioperative dialysis in nondialysis renal failure patients. *Ann Thorac Surg* 87:1085–1089.
134. Reimhold SC, Rutherford JD. Valvular heart disease in pregnancy. *N Engl J Med* 2003;349:52–59.
135. Chandrasekhar S, Cook CR, Colard CD. Cardiac surgery in the parturient. *Anesth Analg* 2009;108:777–785.
136. Arnoni RT, Arnoni AS, Bonini RCA, et al. Risk factors associated with cardiac surgery during pregnancy. *Ann Thorac Surg* 2003;76:1605–1608.
137. Mahli A, Izdes S, Coskun D. Cardiac operations during pregnancy: review of factors influencing fetal outcome. *Ann Thorac Surg* 2000;69:1622–1626.
138. Jilma B, Kamath S, Lip GYH. Antithrombotic therapy in special circumstances. I—pregnancy and cancer. *BMJ* 2003;326:37–40.
139. Engelman R, Shahian D, Shemin R, et al. The Society of Thoracic Surgeons practice guideline series: antibiotic prophylaxis in cardiac surgery, part II: antibiotic choice. *Ann Thorac Surg* 2007;83:1569–1576.

2 Operative Management

BASIC MONITORING

Continuous measurement of the arterial blood pressure is standard during cardiac surgery. Most commonly, a small catheter is inserted into a radial artery by percutaneous technique, a process that is facilitated by the use of a soft-tipped guidewire. Sometimes, particularly in very young pediatric patients, open exposure (cutdown) of the artery is required. In teenagers and adults, an Allen's test is performed before radial artery cannulation to demonstrate adequate ulnar artery collateral flow to the hand (Fig. 2.1); if the test is positive (i.e., inadequate collateral to the hand), that radial artery should not be used (1). If a radial artery is to be used as coronary artery bypass conduit, the monitoring cannula is placed into the contralateral hand. If neither radial artery can be used for whatever reason, a femoral artery is a good second alternative, and because of the size of the artery, percutaneous insertion is usually simple. If aortoiliac disease precludes use of lower extremity arterial pressure monitoring, a brachial or axillary artery monitoring line may be used, although the complication rate may be higher (2).

Following cardiopulmonary bypass (CPB), the radial artery is usually accurate for postoperative monitoring but, at times, may underestimate the true central arterial pressure due to peripheral vasoconstriction, which may be exacerbated by hypothermia or the administration of vasoconstrictor medications (2,3). In some patients, a radial artery monitoring line may not function optimally in the early minutes following CPB, but will improve in a short time. In these circumstances, central aortic pressure can be monitored from the aortic perfusion cannula once bypass is terminated. Most commercially available cannulae or in-line connectors can be obtained with Luer-lock side ports for this purpose. If the difference in monitored blood pressure persists, a femoral artery line can be inserted in the surgical field for postoperative use. In these circumstances, the femoral artery is more reliable than the smaller arteries for pressure measurement (4,5).

Complications of arterial lines are rare if proper techniques of insertion and maintenance are used. The incidence of thrombotic complications is increased by the presence of low cardiac output, hypotension, administration of vasoconstrictor agents, and long duration of use (6,7). Although these factors are related to the individual patient, other factors

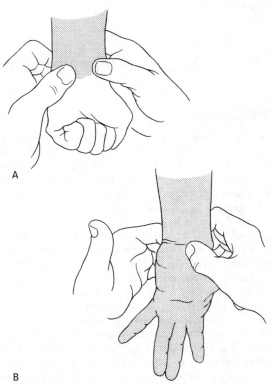

FIGURE 2.1 Arterial line insertion. An Allen's test is used to confirm that the collateral circulation to the hand is intact. The patient is instructed to make a fist, which results in the blanching of the palmar skin. Both ulnar and radial arteries are then manually occluded **(A)**. The patient is instructed to open the hand, and while the radial artery is kept occluded, pressure is removed from the ulnar artery **(B)**. If the perfusion returns to the fingers, adequate collateral circulation via the ulnar artery is intact, and a radial arterial line may be safely inserted.

may contribute to thrombosis, such as multiple attempts at cannulation and large catheter size. The risk of infection of arterial catheters is increased by the use of cutdown rather than percutaneous technique, long duration of use, and inflammation at the catheter site. Femoral arterial catheters may be at somewhat greater risk for infection.

A large-bore cannula or multilumen catheter for central venous pressure measurement, fluid infusion, and drug administration is inserted via the jugular (internal or external) vein with the tip being advanced to the superior vena cava or right atrium. Catheter tip position can be confirmed in the operative field by manual palpation of the superior vena cava; this is particularly important when the catheter is inserted in the left neck or either subclavian position. Proper position is particularly important if central venous pressure is the only filling pressure measurement being used. Peripherally inserted catheters (placed into basilic or cephalic veins) will yield similar measurements of central venous pressure if the catheter tip is properly located and if a continuous fluid infusion device (such as are used with intra-arterial lines) is used (8). During surgery, when the chest is open, catheters may also be inserted directly into the innominate vein or right atrium. In rare circumstances where mechanical valves have been placed in the tricuspid position and where measurement of pulmonary artery (PA) pressure is important, a small-caliber catheter may be inserted into the PA during surgery via a pursestring suture or pledget-reinforced mattress suture in the right ventricular outflow tract. In such circumstances, catheter removal should be done while mediastinal chest tubes are still in place and after coagulation function has normalized.

The internal jugular vein provides safe and direct access for PA catheter insertion (Fig. 2.2). The vein is first located by puncture with a 21- or 22-gauge "exploring" needle; in this manner, an inadvertent puncture of the carotid artery can be managed by holding gentle pressure until there is no risk of hematoma formation. Alternatively, ultrasound can be used to assist in locating the internal jugular vein and distinguishing it from the carotid artery, and using the Trendelenberg position to raise the venous pressure and distend the vein are both useful adjuncts. If the larger Swan–Ganz introducer is mistakenly inserted into the artery, the operation should be postponed unless it is an emergency or urgent, in which case this complication should be managed by open repair of the carotid artery before institution of heparinization and bypass (9). The subclavian vein is an alternative site for PA catheter insertion; the risk of pneumothorax and hemorrhage is higher, but subclavian insertion may be associated with fewer infectious complications (7,10). We avoid using the left-sided central veins as access routes in reoperations and other selected cases in which the innominate vein is at increased risk of injury during the surgical procedure. In addition, if there are multiple implanted pacemaker or internal defibrillator leads passing through the innominate vein, this may also make passing a Swan–Ganz catheter from the left side more difficult.

The technique for PA catheter insertion is outlined in Figure 2.3. Continuous electrocardiographic (ECG) monitoring is mandatory during the insertion of PA catheters as occasional arrhythmias or conduction disturbances may complicate this procedure. These complications may be reduced by passing the catheter through the right ventricle (RV) in an expeditious manner and by avoiding redundant loops of catheter within the cardiac chambers. The development of

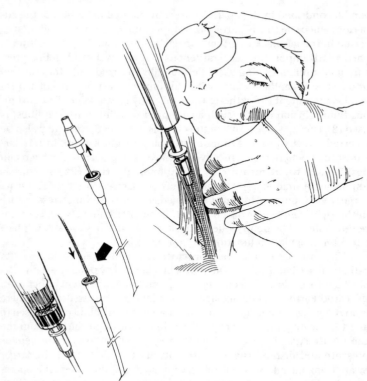

FIGURE 2.2 Technique for internal jugular access. The patient is situated in the Trendelenburg position with the head turned to the side opposite line insertion. After a sterile prep and draping, the left hand is used to localize the carotid artery. A cannula with needle is then directed between the two heads of the sternocleidomastoid muscle to find the vein. After blood return is confirmed from the needle, the cannula is grasped to immobilize it, the needle is withdrawn, and a guidewire is then inserted into the internal jugular vein. The guidewire may be passed into the central venous position, which may sometimes be confirmed by observing that premature ventricular contractions have occurred when the guidewire reaches the right ventricle. The central venous catheter (or Swan–Ganz introducer sheath) may then be introduced over the guidewire. The wire is withdrawn, and central venous position is confirmed by noting that venous blood may be aspirated. If central venous pressures are low, air embolism is a potential risk, and care must be taken not to allow ingress of air when the syringe is removed from the catheter hub.

complete heart block during passage of the PA catheter is more common in patients with left bundle branch block or in patients with *l*-looped ventricular anatomy. In these situations, a separate pacing wire can be inserted before PA catheter placement. Alternatively, a PA catheter that includes a separate port for pacing wire passage can be

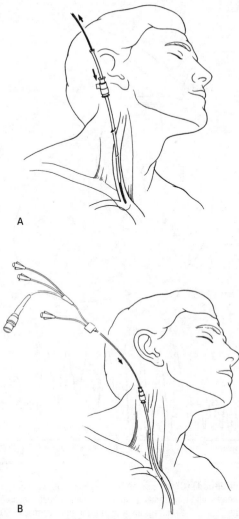

FIGURE 2.3 Swan–Ganz catheter insertion. **(A)** With use of the technique described in Fig. 2.2, an introducer sheath is placed in the internal jugular vein. Such a sheath usually contains a port for intravenous infusion and will usually contain an O ring at the end of the sheath to prevent ingress of air when the Swan–Ganz catheter is not present. **(B)** All ports of the Swan–Ganz catheter are filled with heparinized saline, and the distal port is connected to a physiologic monitor. The Swan–Ganz catheter is inserted into the introducer sheath and advanced initially into the superior vena cava (SVC). (*continued*)

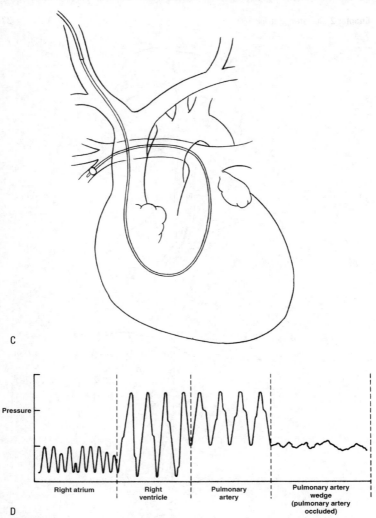

C

D

| Right atrium | Right ventricle | Pulmonary artery | Pulmonary artery wedge (pulmonary artery occluded) |

Pressure

FIGURE 2.3 (Continued) (C) Once present in the SVC, the balloon is inflated, and the catheter is advanced while the pressure monitor is continuously observed. The catheter is passed from the SVC to the right atrium and into the right ventricle. Subsequently, the catheter may be passed into the pulmonary artery and into the pulmonary capillary wedge position. Transit from right atrium to right ventricle and from right ventricle to pulmonary artery can sometimes be facilitated by having the patient take a deep inspiration, which will temporarily bring additional venous return into the heart. **(D)** An example of the hemodynamic tracings obtained during insertion of a Swan–Ganz catheter. The difference between right atrial and right ventricular pressures is often obvious. However, when right ventricular filling pressures are elevated, it may be difficult to distinguish right ventricular from pulmonary artery pressure. A useful guide to note is that during diastole, pulmonary artery pressures will *decrease*.

used or external pacemaker pads can be placed on the chest wall. Ventricular tachycardia or fibrillation is usually manageable by quickly withdrawing the catheter, defibrillation if indicated, and appropriate anti-arrhythmic drugs if needed.

Complications related to PA catheters include infection, air embolism, and PA rupture. PA catheters rarely become infected if removed within 4 days of insertion (7,11). Air emboli are avoided by using standard techniques common to the management of all central venous lines. Rupture of a PA branch is rare but potentially catastrophic. The complication occurs in approximately 0.2% of PA catheter insertions and has a mortality rate of about 50%; it is more common in elderly women and in patients with pulmonary hypertension and in those who are anticoagulated (12). Often, the patient has a warning ("herald") bleed, specifically, an episode of hemoptysis; for the intubated patient, this would be the appearance of blood in the endotracheal tube. If this occurs in the operating room following PA catheter insertion but before surgery has begun, the operation should be postponed, the patient transferred to the intensive care unit, and management carried out as described in Chapter 3. If it occurs during the procedure, manifested commonly during weaning from CPB when PA pressure increases, management may be difficult, especially if massive bleeding develops. Bypass should be reinstituted to temporarily decrease PA pressure. Intraoperative bronchoscopy can confirm the diagnosis, and lobar isolation with a bronchial blocker will usually tamponade the bleeding and protects the remaining lung, particularly if bleeding is from an intraparenchymal lobar branch of the PA. Bypass can then be weaned and heparin reversed. Once coagulation function has been restored, repeat bronchoscopy will confirm control of active bleeding and assist in irrigation and aspiration removal of residual blood from the airway. Generally, 24 hours of bronchial control is needed, after which the blocker should be deflated and the patient observed for recurrent bleeding. Rarely, thoracotomy and lung resection may be required to control the bleeding (13,14).

Transthoracic pressure monitoring lines, placed during the surgical procedure, are used most frequently in infants but may be necessary in older children and adults who have limited venous access. When transvenous access is not possible, insertion of a transthoracic right atrial (RA) or PA catheter will provide necessary pressure measurements. Left atrial (LA) lines may be useful when the pulmonary capillary wedge pressure does not correlate well with the true LA pressure (15); they may be particularly useful for managing right heart failure. During surgery, these lines may be inserted via a pursestring suture in the right superior pulmonary vein, or if this route is used for insertion of a left ventricular vent, the resulting opening provides easy access for insertion of an LA line (Fig. 2.4). LA catheters add the risk of complications including

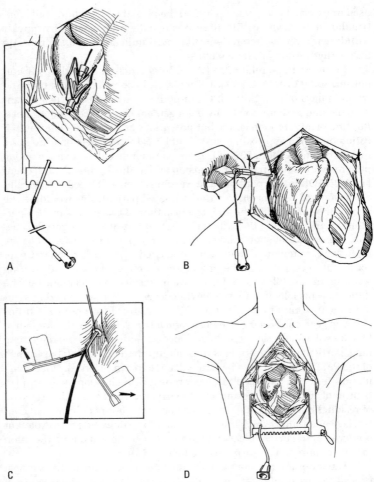

FIGURE 2.4 Intraoperative technique for left atrial line insertion. **(A)** Via a large-bore needle, inserted from inside the epigastric abdominal wall, the left atrial catheter is introduced into the chest. **(B)** With use of a split, "break-away" needle, the end of the left atrial catheter is introduced into the left atrium via the proximal right superior pulmonary vein using a pursestring suture to secure hemostasis at the insertion site. **(C)** The "break-away" needle is then extracted and removed. **(D)** A gentle loop of catheter is left along the right side of the heart to prevent inadvertent extraction of the line when the chest is closed.

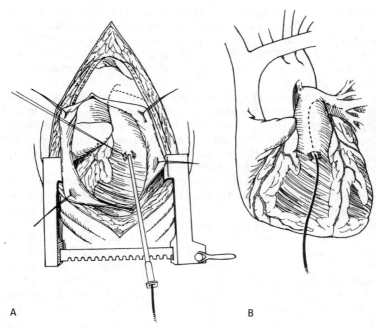

A   B

FIGURE 2.5 Pulmonary artery monitoring line inserted via pursestring suture in the right ventricular outflow tract. Via a pledget-reinforced mattress suture, a catheter is introduced into the right ventricular outflow tract **(A)**, using an introducer or a cannula-over-needle type of intravenous cannula. The introducer is withdrawn, the mattress suture is tightened, and the catheter is exteriorized through a small stab incision **(B)**.

systemic emboli of air and particulate matter, bleeding, and interference with prosthetic mitral valves. Other catheters that are of use include RA and PA lines inserted via a pursestring suture (Fig. 2.5). This approach is particularly useful in neonates and infants for measurement of PA pressure, PA blood sampling, or insertion of thermodilution or oxygen saturation probes. This approach has proved safe, even in relatively hypertensive RVs (16).

Continuous measurement of the patient's temperature is routine and important. This may be accomplished via a probe on the tympanic membrane, in the nasopharynx, and/or in the esophagus. Bladder or rectal probes may also be used but are less accurate, and measurements will lag core temperature during cooling or rewarming, especially in adults. A Swan–Ganz PA catheter also provides continuous determination of the PA blood temperature, but this is not of use during CPB when the lungs are excluded from the circulation. On bypass, arterial and venous blood temperatures are monitored continuously by in-line sensors. Urinary catheters are inserted after induction of anesthesia; periodic determinations of the rate of urine production are recorded before, during, and after CPB, with appropriate interventions being undertaken should the urine output fall below the volume appropriate for the size and age of the patient.

A transcutaneous oxygen saturation monitor probe is attached to the patient's finger. Although useful in detecting sudden changes in peripheral arterial oxygen saturation, it is dependent on tissue perfusion and may be unreliable in low-flow states. Alternatively, they may be placed on an ear lobe where circulation may be better, particularly when peripheral perfusion is compromised.

Nasogastric or orogastric catheters may be inserted after induction of anesthesia, may be deferred until after the procedure is completed, or may not be used at all. If the patient is to remain intubated for a number of hours after surgery or if the abdomen is distended, then stomach drainage may be employed to prevent gastric distension and the likelihood of pulmonary aspiration. Many patients, especially those without risk factors for gastro-esophageal reflux, may be managed without nasogastric tubes, and, in fact, these tubes may be associated with an increased incidence of nosocomial pneumonia (17,18). When a gastric drainage tube is used, it should always be placed to low-level suction.

OTHER MONITORING TECHNIQUES

Flow-directed PA catheters, specifically the *Swan–Ganz catheter*, permit continuous measurement of central venous and PA pressures, estimation of cardiac output, and a port to withdraw blood samples for the determination of mixed venous oxygen saturation. Specially designed PA catheters (and monitors) have a distal sensor that (with a special computer and monitor) provides for continuous real-time determination of the mixed venous oxygen saturation. Other special PA catheters have built-in ports for pacing wire insertion to allow for temporary electrical pacing of the right atrium and the RV. This may be particularly useful in patients with pre-existing sinoatrial node dysfunction, heart block, aortic stenosis, or regurgitation or in reoperations (19). Whereas the use of PA catheters in adults undergoing cardiac surgery is very common, it is not universal or required. At some institutions, PA catheter use is reserved for highly selected patients with excellent results (20–22).

Intraoperative *transesophageal echocardiography* (TEE) has become a commonly performed procedure for both diagnostic and monitoring purposes. At some institutions, TEE is used in the place of a PA catheter for the purpose of monitoring cardiac function during cardiac surgery. The technique has proven to be safe and of considerable value for both routine operations and special situations (23). Direct visualization of the heart with TEE allows for the identification and analysis of several important issues in cardiac operations. These include but are not limited to the following:

1. Presence or absence of patent foramen ovale (PFO), and hence, presence or absence of the risk of air embolization. If a PFO is suspected, a bubble study performed with agitated saline may be needed to confirm the diagnosis. We routinely close PFOs if found at surgery.

2. Adequacy of aortic valve function to permit administration of cardioplegia into the ascending aorta.

3. TEE provides direct visualization of valve anatomy and is particularly useful immediately before mitral valve repair to assess pathologic anatomy in the beating heart. Following repair, the adequacy of valve repair and the dynamics of the anterior mitral leaflet can be determined. In addition, the function and seating of a newly implanted prosthetic valve can be confirmed (24).

4. Detection of atheromatous disease in the descending aorta and aortic arch.

5. Assessment of ventricular distension when operations are conducted without a PA catheter.

6. Monitoring and confirming the adequacy of air removal in open heart operations.

7. Assessment of ventricular (both left and right) contractility and regional function. For example, a new wall motion abnormality following aortic valve replacement could signify compromise of a coronary ostium.

8. Assessment of cardiac chamber filling status, particularly when heart valve operations have altered the relationship between measured filling pressures and actual chamber filling.

9. Monitoring the effects of fluid infusion and administered inotropic and vasoactive drugs.

10. Confirming the diagnosis and assessing the extent of aortic dissections and presence or absence of involvement of the aortic valve. This also includes intraoperative dissections related to cross-clamping or aortic cannulation.

For these reasons, the use of intraoperative TEE has become standard at our hospitals for virtually all procedures. Echocardiographic analysis is performed by cardiac anesthesia specialists, occasionally with input from cardiologists for particularly complex valve problems or for analysis of unexpected findings. Although safe for use in the majority of patients, there remains a small incremental risk to the use of TEE

(25). Patients with known esophageal pathology or hiatus hernia may pose an increased risk for use of TEE, particularly for transgastric viewing.

NEUROLOGIC MONITORING DURING CARDIAC SURGERY

It is well recognized in adult and pediatric heart surgery that neurologic complications can occur during hypothermic circulatory arrest or as a result of perfusion mishaps. For the purpose of monitoring cerebral oxygen delivery during CPB and/or during circulatory arrest, near infrared spectroscopy has been adopted for relatively simple intraoperative use (INVOS™, Somanetics, Inc.). This technique uses light-emitting diode generated light that is aimed through the anterior scalp and frontal bone and records reflected light from both left and right frontal lobe areas. Although the technique does not measure actual oxygen tension or saturation, it provides comparison to starting levels of oxygenation as well as left–right comparison. Although definitive studies demonstrating its utility in cardiac surgery are lacking, some clinical evidence suggests that it might have value in certain settings, particularly in pediatric heart surgery (26,27), for operations performed under circulatory arrest, or when selective antegrade cerebral perfusion is employed.

PACING AND ARRHYTHMIAS

Unexpected sinus bradycardia occurring during induction of anesthesia or in the earliest stages of the operation can be treated pharmacologically (see Chapter 4). Alternatively, the heart can usually be electrically paced via a pacing port Swan–Ganz catheter. It should be remembered that although bradycardia may be a response to anesthesia, it may also be indicative of a more serious problem such as hypoxia or myocardial ischemia.

Patients with previously placed permanent pacemakers should be evaluated before operation; the pacemaker manufacturer and model should be known, and a copy of a recent pacemaker interrogation should be available in the operating room. Electrocautery and defibrillation may affect the performance of the pacemaker in a variety of undesirable ways, such as reversion to a backup mode or damage to the sensing and pulse generator circuits. Although modern pacemaker electronics permit safe and uneventful operation in most cases, certain precautions should be employed. These include placing the cautery ground plate as far from the pacemaker as possible, using the lowest possible cautery intensity, and keeping the appropriate pacemaker programmer in the operating room throughout the procedure. Patients who are pacemaker-dependent and in whom electrocautery results in pacer suppression and bradycardia or asystole can be managed by placement of a magnet over the pacemaker generator, which will revert the generator into a fixed-rate mode. Many pacemakers implanted today are rate-responsive models that monitor and respond to physiologic parameters such as minute ventilation or muscle activity. Prior to surgery, pacemakers should be interrogated so that behavior with a magnet applied will be known in advance (28).

ANESTHESIA

Narcotics are an important component of the anesthetic management of patients who are undergoing cardiac surgery because they have minimal effects on cardiac function and limited interaction with other agents. Synthetic narcotic agents such as fentanyl and sufentanil provide rapid induction and emergence from anesthesia with few effects on hemodynamics, even in patients with critical cardiac disease (29).

Narcotics alone are not always adequate to prevent hemodynamic responses to operative stimuli, particularly in children. In addition, in contemporary practice, less narcotic is being used to permit more rapid emergence and extubation following surgery. For this reason, inhalation agents (such as isoflurane, desflurane, or sevoflurane) are often added as needed, particularly during periods of greater surgical stimulation or to help control peripheral vascular resistance. The inhalational anesthetic agents are short acting, provide for early extubation, and are cost-effective (30). They can also be readily titrated up and down as needed to control blood pressure. They are, however, used with care due to a mild direct negative inotropic effect (particularly at higher concentration) and a positive chronotropic effect that may increase oxygen consumption requirements. Because inhalation agents are potent vasodilators, the net effect on cardiac output may, however, be beneficial. Inhalation agents may also be added to the oxygenator gas flow during CPB; this is particularly useful for management of hypertension during bypass. Nitrous oxide is used infrequently because of its negative effects on cardiac output and blood pressure, its relative anesthetic impotency, and its ability to worsen any potential air embolism.

Intravenously administered sedatives such as the benzodiazepines are frequently added, particularly when lower doses of narcotics are used. In patients taking benzodiazepines on a chronic basis, higher doses of these medications are required to prevent procedure recall. Ketamine is used in children, particularly by intramuscular administration because of its rapid hypnotic and analgesic effects without depression of respiratory or cardiovascular function. For this reason, ketamine may also be useful for induction of severely unstable patients such as those with tamponade or with massive pulmonary embolus. Muscle relaxants including vecuronium and cisatricurium are particularly useful after induction of general anesthesia to reduce the muscular rigidity associated with agents such as fentanyl that may make ventilation difficult.

For patients who undergo surgery with reduced narcotic dosing, propofol infusion (25 to 30 μg/kg/min) may be used during the early postoperative period to maintain deep sedation until body temperature has normalized and surgical bleeding has stopped. When infusion is discontinued, this short-acting agent permits rapid wake-up and extubation.

At some hospitals, spinal and epidural techniques are used in conjunction with narcotic and inhalational agents for adults undergoing cardiac operations (31).

CONDUCT OF THE OPERATION

The patient should be properly positioned to allow access to all fields of interest. For coronary bypass operations, this includes adequate exposure of the saphenous vein harvest sites. A circumferential leg prep permits harvesting of greater or lesser saphenous veins, if needed. In patients with superficial varicosities, or in patients who are obese where saphenous veins cannot be palpated, preoperative ultrasound vein mapping is useful to identify vein diameter and to identify varices. In circumstances where additional arterial conduits are desired, such as in young patients or when a lower extremity vein is not available, the radial artery can be used. If use of this conduit is a possibility, the selected extremity must be kept free of intra-arterial and intravenous lines and should be included in the surgical field. In general, the radial artery is harvested from the nondominant arm. The integrity and function of the palmar arch are confirmed by the preoperative Allen's test and by measuring the distal index finger oxygen saturation with an oximetry probe during manual compression of the radial pulse. In addition to a negative Allen's test, fingertip oximetry should show a saturation of at least 95% during radial pulse compression to harvest the radial artery. We also continuously measure the index fingertip oximetry during the radial artery harvesting process.

Careful positioning of the patient is important to avoid peripheral nerve complications, which may result from hyperabduction of the shoulders or inadequate cushioning of the arms or legs. All arterial and venous lines must be secure and accessible to the anesthesiologist. Connections must be securely tightened and any stopcocks properly capped to avoid contamination. The patient's body hair is clipped (not shaved) within a few hours prior to being brought to the operating room (32). The skin is prepared with disinfectant soap by experienced personnel after all other manipulation of the patient has ceased. During the skin preparation, it is poor technique to permit members of the team to start intravenous lines, insert nasogastric tubes, attach cautery ground plates, or otherwise risk contamination. Extreme caution must be used with alcohol-containing skin prep solutions to avoid excessive solution and pooling that can create a fire risk.

In selected cases, including all reoperations, we apply adhesive external defibrillator pads to the lateral chest walls; these permit the transthoracic administration of direct current countershock before the heart has been adequately exposed (33). In all cases, internal defibrillator paddles must be readily available to the surgeon and should be tested at the outset to ensure proper function. The pump oxygenator is primed and available to be present in the operating room no later than during induction of anesthesia. Sudden hemodynamic deterioration may require emergency cannulation and establishment of bypass. The perfusionist is also in attendance throughout this period.

Although the cosmetic benefits of a small incision may be appealing, it is important to make a large enough incision to perform the operation without compromising the surgical endpoint. In recent years, with the emphasis on less invasive approaches to cardiac surgery in appropriate cases, uses of alternatives to a standard full sternotomy have become more commonplace. Partial upper and lower sternotomies can be used for aortic valve surgery (34), mitral valve surgery (35), and correction of some types of congenital heart defects (36). These are illustrated in Figure 2.6. When a lower partial sternotomy is utilized, particularly in children, access to the ascending aorta and superior vena cava can be enhanced substantially by retracting the upper sternum anteriorly, as shown in Fig. 2.7. At times, a right anterolateral thoracotomy incision can be used, particularly for mitral and tricuspid valve operations or atrial septal defects; in these situations, the right inguinal area should be prepped in the field in the event that arterial or venous access is needed for bypass. Occasionally, coronary bypass procedures involving the left circumflex artery only are performed through a left lateral thoracotomy incision (37). A bilateral inframammary incision provides a cosmetically pleasing full median sternotomy, albeit with some compromise of exposure; this approach is now rarely used (38).

Operations performed on patients who have previously undergone a sternotomy incision ("redos") require special considerations (39–41). Adhesions between the heart, great vessels, sternum, and other surrounding structures can complicate re-entry into the chest with risk of damage to the heart (especially the RV) and/or previously placed bypass grafts (especially mammary artery grafts). The surgeon should review previous operative report(s) and anesthesia records. The lateral chest x-ray film is reviewed to prepare for any particularly hazardous anatomy; if present, the location of the previously placed internal mammary artery pedicle is usually identifiable by the hemostatic clips that were attached to it. Coronary angiography may provide a clue to determine whether the RV is densely adherent to the back of the

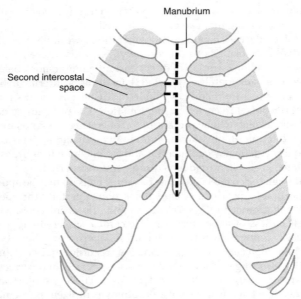

FIGURE 2.6 The dotted lines indicate two options for partial sternotomy. The upper partial sternotomy may be used for procedures such as aortic valve replacement, while the lower partial sternotomy is used for operations on the mitral and tricuspid valves, as well as for congenital cardiac procedures requiring access through the atria. A vertical osteotomy is made, and in either case, a short transverse osteotomy on the right side of the second interspace completes the partial sternotomy. In most cases, retraction can be accomplished without having to divide or damage the right internal mammary artery.

sternum or not. The appearance and motion of RV marginal branches during the cardiac cycle should be observed. If the opacified branches move freely underneath the sternal midline, then it is likely that the RV is not densely adherent. Finally, preoperative CT scanning may be needed and may be of particular value to plan a reoperation when aortic enlargement, RV dilation, or patent bypass grafts are present (42).

For patients who have hazardous anatomy (such as a patent internal mammary artery that is close to the posterior aspect of the sternum), we usually place a cannula into one of the femoral arteries to be available for access should expeditious cannulation be required. When there have been multiple previous operations, cardiomegaly, elevated RA pressures, or other circumstances that cause even greater concern (e.g., ascending aortic aneurysm or false aneurysm), isolation of the femoral artery and vein (via a groin cutdown incision) before making the sternotomy incision permits rapid cannulation if problems arise. In rare cases, CPB may

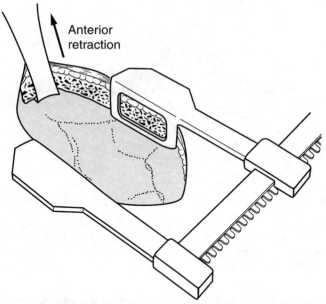

FIGURE 2.7 When partial sternotomies are utilized, visibility can often be enhanced by anterior retraction on the sternum utilizing a retractor that is fixed to the side of the operating table.

be established via the femoral route before attempting posterior sternal division; this is frequently the most prudent approach in reoperations when there is severe tricuspid regurgitation with significant elevation of RA pressure (>20 mm Hg). Bypass may be instituted with mild hypothermia to permit continued ejection of the heart, and bypass flow can be temporarily reduced to decompress the right heart for the posterior sternotomy. Right heart decompression can also be achieved by using a long, thin-walled venous drain that has been advanced over a guidewire from the femoral vein into the right atrium, as confirmed by echocardiography.

Sternal re-entry is made safer by using an oscillating (cast-cutter) saw with the first assistant elevating the sternum anteriorly (Fig. 2.8). Another useful maneuver is to leave the posterior portion of the sternal wires in place while the oscillating saw is applied. In this fashion, 1 or 2 mm of additional space may be available for safe passage of the saw blade. After the sternal bone is divided, the table-mounted internal mammary artery retractor is useful for elevating the sternal half while dissecting the underlying tissues from the bone.

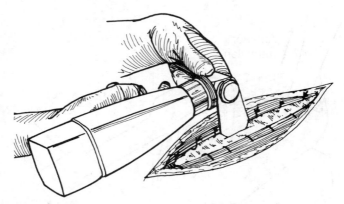

FIGURE 2.8 In reoperations for cardiac surgery, the redo sternotomy is generally performed with an oscillating saw. The major concern is adherence of cardiac structures to the posterior table of the sternum. One approach to prevent injury to the aorta or right ventricle is shown: After cutting old sternal wires, they are left in place and used as a guide to the depth of penetration by the oscillating saw, thus decreasing the risk of injuring the aorta or right ventricle.

ANTICOAGULATION FOR CARDIOPULMONARY BYPASS

Heparin

Contact between the patient's blood and the nonendothelialized surface of the heart–lung machine is a powerful stimulus for thrombin generation and clot formation; therefore, complete anticoagulation of the blood is required for safe extracorporeal perfusion. Except for very special circumstances, this is accomplished by the administration of a large dose of unfractionated heparin. Heparin is an anionic, sulfated glycosaminoglycan derived from the mast cells of either porcine intestine or bovine lung (43). Unfractionated heparin is a heterogeneous mix of molecules with a mean molecular mass of 15,000 Da. In the United States, heparin potency is described in terms of USP units. USP units are not, however, equivalent to international units (IU). In the United States, the required potency of heparin is 140 USP U/mg of heparin (44). Thus, a dose of 3 mg/kg of body weight (a loading dose used at some institutions) is equivalent to 420 USP U/kg. Heparin acts to catalyze the rate at which the endogenous anticoagulant antithrombin III neutralizes thrombin and activated coagulation factor X (Xa). In order for heparin to be effective, therefore, sufficient antithrombin III must be present because heparin alone has little or no anticoagulant activity. There is considerable variation in responsiveness to heparin. The degree of anticoagulation may be monitored by a number of different tests, although the activated clotting time (ACT) is by far the one most commonly used (45). The patient's ACT is measured before and after administration of heparin. The ACT is a rather crude but global measure of clotting function. In the ACT tube is an activator substance, typically either celite (diatomaceous earth) or kaolin (clay), that acts to accelerate the blood coagulation. The ACT is, however, affected by other factors besides the presence of heparin, including hypothermia, extreme hemodilution, thrombocytopenia, and antithrombin III deficiency.

A commonly used heparin loading dose is 450 U/kg of body weight, although variation among institutions exists. The minimum ACT duration required to eliminate thrombin formation during CPB is not known and is likely not the same for all patients. The ACT duration of 450 seconds is a commonly used minimum threshold considered necessary for safe extracorporeal perfusion; thus, an ACT of 450 seconds is achieved before instituting CPB. The ACT is checked every 30 minutes on bypass and maintained above the selected minimum duration by additional heparin doses.

Other methods to monitor anticoagulation for CPB are available; a common one is the heparin concentration assay, which uses an automated protamine titration method (45,46). Although quite useful, it must be remembered that measuring the direct heparin concentration may not reflect the true coagulation status of the blood. In the circumstance of antithrombin deficiency (heparin resistance; see following discussion), clotting can still occur despite the presence of adequate heparin levels; therefore, concomitant measurement of the ACT is recommended even when heparin concentration assays are utilized.

Protamine

Heparin is neutralized by the administration of protamine, a strongly cationic protein derived from salmon sperm. Although generally safe, occasional adverse reactions to protamine do occur.

Not infrequently, protamine infusion produces mild hypotension by a direct vasodilation effect (47,48). This is due to the release of histamine from mast cells in response to the alkaline nature of protamine. The severity of the hypotensive response is directly related to the rate at which the protamine is infused and is increased in hypovolemic patients. Slow infusion will prevent the development of the hypotensive response to protamine.

More importantly, however, protamine may cause one of two types of hemodynamic response associated with profound systemic hypotension (49). The first type is a nonimmunologic reaction related to complement activation and thromboxane release (50). This causes severe bronchospasm and pulmonary vasoconstriction. Systemic pressure falls as a result of poor pulmonary venous return. Although this response is usually short-lived, support of the circulation sometimes requires reheparinization and placing the patient back on CPB. After several minutes of stabilization, the patient may again be separated from bypass. Because this is not a true allergic response, protamine may be safely readministered, although we prefer to infuse it into the aortic root at a very slow rate. The second type of protamine reaction is a true immune-mediated anaphylactic response that may be fatal (48,49). This is usually characterized by bronchospasm, pulmonary hypertension, hypoxemia, left heart failure, and complete circulatory collapse. Resumption of CPB may be lifesaving. Treatment usually requires α-adrenergic vasoconstrictor agents (norepinephrine, phenylephrine), although vasodilators (nitroglycerin, milrinone) may also be useful to combat the pulmonary hypertension. Treatment with steroids (methylprednisolone 30 mg/kg IV) and histamine antagonists (diphenhydramine 25 to 50 mg IV) may help prevent a second reaction on re-exposure, and protamine infusion into the left side of the circulation may reduce histamine release. If the reaction was severe and life-threatening, protamine should not be readministered. Risk factors for serious protamine reactions include NPH insulin use, fish allergy, and history of nonprotamine medication allergy (51).

Protamine neutralizes heparin and normalizes the ACT. The dose of protamine required for reversal of heparin may be calculated by measuring the circulating heparin or by administering a dose based on the total dose of heparin that was administered during the procedure, followed by confirmation that the ACT has returned to baseline. A commonly used dose is 0.5 to 0.75 mg of protamine/100 U of heparin administered during the procedure. It should be administered slowly, over at least 5 minutes. The ACT is then rechecked and further protamine is given if it has not returned to baseline. Excess protamine is avoided, as it is associated with impaired platelet function, prolongation of the ACT, and increased bleeding (52,53).

Heparin Resistance

Occasional patients do not achieve the ACT minimum threshold despite large doses of heparin (such as 600 U of heparin/kg of body weight). This condition of reduced heparin responsiveness or "heparin resistance" is more common in patients who have received heparin preoperatively (a common therapy for unstable angina) and patients who are on an intra-aortic balloon pump before surgery (54). If the initial heparin-loading dose does not achieve adequate prolongation of the ACT, an additional dose of 100 to 150 U/kg is administered. If this still does not adequately prolong the ACT, antithrombin III deficiency must be suspected and treated. Fresh frozen plasma (2 U for an adult) or antithrombin concentrate (500 to 1,000 U) is administered, and the ACT is rechecked before institution of bypass (55,56).

Heparin-Induced Thrombocytopenia

Patients treated with heparin may develop thrombocytopenia with two distinct forms of heparin-induced thrombocytopenia (HIT) being recognized. Type I is an acute and mild reduction in the platelet count that occurs as a direct agglutinating effect of heparin; this is not associated with thrombosis and resolves even with continued heparin treatment. Type II is immune-mediated. IgG antibodies react with heparin–platelet factor 4 complexes, and these complexes then bind platelets, causing platelet activation, aggregation (resulting in thrombosis), and consumption (resulting in thrombocytopenia). This subject is also discussed in Chapter 5. Patients with HIT type II who require cardiac surgery (during which heparin is to be administered) are at considerable risk for complications when re-exposed to heparin. Thus, intraoperative anticoagulation is problematic (57). There are three options for such patients. Surgery can be delayed until IgG antibody levels decrease; this usually requires at least 3 months.

Platelet function antagonists such as tirofiban or prostaglandin may be used in conjunction with unfractionated heparin to minimize platelet activation until heparin can be fully reversed after surgery (58). Although this approach has been used in patients with HIT without thrombosis, we have been very cautious and have avoided its use in patients with HIT and the thrombosis syndrome.

Finally, direct thrombin inhibitors may be used. Although none of these agents have been approved yet, recombinant hirudin and lepirudin and the low-molecular-weight heparinoid danaparoid have been used with success (59,60). Another direct thrombin inhibitor that has been the subject of a clinical trial for this indication is bivalirudin (61). This agent has a short half-life and is eliminated primarily by proteolytic cleavage; it is approved for use in interventional cardiology. Keeping its short half-life (25 minutes) and method of elimination in mind, a protocol for its use in cardiac surgery has been developed. A bolus dose of 1 mg/kg is administered to the patient, 50 mg is put into the CPB prime, and a continuous infusion of 2.5 mg/kg per hour is started. We use an ACT target of 400 to 450 seconds with this agent. Keeping its method of elimination in mind, certain principles of intraoperative management are important. Hemofiltration should be avoided, as this can eliminate the agent. Any blood in a cardiotomy reservoir or in the surgical field must be kept aspirated into the bypass circuit, as "standing" blood can undergo degradation of bivalirudin and loss of anticoagulation. ACT should be monitored and the bivalirudin dose adjusted to keep the ACT in the 400 to 450 second range to minimize the time needed for the drug's effect to disappear after surgery. The infusion should be terminated approximately 15 minutes before the anticipated end of the bypass run and the ACT frequently checked. Once it diminishes to less than 400 seconds, bypass should be terminated. The blood left in the bypass circuit should be infused back into the patient as soon as possible or processed through a cell saver device. The anticoagulant effect of the agent will then diminish with a half-life of 25 to 30 minutes. Meticulous surgical hemostasis should be ensured, as often 2 or 3 hours are required to establish good clotting function.

TECHNIQUES OF EXTRACORPOREAL CIRCULATION (PERFUSION)

The ascending aorta is usually preferred for arterial cannulation but does carry the risk of embolization of atherosclerotic material to the head vessels. When selecting a cannulation site, the aorta should be palpated to exclude large plaques (Fig. 2.9). Intraoperative epiaortic ultrasound may be used to quickly examine the potential sites for cannulation and cross-clamp application (62). Use of this technique will, on occasion, reveal the presence of soft plaque that was not detected by palpation (Fig. 2.10). If this is encountered, the site for cannulation will need to be altered to reduce the chance of plaque embolization. The ascending aorta is cannulated, with care being taken to ensure that the cannula's flow is not directed into the innominate artery. See also the discussion of perioperative stroke in Chapter 5.

Femoral or external iliac artery access is required for a variety of aortic arch procedures, as well as for patients with severe ascending aortic disease that may make direct aortic cannulation hazardous. In patients with aortoiliac disease and ascending aortic or arch atherosclerosis, an alternative approach that is sometimes useful is cannulation of the axillary artery, as shown in Figure 2.11 (63–66). This approach is particularly useful for the operative management of aortic dissection and for arch replacement, as it permits selective antegrade cerebral perfusion.

The technique of venous cannulation depends on the planned procedure. For operations that involve the coronary arteries, aorta, or aortic valve only, usually a dual-stage cannula placed in the right atrium provides adequate drainage. For operations involving the right heart chambers, bicaval (superior and inferior) cannulation with separate cannulas and use of caval tourniquets are required to prevent air from entering the bypass circuit. For mitral valve operations, either RA or bicaval cannulation may be used, although we usually use the latter method. For mitral valve procedures via a small right thoracotomy incision (so-called "minimally invasive"), arterial and venous cannulation

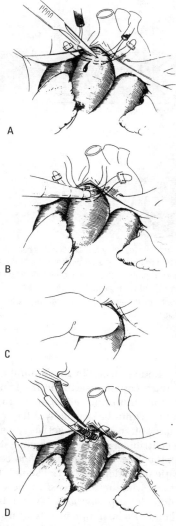

FIGURE 2.9 The aorta is palpated to ensure that the site selected for cannulation does not contain palpable plaque. **(A)** Two concentric pursestring sutures are placed around the selected site. An aortotomy is made with a no. 11 or 15 scalpel blade. **(B)** Particularly if some aortic atherosclerosis is present, it may be necessary to dilate the aortotomy site with a tapered dilator. **(C)** After making the aortotomy, temporary control is achieved with gentle digital pressure. **(D)** The aortic cannula is introduced, making sure that the tip is facing downstream, aortic pursestring sutures are tightened, and the pursestring suture tourniquets are secured to the cannula using heavy silk ligatures.

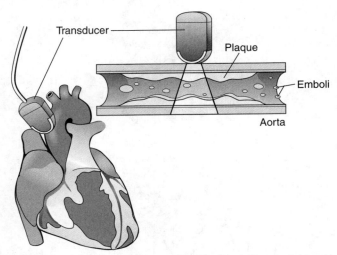

FIGURE 2.10 Epiaortic and transesophageal echocardiographic scanning provides an additional level of protection to older patients who may face higher risks of brain injury due to a greater likelihood of embolization secondary to aortic atheroma. (From Hammon JW, Stump DA, Kon ND, et al. Risk factors and solutions for the development of neurobehavioral changes after coronary bypass grafting. *Ann Thorac Surg* 1997;63: 1613–1618, with permission).

are performed via catheters placed in the femoral artery and vein. A long, thin-walled cannula can be inserted in the femoral vein and advanced into the right atrium under echocardiographic guidance. A small bore, thin-walled cannula is usually adequate to completely empty the right atrium, often aided by active venous drainage, augmenting flow with a centrifugal pump or vacuum assistance. Occasionally, the right internal jugular or innominate vein can be used for venous drainage. In patients undergoing atrial septal defect repair via a partial lower sternotomy with limited access to the superior vena cava, an alternative technique for superior vena cava cannulation is to cannulate with a cuffed endotracheal tube inserted through a pursestring suture in the RA free wall. The cuff can be inflated in lieu of a caval tourniquet. For operations in which the right heart is not readily accessible (difficult reoperations) or in which it is desired to institute CPB before opening the chest (such as in the case of a substernal aortic aneurysm), then femoral vein cannulation is performed; when this is necessary, the right femoral vein usually provides the easiest access to the inferior vena cava and the atrium. In patients having small incision

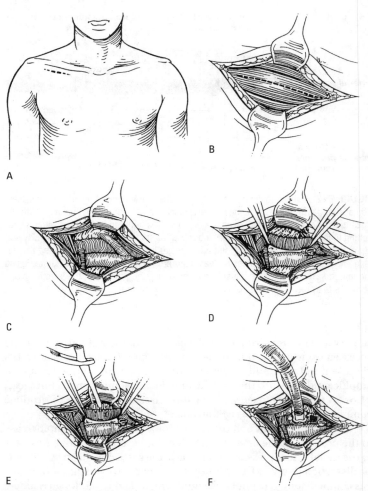

FIGURE 2.11 Surgical technique of axillary artery cannulation. **(A)** Site of incision below and parallel to clavicle. **(B)** After incision of skin and subcutaneous tissue, before division of pectoralis major muscle in the direction of its fibers. **(C)** After the clavipectoral fascia is incised and the pectoralis minor muscle is retracted laterally, the axillary artery is identified above the axillary vein. **(D)** The crossing vein is divided, and proximal and distal control of the subclavian artery is obtained. **(E)** Placement of pursestring suture and tourniquet. **(F)** Cannulation of axillary artery with right-angled cannula. (From Sabik JF, Lytle BW, McCarthy PM, et al. Axillary artery: an alternative site of arterial cannulation for patients with extensive aortic and peripheral vascular disease. *J Thorac Cardiovasc Surg* 1995;109:885–890, with permission).

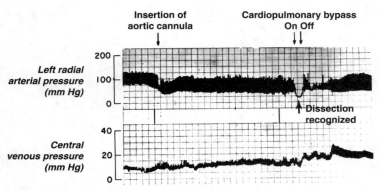

FIGURE 2.12 Hemodynamic tracings from a patient in whom iatrogenic aortic dissection occurred with the aortic cannula being placed initially in a false channel. With the institution of cardiopulmonary bypass, perfusion was initiated in the false channel, resulting in loss of perfusion to the left subclavian artery. The dissection was quickly recognized, bypass was terminated, and with the cardiac output directed into the true lumen, the left radial arterial pressure was restored. The patient was recannulated using the femoral artery, bypass was instituted, and during the procedure, the iatrogenic dissection site at the ascending aortic cannulation was repaired.

surgery and not requiring bicaval cannulation, the right atrium can be accessed using a long, thin-walled venous cannula that can be inserted via a femoral vein and directed using a guidewire and echocardiographic guidance into the right atrium. Small caliber venous lines (e.g., 21 or 23 Fr) can be used with vacuum-assisted drainage to produce complete drainage of the right atrium.

After cannulation and the institution of bypass, a sudden increase in the pressure in the arterial perfusion line associated with a decrease in the radial artery pressure should raise the suspicion of iatrogenic aortic dissection (Fig. 2.12). In this event, it is mandatory to discontinue bypass immediately, recannulate in another site, and repair the dissection, usually by an interposition graft. Intraoperative TEE can be very useful in making the diagnosis of aortic dissection. This is also a risk in off-pump surgery where instrumentation of the aorta with side-biting clamps can produce this complication.

Patients undergoing repair of acute ascending aortic dissection may pose additional risks and considerations regarding arterial cannulation. In these patients, there can be multiple re-entry points in the descending and abdominal aorta, and retrograde (femoral artery) cannulation can result in perfusion of the false lumen and visceral branch obstruction. For this reason, on completion of the distal aortic anastomosis, we prefer to move the perfusion site from the femoral artery to the implanted aortic graft to re-establish antegrade perfusion as early as possible.

Myocardial Protection

Myocardial protection is a broad concept that includes a number of measures performed to limit injury to the heart muscle. One essential component of myocardial protection is ventricular decompression. The left ventricle (LV) may become distended during CPB, most commonly during ventricular fibrillation; this may impair myocardial perfusion, particularly in the subendocardial region (67). This will occur in patients with aortic valve insufficiency or a large amount of bronchial artery return. Prevention of this complication requires venting of the LV. Venting is particularly important in patients with depressed ventricular function to keep the heart decompressed during reperfusion, rewarming, and stabilization of cardiac function before weaning bypass. This is accomplished by placing a cannula in one of several locations: directly into the LV via the right superior pulmonary vein, in the aortic root, or into the PA (68). If necessary, particularly when a mechanical mitral prosthesis is present, the ventricle can be vented by insertion of a small-bore cannula directly into the apex of the LV. Irrespective of venting technique, in addition to metabolic protection, avoidance of distension is an important component of myocardial protection.

Hypothermia

The use of hypothermia for heart surgery may be the single most important component of myocardial protection. Hypothermia protects the myocardium by reducing its energy demands and increasing its buffering capacity (69). It also reduces the oxygen and metabolic requirements of the brain and other organs. The myocardial protection provided by systemic hypothermia is superior to that of cold cardioplegia alone, possibly due to better maintenance of myocardial cooling (70). Early in the development of cardioplegia, substantial systemic cooling was used (25°C); recent trends, however, have evolved toward using lesser degrees of cooling (28 to 32°C).

Topical cardiac hypothermia is also used in the form of cold saline or iced slush. The addition of topical hypothermia provides improved myocardial protection, particularly when coronary stenoses prevent the even distribution of cardioplegia (71). It may also be of value to supplement protection of the RV, which may more be subject to rewarming in the surgical field due to ambient air temperature and overhead lighting. Care is required in the use of topical hypothermia because of the risk of phrenic nerve paresis associated with excessively cold temperatures (72). An insulation pad may help to protect the phrenic nerve when iced slush is liberally used.

Cardioplegia

In the early years of this specialty, cardiac operations were performed using intermittent aortic cross-clamping or fibrillation arrest. Thus, the heart was subjected to potentially deleterious periods of ischemia, and the aorta was subjected to multiple applications of the cross-clamp that could increase the chance of plaque embolization or dissection. In contemporary practice, cardioplegia solution most frequently is used to electromechanically arrest and protect the heart (73,74). A variety of cardioplegia additives have been proposed to enhance myocardial protection, including calcium channel blockers, metabolic substrates, free radical scavengers, oxygen, and red blood cells. Most often, cardioplegia solution is administered to the heart at a low temperature to reduce the myocardial oxygen consumption and to allow for total cessation of coronary blood flow between doses, thereby providing a bloodless field for the surgeon. In this fashion, the heart is arrested with cold hyperkalemic cardioplegia (usually with blood), and then maintenance doses of cold normokalemic or hyperkalemic solution are given at 20- to 30-minute intervals. Alternatively, warm hyperkalemic-oxygenated blood cardioplegia may be administered continuously to the heart (75–77). This technique may, however, obscure the surgeon's vision and require local coronary vessel occlusion (to sew the bypass grafts), thereby leading to brief periods of local ischemia. The superiority and safety of warm continuous cardioplegia over other methods have not been firmly established (74,78). We sometimes use this myocardial protection strategy in patients with poor LV function or when surgery is needed in the setting of acute ischemia.

Cardioplegia may be administered by three different methods: (a) infusion into the aortic root, (b) direct cannulation of the coronary arteries and/or bypass grafts, and (c) retrograde perfusion via the coronary sinus (79). Any of these routes may be satisfactory in some cases, whereas a particular technique may be optimal in others; therefore, the surgeon should be familiar with all of these methods. Whereas some surgeons use retrograde cardioplegia routinely, others use the technique selectively for circumstances such as reoperations, when there is tight stenosis of the left main or left anterior descending coronary artery, when the left main coronary artery cannot be cannulated during aortic valve replacement, and for aortic and mitral valve procedures. Retrograde cardioplegia may not provide optimal protection of the RV. Thus, if it is used, it is important that some antegrade cardioplegia is given into the right coronary artery.

Cardioplegia should be administered immediately after aortic cross-clamping to reduce myocardial ischemia. Furthermore, the surgeon must be aware that standard surface ECG monitors may be an insensitive method of monitoring electrical cardiac arrest. Low-level myocardial activity (and hence, increased myocardial oxygen consumption) may occur despite a "flat-line" ECG. Such activity during cross-clamping can compromise myocardial protection.

Profound Hypothermia and Circulatory Arrest

Many operations in small infants and certain adult procedures, especially those involving the distal ascending aorta and aortic arch, are performed using profound core cooling and circulatory arrest. This provides a completely bloodless field and access to all major intrathoracic vessels. Core cooling to 16 to 18°C is performed. Some studies have suggested that cerebral protection is optimized if deeper cooling is used and arrest times are kept to <30 minutes (80). Some degree of hemodilution (hematocrit 26% to 28%) is an important part of the profound hypothermia technique to avoid red blood cell sludging in the capillaries, which can lead to a "no reflow" phenomenon. Rewarming is performed gradually (81). Hypothermia interferes with coagulation factors, causes platelet dysfunction, and activates vasoactive peptides (kinins). The result is impaired hemostasis, and postoperative bleeding is a more frequent problem in procedures that employ deep hypothermic circulatory arrest. Cerebral oximetry may have its greatest value in the monitoring of brain oxygenation during circulatory arrest.

Separation from Cardiopulmonary Bypass

Preparation for terminating extracorporeal circulation begins even before all technical maneuvers are completed. Among the most important considerations is removal of air from the heart. Despite great care in avoiding air embolism, there is an almost unavoidable introduction of microbubbles into the circulation, beginning with aortic cannulation (82). The use of arterial line filters may reduce this problem (83). In the case of intracardiac surgery, carbon dioxide gas, which is much more soluble than the nitrogen in air and denser than air, can be flooded onto the surgical field during a procedure to displace air, thus helping to minimize the formation of bubbles that persist in the circulation (84,85). If this technique is used, additional attention must be paid to blood–gas management to avoid hypercarbia from gas absorption or entrainment by cardiotomy suction (86). In general, if carbon dioxide is used in the surgical field, gas flow in the CPB circuit must be increased to avoid hypercarbia.

Although a steep Trendelenburg position can be used at the time of aortic cross-clamp removal to minimize the passage of air into the carotid arteries, experimental evidence raises questions as to the efficacy of this maneuver (87). Additional methods of removing air from the heart include vigorous ballottement of the heart while filling it with blood before cross-clamp removal, ventilation of the lungs, suction of the aortic root and the left ventricular vent, and elevation and aspiration of the LV apex (88).

The ejection of air from the heart during separation from bypass may be first manifest by right heart dysfunction and, depending on the dominance of the coronary circulation, inferior wall ischemia due to the anterior nature of the origin of the right coronary artery ostium. In such instances, bypass should be reinstituted, perfusion pressure increased, and sufficient time permitted for air to transit the myocardium and RV function and the electrocardiogram to normalize.

Even after meticulous efforts to remove air, cardiac microbubbles can be detected by echocardiography in 75% of patients undergoing intracardiac operations and in 10% of patients undergoing coronary bypass surgery (89,90). The effect of these small bubbles on postoperative neurologic status is uncertain.

Massive air emboli are rare in contemporary cardiac surgery. CPB circuits incorporate multiple safety systems to avoid massive air embolism, including photoelectric blood-level detectors, air-activated ball valves, and automatic shut-off devices. Nevertheless, significant air embolism may still occur. When such a catastrophe happens, the pump should be stopped and the aorta should be vented with the patient in the Trendelenburg position. Reversal of cerebral flow has been proposed by some surgeons (91). Others have advocated hypothermia, steroids (dexamethasone 10 mg IV), barbiturates (thiopental 10 mg/kg IV), and hyperbaric oxygen therapy (92,93). In general, when antegrade flow is restored in such circumstances, measures to temporarily decrease cerebral metabolic rate, such as hypothermia and use of barbiturates, may be of value to minimize ischemic injury during the transit of air through the cerebral microcirculation.

Rhythm

Separation from bypass requires a stable cardiac rhythm. In many cases, the heart must be electrically defibrillated to achieve this. Defibrillation should be accomplished with the lowest energy possible because myocardial injury can result from defibrillation, although this occurs only after multiple applications of high-energy shocks (94). Many well-perfused and well-decompressed fibrillating hearts on bypass can be successfully defibrillated with a single shock of 2.5 J, particularly with contemporary defibrillators that deliver biphasic shock waveforms. If ventricular fibrillation recurs, a bolus dose of lidocaine (2 mg/kg) has been shown to reduce the incidence of ventricular fibrillation during reperfusion (95).

Adequate coronary perfusion pressure, higher systemic vascular resistance, physiologic temperature, and serum potassium in the high-normal range facilitate defibrillation. When initial defibrillation attempts fail, increasing defibrillation energy and decreasing left ventricular volume by venting or by manual compression of the heart are two techniques to improve the results of countershock. In addition, increasing aortic perfusion pressure may help achieve successful defibrillation. For the difficult-to-defibrillate heart, we have found that a single bolus dose of esmolol (adult dose 50 to 100 mg) may be of value. For the heart that defibrillates but then repeatedly refibrillates, the use of lidocaine (1 to 2 mg/kg bolus, then infusion 1 to 2 mg/kg per minute for adults) or amiodarone [adult dose 150-mg load over 10 minutes (which can be repeated if needed), then 1 mg per minute for 6 hours] may help sustain normal rhythm.

Most arrhythmias that occur during cardiac operations are due to the operative manipulations, pre-existing cardiac abnormalities, or myocardial ischemia. Diagnosis of arrhythmias is usually easy with the heart under direct observation. For example, whereas atrial fibrillation, atrial flutter, supraventricular tachycardia, and junctional rhythm may be difficult to distinguish using the surface ECG, they are usually readily discerned by simply inspecting the heart.

Atrial fibrillation may cause reduced cardiac performance during and after separation from CPB. When this occurs, electrical defibrillation of the atria should be attempted. To cardiovert atrial fibrillation, the defibrillator electrodes should be positioned on the atria insofar as possible. Low-level energy (2 to 5 J) should be used as a starting point. If the patient is not on bypass, the defibrillator *must be synchronized* to not discharge during the T-wave of the ECG to avoid causing ventricular fibrillation. Even in patients in whom atrial fibrillation has been present for several months preoperatively, sinus rhythm can sometimes be established for at least a portion of the early postoperative period. When sinus rhythm is established, atrial pacing may help to maintain this rhythm. If ventricular function permits and if catecholamine inotropic agents are not needed, low-level β-blockade, combined with atrial or atrioventricular pacing, not only may control atrial arrhythmias, but also may be of value in patients with ventricular irritability or recurrent ventricular fibrillation.

For patients with poor ventricular function, atrial and ventricular arrhythmias may be a serious issue following CPB and in the postoperative period. In this patient group, short-term amiodarone therapy has been used with increasing frequency (96,97). If needed, a loading

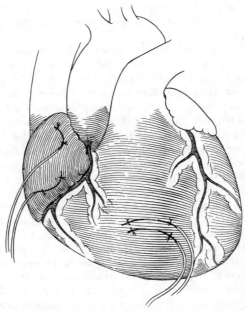

FIGURE 2.13 Placement of temporary atrial and ventricular pacing wires at the end of the operation.

dose is administered (150 to 300 mg) followed by an intravenous infusion (1 mg per minute for 6 to 12 hours, followed by 0.5 mg per minute). See Chapter 5 for further discussion of postoperative rhythm management.

Temporary pacing wires are placed on the right atrium and RV (Fig. 2.13) and can be used for diagnostic or therapeutic pacing purposes. In patients receiving bicaval cannulation for CPB, atrial-pacing wires can be placed under the pursestring sutures used to secure the atrial cannulation sites. Alternatively, commercially available single bipolar wires can be utilized.

Temporary cardiac pacing is frequently helpful in maintaining an adequate heart rate, treating arrhythmias, and augmenting cardiac output. Placement of temporary ventricular-pacing wires at the time of cardiac surgery is standard. Patients with normal cardiac function as well as those with myocardial impairment benefit from the atrioventricular synchrony that a pacemaker provides (98,99). As a routine measure, we place pacing wires on the right atrium and on the RV to permit sensing and pacing of the atria and ventricles (100). These wires may also be used after the chest is closed in the accurate diagnosis of postoperative arrhythmias by permitting recording of atrial electrograms (101). Atrial electrograms can be recorded in unipolar fashion using the precordial lead on one of the atrial wires or for higher resolution, recording in bipolar fashion using the arm leads on each wire and recording Lead I of the ECG.

Wires used most commonly for temporary postoperative pacing are made of multifilament braided or twisted stainless steel wire with an attached needle to permit insertion into ventricular muscle. Although this type of pacing lead provides sufficient reliability for most patients who undergo cardiac surgery, if pacing, particularly ventricular pacing, is expected to be needed for more than a few days, then temporary pacing leads with discrete solitary alloy electrodes provide greater reliability over more extended periods of time (102,103). Many institutions use leads with discrete electrodes routinely rather than plain wires. Bipolar temporary pacing leads are also available that have two discrete (4-mm) electrodes on the same lead that are separated by a distance thought to be optimal for electrical pacing and sensing. Bipolar lead performance is generally considered to be superior to unipolar leads, particularly in the atrium.

Contemporary external pacers are capable of atrial sensing. Thus, physiologic "tracking" of the atria is possible, resulting in the benefits of atrioventricular synchrony without having to overdrive a native atrial rate such as AAI or DDD mode (see Chapter 5). The sensed atrial electrical potential is of smaller amplitude than sensed ventricular potentials, and spurious sensing and inappropriate ventricular pacing may occur because of electrical noise in the environment. To avoid this, bipolar atrial electrodes are placed 1- to 2-cm apart on the atrium, so that the amount of atrial muscle depolarizing between the two electrodes creates a signal of sufficient amplitude for the pacer to sense. If an external DDD pacer is to be used, atrial lead position should be optimized before the chest is closed to ensure that dependable atrial sensing is obtained.

Weaning from Bypass

After the placement of pacing wires, restoration of a satisfactory native or paced rhythm, and rewarming of the patient to at least 35°C, ventilation is resumed. At this point, the surgeon determines that satisfactory lung expansion occurs with ventilation, that there is no closed pneumothorax, and that ventilation compromises no structures (e.g., places tension on an internal mammary artery graft). Failure to achieve adequate ventilation may require repositioning or clearing the endotracheal tube. Mucous plugs or blood clots may create a ball-valve effect on the end of the endotracheal tube, and this may not be resolved by passage of a suction catheter. Complete endotracheal tube removal and insertion of a new tube on bypass may be required when ventilation is unsatisfactory. Rarely, bronchoscopy must be performed to establish a clear tracheobronchial tree. Pleural effusions are drained, and pleural tubes may be inserted before weaning from bypass, so that optimum lung expansion is ensured.

During the terminal phases of rewarming on bypass, systemic vascular resistance, and hence the systemic arterial pressure, may be low. This vasodilation is due to anesthesia, hemodilution (with resultant low blood viscosity), and preoperative use of antihypertensive and vasodilator medications. Knowledge of the prebypass cardiac output can help determine what, if any, intervention is needed to increase systemic vascular resistance before weaning bypass. In general, at a bypass flow equivalent to prebypass cardiac output, the desired mean blood pressure will vary according to the type of patient undergoing surgery. For example, patients with normal coronary arteries having surgery for lesions such as atrial septal defect or mitral valve pathology can be weaned from bypass with initially lower systemic pressures (e.g., mean pressure 60 to 70 mm Hg), whereas other patients such as those with coronary artery disease or with left ventricular hypertrophy may need higher systemic pressure to obtain stable hemodynamics (e.g., mean pressure 70 to 80 mm Hg or even greater). Phenylephrine and norepinephrine are two agents commonly used to increase the systemic vascular resistance.

Weaning from CPB requires adequate filling of the heart. With guidance from the surgeon, the perfusionist inhibits the venous return from the patient to the bypass apparatus and progressively transfers the fluid volume into the patient. During weaning from bypass, systemic arterial pressure and cardiac filling pressures are observed as the blood volume in the patient is gradually increased. In addition to information from invasive monitoring, adequate filling is also confirmed by observation of ventricular size and motion and by palpation of the PA and aorta. TEE assists in monitoring left ventricular filling and is particularly useful in patients with left ventricular hypertrophy or for patients with right heart dysfunction (104). Caution must be used in attempting to infer left ventricular end-diastolic pressure or left ventricular volume from PA diastolic or pulmonary capillary wedge pressures; the latter are at best unreliable guides to the former (105). Knowledge of prebypass filling pressures can often serve as a preliminary guide to filling pressures during weaning from bypass. TEE can also be used after weaning from bypass to determine the relationship between hemodynamic measurements and ventricular filling. If ventricular performance was reasonably good preoperatively and an effective operation has been performed with good myocardial protection, CPB can usually be terminated without difficulty.

If the patient does not manifest adequate perfusion after achieving adequate cardiac-filling pressures, the surgeon must attempt to determine a cause. In the absence of a definable, remediable condition, poor myocardial performance may require a return to CPB for an additional period of reperfusion before a second attempt to separate. During this time, the use of inotropic agents and afterload reduction may be initiated and often make it possible to separate the patient from bypass. At this point, TEE is extremely useful to examine global and regional ventricular function and valve function (106). In a systematic way, TEE can evaluate the results of the surgical repair, determine that valve function is satisfactory, and that regional and global myocardial function is adequate. If mechanical heart valve(s) have been implanted, their function and seating can be confirmed. The information gained from TEE should be approximately consistent with that obtained by examination in the surgical field and that obtained by invasive monitoring. Residual valve dysfunction, such as a paravalvular leak around a prosthetic valve or regurgitation through a repaired valve, should be resolved. This may require another period of aortic cross-clamping and cardioplegia. It may require replacement of a valve that was subjected to attempted repair. If the cause of failure to wean from bypass is poor ventricular function, inotropic support should be increased, with increasing doses of β-agonists (epinephrine and/or norepinephrine) and, if required, the addition of milrinone. If function is still inadequate, an intra-aortic balloon pump is placed. If hemodynamics are not stable and improving after weaning a marginal patient from CPB, mechanical support should be considered, first with an intra-aortic balloon pump. If this is inadequate, single-ventricle or biventricular cardiac assist may be required. Chapter 8 discusses mechanical support of the heart in more detail.

Right Heart Failure

RV failure is a particular issue in certain cardiac surgical settings: cardiac transplantation, congenital heart disease, mitral valve disease with pulmonary hypertension, coronary artery disease, and following institution of left heart support (left ventricular assist device, LVAD). In these settings, it can be a source of major morbidity and mortality and requires additional management strategies (107).

When physiologically significant RV failure occurs, RA pressure exceeds LA pressure, often with low LA pressure due to the inability of the right heart to provide left heart filling. A minimal degree of RV failure or even mismatch between RV function and RV afterload can be defined when RA pressure $\geq$ LA pressure, as is frequently the case following cardiac transplantation. Although this might not signify overt RV failure, it does suggest the need for clinical vigilance, particularly during emergence from anesthesia.

For these reasons, when RV failure or a potential risk is noted (such as following cardiac transplantation), an LA pressure monitoring line should be provided to monitor continuously the relationship between right- and left-sided filling pressures.

In recent years, the introduction of inhaled nitric oxide (iNO) gas has provided a major tool for minimizing pulmonary vascular resistance, even when potent systemic vasoconstrictors are in use.

Before iNO is instituted, simple measures should already be in place:

1. The patient should be well oxygenated.
2. The patient should be deeply anesthetized.
3. Hypercarbia should be assiduously avoided.
4. Pleural spaces should be free of blood and effusion.
5. Ventilation should be adjusted to minimize mean airway pressure (i.e., no PEEP, short I:E ratio).

If these measures are in place and systemic hemodynamics are optimized, iNO is begun at 10 ppm and advanced by 5 ppm increments up to 40 ppm if needed. Although greater concentrations of iNO have been used, if there is no clinically apparent improvement, iNO will not likely be effective.

Experimental physiology studies suggest that approximately half of overall RV function is derived from the RV free wall and half from the interventricular septum. In the setting of cardiac surgery, RV protection must be optimum, particularly for surgery in settings where RV failure is anticipated to be a risk. In the setting of concomitant coronary artery disease, the integrity of the RV blood supply must be considered. This is the typical setting where revascularization of RV marginal arteries may need to be included in the revascularization plan, not only for long-term perfusion but also for delivery of cardioplegia during a cardiac surgical procedure.

A particular clinical setting that deserves special mention is the patient who has sustained an acute right coronary territory infarction with proximal occlusion of the right coronary artery. If the infarction includes the RV, this type of patient will sometimes decompensate, even with opening the pericardium at surgery. To the extent possible, such patients should be temporized until RV healing and recanalization of the RV blood supply occur.

Systemic perfusion pressure must be maintained to ensure adequate RV free wall perfusion. This physiologic management principle also pertains to maximizing the contribution of the interventricular septum to overall RV function. To this end, a strategy must be devised in each patient with RV failure to wean from CPB with as much developed LV pressure as possible. In the case of cardiac transplantation, this might be achieved merely by systemic vasoconstriction. In these patients, pre-transplantation heart failure management regimens may include substantial use of vasodilator drugs. In these circumstances, vasopressin or high doses of agents such as norepinephrine may be needed, particularly during the early postoperative hours.

In the case of patients being placed on LV assist, however, clinical management of right heart failure may be more complex. Most LVAD devices, when used in their "automatic" modes, will maximally reduce LV preload, and hence, LV developed pressure. In this setting, it is sometimes useful and effective to decrease LVAD flow sufficiently to allow some left-heart filling and hence, LV developed pressure.

Decannulation

After separation of the patient from CPB and reinfusion of the appropriate fluid volume from the bypass circuit, the venous and arterial cannulas are removed, and the previously placed pursestring sutures are secured. Before removal of the arterial cannula, protamine administration should be started. Thus, as discussed previously, if a serious protamine reaction occurs, it is easy to readminister heparin and return to full CPB to resuscitate the patient. The protamine dose should be given slowly, and if hemodynamics are stable after the first 25 to 50 mg is given, decannulation can proceed. At some hospitals, removal of the arterial cannula is delayed until just after all of the protamine has been given to the patient.

After successful weaning from CPB, protamine administration, and decannulation, blood remaining in the bypass circuit is usually hemoconcentrated by recirculation through a hemofilter or through a cell-saver device. The concentrated product is then returned to the patient.

CORONARY BYPASS SURGERY WITHOUT CARDIOPULMONARY BYPASS

CPB results in a systemic ("whole-body") inflammatory response with resultant capillary leakage, organ edema, and coagulopathy (108–110). In recent years, the development of devices to stabilize the beating heart, combined with better pharmacologic control of hemodynamics during cardiac surgery, has led to the ability to perform coronary bypass surgery with the heart beating and without the use of CPB ("off pump") (111–114). With the use of pericardial retraction sutures, fluid administration, and control of heart rate and blood pressure, it is possible to retract the heart while it is beating so as to gain access to any myocardial territory for placement of distal anastomoses. Although practices vary widely, patients are heparinized (150 to 400 U/kg) during the procedure. Proximal and distal control is obtained of the coronary artery being grafted, usually in conjunction with a device to produce localized immobilization. Off-pump revascularization strategies usually call for placing the first bypass graft to the artery supplying the myocardial territory most at risk for ischemia, followed by the remainder of planned anastomoses. The technique is used for multivessel revascularization, including techniques that base all bypasses on the mammary arteries, thus obviating the need to place a clamp on the aorta. Although CPB is not utilized, considerable fluid administration may be required during off-pump surgery to maintain the systemic blood pressure. This may result in significant fluid gain. Practices vary widely with respect to heparin neutralization; we generally administer a full CPB dose of heparin (420 U/kg) and partially reverse the heparin with a small dose of protamine (50 to 75 mg). Aspirin is administered early after surgery. In addition, as CPB is not utilized, excessive intra-operative hypothermia can be a concern, and the operating room temperature should be increased and/or or a warming blanket should be utilized during off-pump surgery.

Theoretically, off-pump coronary bypass procedures should obviate the potential risks of CPB and may be of particular value in high-risk patients such as those with cerebrovascular disease, aortic atherosclerosis, or renal failure. Studies have demonstrated the safety and efficacy of this technique. Potential benefits include reductions in blood transfusions, stroke, and encephalopathy (115–119). The technique may be particularly useful for higher-risk patients, especially those with atherosclerosis involving the ascending aorta. Potential disadvantages include incomplete myocardial revascularization with a possible increased need for future coronary interventions (120,121).

Graft Patency Following Coronary Bypass Surgery

Whether coronary bypass surgery is performed with bypass and cardioplegia or off bypass, achievement of long-term graft patency is a major goal in the surgical treatment of coronary artery disease. To this end, determining the technical adequacy of bypass graft anastomoses at the time of operation is important. Measurement of bypass graft flow and its phasic pattern can predict both short- and intermediate-term patency (122). In surgical facilities equipped for hybrid procedures, immediate postprocedure angiography can document anastomotic quality and patency (123). This may be of particular value in off-pump bypass surgery.

Pericardial Closure

Some surgeons believe it is desirable to reapproximate the pericardium in patients in whom future reoperation may be possible; in practice, this includes all but the very elderly. Pericardial closure may diminish the formation of adhesions, although this point is debatable. It certainly interposes some tissue between the sternum and the anterior wall of the heart, which may increase the safety of subsequent resternotomy. When the pericardium cannot be closed, approximation of opposite pleural membranes may be performed instead. Alternatively, even closure of the thymic remnant over the aorta may diminish the risk of future resternotomy. Other surgeons have questioned the value of pericardial closure, with some studies suggesting possible adverse hemodynamic consequences. In most practices, the pericardium is not closed if coronary bypass grafting has been performed. In other patients, it is closed if it is tolerated hemodynamically. For the patient in whom the native pericardium cannot be approximated or is absent, a variety of pericardial substitutes have been advocated, including bovine pericardium, silicone rubber, and polytetrafluoroethylene (124–127). Use of these materials has uncertain benefits; dense adhesions between the prosthesis and the epicardium, severe inflammatory reactions, pericardial effusions, and calcification have been described (128,129).

Closure of the Chest

Large tubes are positioned in the mediastinum before the chest is closed (Fig. 2.14). Conventionally, one tube lies on top of the diaphragm and another behind the sternum. Use of large ($\geq$32 Fr) tubes may reduce the possibility of tube obstruction due to clots and consequent tamponade. Additionally, the pleural spaces should be drained if they have been entered or if pleural effusions are present. We use Blake Silastic drains for this purpose, as they can remain in the patient yet permit ambulation. Patients who have had their internal mammary arteries mobilized will sometimes drain serosanguineous fluid for a few days, and the presence of the drain prevents pleural effusion accumulation. These are also useful in patients undergoing surgery in the setting of severe heart failure, where pleural effusions are present before surgery and will tend to reaccumulate in the first few postoperative days unless drainage is provided.

Closure of the chest must never be performed in a casual fashion. Lack of sternal stability is a principal cause of wound complications (130–132). The increased operative mortality associated with sternal wound infections dictates a precise and standardized approach to sternotomy closure to minimize the frequency of this dreaded complication. Excellent results have been obtained by surgeons using a wide variety of materials for sternal reapproximation, including wires, sutures, and metal bands (133). Patients at high risk for sternal instability include patients who are obese, patients with chronic obstructive lung disease,

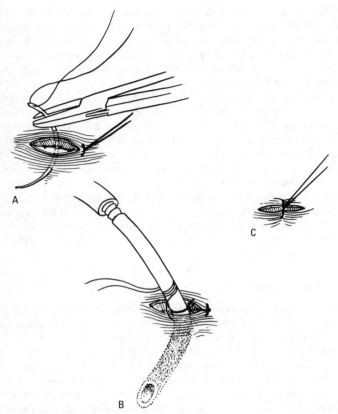

FIGURE 2.14 Mediastinal tubes are secured to the skin with heavy silk suture. In addition, a heavy silk suture may be placed for subsequent closure of the chest tube insertion incision **(A)**. The suture is not tied at the time of chest tube insertion, but the excess suture is wrapped around the chest tube **(B)**. After chest tube removal, the suture is tied down to reapproximate the skin edges **(C)**.

and patients with impaired mobility who must use crutches or significant traction with their arms to ambulate. In these situations, use of extra wires, double wires, or sternal bands may help confer additional sternal stability and integrity of the closure.

The patient who is obese and the patient who is cachectic share a common risk of sternal wound problems, the former because of the increased force applied to the line of closure and the latter because of decreased tissue strength. To a greater degree than patients of normal habitus, these individuals require particular attention to hemostasis, careful approximation of tissues, and avoidance of dead space. It is, at times, helpful to perform the "sternal weave" technique to reinforce the fragile or narrow sternum or the sternum with multiple transverse fractures (131).

Proper closure of the abdominal fascia must not be neglected. Incisional hernia has been reported in 4% of patients undergoing median sternotomy, and up to one third of these may be sufficiently symptomatic to require operative repair. Hernia is most common in male patients, patients who are obese, and patients with complicated postoperative courses (134). Limiting the incision inferiorly to the level of the mid-xiphoid process helps to reduce the incidence of incisional hernia.

Special Problems in Chest Closure

At times, myocardial edema, acute cardiac dilatation, or other problems may make closure of the sternum impossible. On these occasions, closure of the skin alone or coverage with a silicone rubber sheet may be performed (135). Struts may be cut from chest tubes to hold the sternal edges apart. In 1 to 4 days, the patient may be returned to the operating room for sternal approximation and complete wound closure when cardiac edema has subsided. This procedure does not increase the risk of mediastinitis or sternal osteomyelitis.

Postoperative sternotomy wound infection and mediastinitis are a major source of morbidity and mortality. These issues are discussed in detail in Chapter 5.

TRANSPORT OF THE PATIENT

Movement of the postoperative patient from the operating room to the recovery area or intensive care unit is potentially hazardous. Narcotic anesthesia minimizes hemodynamic changes during this critical period (136). Safe transport of the patient from the operating room requires careful attention to all intravascular catheters, infusion devices, and drainage tubes. The patient's ECG, blood pressure, and, ideally, oxygen saturation are monitored continuously with a battery-powered transport monitor. A portable defibrillator also accompanies the patient. Adequate ventilation and oxygenation must be ensured. If the patient is awakening, additional sedation may be necessary to avoid thrashing, which may cause disconnection of a life-supporting piece of equipment or hemodynamic instability. For patients intended for early extubation, propofol is an excellent agent for short-term supplementation of anesthesia. For our pediatric patients, we arrange for the postoperative nurse to come to the operating room to assist in transport. This measure facilitates proper organization and rapid reconnection of essential monitors and drugs on arrival in the intensive care unit.

References

1. Cable DG, Mullany CJ, Schaff HV. The Allen test. *Ann Thorac Surg* 1999;67: 876–877.
2. Bazarel MG, Welch M, Golding LAR, et al. Comparison of brachial and radial arterial pressure monitoring in patients undergoing coronary bypass surgery. *Anesthesiology* 1990;73:28–45.
3. Dorman T, Breslow MJ, Lipsett PA, et al. Radial artery pressure monitoring underestimates central artery pressure during vasopressor therapy in critically ill surgical patients. *Crit Care Med* 1998;26:1646–1649.
4. Mohr R, Lavee J, Goor DA. Inaccuracy of radial artery pressure measurement after cardiac operations. *J Thorac Cardiovasc Surg* 1987;94:286–290.
5. Augoustides J, Weiss SJ, Pochettino A. Hemodynamic monitoring of the postoperative adult cardiac surgery patient. *Semin Thorac Cardiovasc Surg* 2000;12:309–315.
6. Gardner RM, Schwartz R, Wong HC, et al. Percutaneous indwelling radial-artery catheters for monitoring cardiovascular function. Prospective study of the risk of thrombosis and infection. *N Engl J Med* 1974;290:1227–1231.
7. Bowdle TA. Complications of invasive monitoring [review]. *Anesthesiol Clin North America* 2002;20:571–588.
8. Black IH, Blosser SA, Murray WB. Central venous pressure measurements: peripherally inserted catheters versus centrally inserted catheters. *Crit Care Med* 2000;28:3833–3836.
9. McEnany MT, Austen WG. Life-threatening hemorrhage from inadvertent cervical arteriotomy. *Ann Thorac Surg* 1977;24:233.
10. Pearson ML, Hierholzer WJ, Garner JS, et al. Guidelines for prevention of intravascular-device-related infections. *Infect Control Hosp Epidemiol* 1996;17: 438–473.
11. Kac G, Durain E, Amrein, et al. Colonization and infection of pulmonary artery catheter in cardiac surgery patients: epidemiology and multivariate analysis of risk factors. *Crit Care Med* 2001;29:971–975.
12. Mullerworth MH, Angelopoulos P, Couyant MA, et al. Recognition and management of catheter-induced pulmonary artery rupture. *Ann Thorac Surg* 1998;66:1242–1245.
13. Urschel JD, Myerowitz PD. Catheter-induced pulmonary artery rupture in the setting of cardiopulmonary bypass. *Ann Thorac Surg* 1993;56:585–589.
14. Sirivella S, Gielchinsky I, Parsonnet V. Management of catheter-induced pulmonary artery perforation: a rare complication in cardiovascular operations. *Ann Thorac Surg* 2001;72:2056–2059.
15. Raper R, Sibbald WJ. Misled by the wedge? The Swan–Ganz catheter and left ventricular preload. *Chest* 1986;89:427–434.
16. Gold JP, Jonas RA, Lang P, et al. Transthoracic intracardiac monitoring lines in pediatric surgical patients: a ten-year experience. *Ann Thorac Surg* 1986;42: 185–191.
17. Russell GN, Ip Yam PC, Tran J, et al. Gastroesophageal reflux and tracheobronchial contamination after cardiac surgery: should a nasogastric tube be routine? *Anesth Analg* 1996;83:228–232.
18. Leal-Noval SR, Marquez-Vacaro JA, Garcia-Curiel A, et al. Nosocomial pneumonia in patients undergoing heart surgery. *Crit Care Med* 2000;28:935–940.
19. Risk CS, Brandon D, D'Ambra MN, et al. Indications for the use of pacing pulmonary artery catheters in cardiac surgery. *J Cardiothorac Anesth* 1992; 6:275–279.

20. Pulmonary Artery Catheter Consensus Conference Participants. Pulmonary Artery Catheter Consensus Conference: consensus statement. *Crit Care Med* 1997;25:910–925.

21. Schwann TA, Zacharias A, Riorda CJ, et al. Safe, highly selective use of pulmonary artery catheters in coronary artery bypass grafting: an objective patient selection method. *Ann Thorac Surg* 2002;73:1394–1402.

22. Tuman KJ, McCarthy RJ, Spiess BD, et al. Effect of pulmonary artery catheterization on outcome in patients undergoing coronary artery surgery. *Anesthesiology* 1989;70:199–206.

23. Eltzschig HK, Rosenberger P, Löffler M, et al. Impact of intraoperative transesophageal echocardiography on surgical decisions in 12,566 patients undergoing cardiac surgery. *Ann Thorac Surg* 2008;85:845–853.

24. Morehead AJ, Firstenberg MS, Shiota T, et al. Intraoperative echocardiographic detection of regurgitant jets after valve replacement. *Ann Thorac Surg* 2000;69:135–139.

25. Percy M, McNicol L, Dinh DT, et al. Major complications related to the use of transesophageal echocardiography in cardiac surgery. *Cardiothorac Vasc Anesth* 2009;23:62–65.

26. Ricci M, Lombardi P, Schultz S, et al. Near-infrared spectroscopy to monitor cerebral oxygen saturation in single-ventricle physiology. *J Thorac Cardiovasc Surg* 2006;131:395–402.

27. Hirsch JC, Charpie JR, Ohye RG, et al. Near-infrared spectroscopy: what we know and what we need to know—a systematic review of the congenital heart disease literature. *J Thorac Cardiovasc Surg* 2009;137:154–159.

28. Bourke M. The patient with a pacemaker or related device. *Can J Anaesth* 1996;43:R24–R41.

29. Sanford TJ Jr, Smith T, Dec-Silver H, et al. A comparison of morphine, fentanyl, and sufentanyl anesthesia for cardiac surgery: induction, emergence, and extubation. *Anesth Analg* 1986;65:259–266.

30. Engoran MC, Kraras C, Garzia F. Propofol-based versus fentanyl-isoflurane-based anesthesia for cardiac surgery. *J Cardiothorac Vasc Anesth* 1998;12:177–181.

31. Goldstein S, Dean D, Kim SJ, et al. A survey of spinal and epidural techniques for adult cardiac surgery. *J Cardiothorac Vasc Anesth* 2001;15:158–168.

32. Ko W, Lazenby D, Zelano JA, et al. Effects of shaving methods and intraoperative irrigation on suppurative mediastinitis after bypass operations. *Ann Thorac Surg* 1992;53:301–305.

33. Bojar RM, Payne DD, Rastegar H, et al. Use of self-adhesive external defibrillator pads for complex cardiac surgical procedures. *Ann Thorac Surg* 1988;46: 587–588.

34. Brown ML, McKellar SH, Sundt TM, et al. Ministernotomy versus conventional sternotomy for aortic valve replacement: A systematic review and meta-analysis. *J Thorac Cardiovasc Surg* 2009;137:670–679.

35. McClure RS, Cohn LH, Wiegerinck E, et al. Early and late outcomes in minimally invasive mitral valve repair: an eleven-year experience in 707 patients. *J Thorac Cardiovasc Surg* 2009;137:70–75.

36. Doty DB, DiRusso GB, Doty JR. Full-spectrum cardiac surgery through a minimal incision: mini-sternotomy (lower half) technique. *Ann Thorac Surg* 1998;65:573–577.

37. Pratt JW, Williams TE, Michler RE, et al. Current indications for left thoracotomy in coronary revascularization and valvular procedures. *Ann Thorac Surg* 2000;70:1366–1370.

38. Brutel de la Rieviere A, Brom GH, Nron AG. Horizontal submammary skin incision for median sternotomy. *Ann Thorac Surg* 1981;32:101–104.
39. Dobell ARC, Jain AK. Catastrophic hemorrhage during redo sternotomy. *Ann Thorac Surg* 1984;37:273–278.
40. Loop FD. Catastrophic hemorrhage during sternal reentry. *Ann Thorac Surg* 1984;37:271–272.
41. Machiraju VR. How to avoid problems in redo coronary artery bypass. *J Cardiac Surg* 2001;17:20–25.
42. Gasparovic H, Rybicki FJ, Millstine J, et al. Three dimensional computed tomographic imaging in planning the surgical approach for redo cardiac surgery after coronary revascularization. *Eur J Cardiothorac Surg* 2005;28:244–249.
43. Hirsh J, Anand SS, Halperin JL, et al. Guide to anticoagulant therapy: heparin. *Circulation* 2001;103:2994–3018.
44. McEvoy GK, ed. *AHFS drug information 2002.* Bethesda: American Society of Health-System Pharmacists, 2002:1444.
45. Despotis GJ, Gravlee G, Filos K, et al. Anticoagulation monitoring during cardiac surgery. *Anesthesiology* 1999;91:1122–1151.
46. Despotis GJ, Joist JH, Hogue WCW, et al. The impact of heparin concentration and activated clotting time monitoring on blood conservation. *J Thorac Cardiovasc Surg* 1995;110:46–54.
47. Shapira N, Schaff HV, Piehler JM, et al. Cardiovascular effects of protamine sulfate in man. *J Thorac Cardiovasc Surg* 1982;84:505–514.
48. Ravi R, Frost EAM. Cardiac surgery in patients with protamine allergy. *Heart Dis* 1999;5:289–294.
49. Porsche R, Brenner ZR. Allergy to protamine sulfate. *Heart Lung* 1999;28:418–428.
50. Morel DR, Zapol WM, Thomas SJ, et al. C5a and thromboxane generation associated with pulmonary vaso- and broncho-constriction during protamine administration. *Anesthesiology* 1987;66:597–604.
51. Kimmel SE, Sekeres MA, Berlin JA, et al. Risk factors for clinically important adverse events after protamine administration following cardiopulmonary bypass. *J Am Coll Cardiol* 1998;32:1916–1922.
52. Despostis GJ, Joist JH. Anticoagulation and anticoagulation reversal with cardiac surgery involving cardiopulmonary bypass: an update. *J Cardiothorac Vasc Anesth* 1999;13(suppl 1):18–29.
53. Mochizuki T, Olson PJ, Szlam F, et al. Protamine reversal of heparin affects platelet aggregation and activated clotting time after cardiopulmonary bypass. *Anesth Analg* 1998; 87:781–785.
54. Staples MH, Dunton RF, Karlson KJ, et al. Heparin resistance after preoperative heparin therapy or intraaortic balloon pumping. *Ann Thorac Surg* 1994;57:1211–1216.
55. Lemmer JH, Despotis GJ. Antithrombin III concentrate to treat heparin resistance in patients undergoing cardiac surgery. *J Thorac Cardiovasc Surg* 2002;123:213–217.
56. Williams MR, D'Ambra AB, Beck JR, et al. A randomized trial of antithrombin concentrate for treatment of heparin resistance. *Ann Thorac Surg* 2000;70: 873–877.
57. Follis F, Schmidt CA. Cardiopulmonary bypass in patients with heparin-induced thrombocytopenia and thrombosis. *Ann Thorac Surg* 2000;70: 2173–2181.
58. Koster A, Meyer O, Fischer T, et al. One-year experience with the platelet glycoprotein IIb/IIIa antagonist tirofiban and heparin during cardiopulmonary

bypass in patients with heparin-induced thrombocytopenia type II. *J Thorac Cardiovasc Surg* 2001;122:1254–1255.

59. Koster A, Hansen R, Kuppe H, et al. Recombinant hirudin as an alternative to anticoagulation during cardiopulmonary bypass in patients with heparin-induced thrombocytopenia type II: a 1-year experience in 57 patients. *J Cardiothorac Vasc Anesth* 2000;14:243–248.

60. Miller L, Nicest R, Magna NIH. Successful cardiopulmonary bypass surgery with Organ in patients with heparin induced thrombocytopenia. *Thromb Haemost* 1997;78(suppl):446.

61. Koster A, Dyke CM, Aldea G, et al. Bivalirudin during cardiopulmonary bypass in patients with previous or acute heparin-induced thrombocytopenia and heparin antibodies: results of the CHOOSE-ON Trial. *Ann Thorac Surg* 2007;83:572–577.

62. Royse C, Royse A, Blake D, et al. Screening the thoracic aorta for atheroma: a comparison of manual palpation, transesophageal and epiaortic ultrasonography. *Ann Thorac Surg* 1998;4:347–350.

63. Leyh RG, Bartels C, Motzold A, et al. Management of the porcelain aorta during coronary artery bypass grafting. *Ann Thorac Surg* 1999;67:986–988.

64. Barbeau YR, Westbrook BM, Charlesworth DC, et al. Arterial inflow via an axillary artery graft for the severely atheromatous aorta. *Ann Thorac Surg* 1998;66:33–37.

65. Sabik JF, Lytle BW, McCarthy PM, et al. Axillary artery: an alternative site of arterial cannulation for patients with extensive aortic and peripheral vascular disease. *J Thorac Cardiovasc Surg* 1995;109:885–890.

66. Whilark JD, Goldman SM, Sutter FP. Axillary artery cannulation in acute ascending aortic dissections. *Ann Thorac Surg* 2000;69:1127–1128.

67. Lucas SK, Schaff JT, Flaherty JT, et al. The harmful effects of ventricular distension during postischemia reperfusion. *Ann Thorac Surg* 1981;32:486–494.

68. Little AG, Lin CY, Wernly JA, et al. Use of the pulmonary artery for left ventricular venting during cardiac operations. *J Thorac Cardiovasc Surg* 1984;87: 532–538.

69. Lange R, Cavanaugh AC, Zierler M, et al. The relative importance of alkalinity, temperature, and the washout effect of bicarbonate-buffered, multidose cardioplegic solution. *Circulation* 1984;70(suppl I):I75–I83.

70. Grover FL, Fewel JG, Ghidoni JJ, et al. Does lower systemic temperature enhance cardioplegic myocardial protection? *J Thorac Cardiovasc Surg* 1981;81: 11–20.

71. Lazar HL, Rivers S. Importance of topical hypothermia during heterogeneous distribution of cardioplegic solution. *J Thorac Cardiovasc Surg* 1989;98: 251–257.

72. Efthimiou J, Butler J, Woodham C, et al. Diaphragm paralysis following cardiac surgery: the rope of phrenic nerve cold injury. *Ann Thorac Surg* 1991;52: 1005–1008.

73. Gay WA Jr, Ebert PA. Functional, metabolic, and morphologic effects of potassium-induced cardioplegia. *Surgery* 1973;74:284–290.

74. Buckberg GD. Update on current techniques of myocardial protection. *Ann Thorac Surg* 1995;60:805–814.

75. Lichtenstein SV, Ashe KA, el Delati H, et al. Warm heart surgery. *J Thorac Cardiovasc Surg* 1991;101:269–274.

76. Salerno TA, Houck JP, Barrozo CA, et al. Retrograde continuous warm cardioplegia: a new concept in myocardial protection. *Ann Thorac Surg* 1991;51: 245–247.

77. Mauney MC, Kron IL. The physiologic basis of warm blood cardioplegia (review). *Ann Thorac Surg* 1995;60:819–823.

78. Martin TD, Craver JM, Gott JP, et al. Prospective randomized trial of retrograde warm blood cardioplegia: myocardial benefit and neurologic threat. *Ann Thorac Surg* 1994;57:298–304.

79. Solorano J, Taitelbaum G, Chiu RC. Retrograde coronary sinus perfusion for myocardial protection during cardiopulmonary bypass. *Ann Thorac Surg* 1978;25:201–208.

80. McCollough JN, Zhang N, Reich DL, et al. Cerebral metabolic suppression during hypothermic circulatory arrest in humans. *Ann Thorac Surg* 1999;67: 1895–1899.

81. Gfrigore AM, Grocott HP, Matthew JP, et al. The rewarming rate and increased peak temperature alter neurocognitive outcome after cardiac surgery. *Anesth Analg* 2002;94:4–10.

82. Padayachee TS, Parsons S, Theobold R, et al. The detection of microemboli in the middle cerebral artery during cardiopulmonary bypass: a transcranial Doppler ultrasound investigation using membrane and bubble oxygenators. *Ann Thorac Surg* 1987;44:298–302.

83. Padayachee TS, Parsons S, Theobold R, et al. The effect of arterial filtration on reduction of gaseous microemboli in the middle cerebral artery during cardiopulmonary bypass. *Ann Thorac Surg* 1988;45:647–649.

84. Frados A. Carbon dioxide field flooding: a retrospective study. *J Extracorporeal Technol* 2001;32:91–93.

85. Svenarud P, Persson M, van der Linden J. Effect of CO_2 insufflation on the number and behavior of air microemboli in open-heart surgery. A randomized clinical trial. *Circulation* 2004;109:1127–1132.

86. Nadolny EM, Svensson LG. Carbon dioxide field flooding techniques for open heart surgery: monitoring and minimizing potential adverse effects. *Perfusion* 2000;15:151–153.

87. Butler BD, Laine GA, Leiman BC, et al. Effect of the Trendelenburg position on the distribution of arterial air emboli in dogs. *Ann Thorac Surg* 1988;45: 198–202.

88. Oka Y, Inoue T, Hong Y, et al. Retained intracardiac air. Transesophageal echocardiography for definition of incidence and monitoring removal by improved techniques. *J Thorac Cardiovasc Surg* 1986;91:329–338.

89. Oka Y, Moriwaki KM, Hong Y, et al. Detection of air emboli in the left heart by M-mode transesophageal echocardiography following cardiopulmonary bypass. *Anesthesiology* 1985;63:109–113.

90. Topol EJ, Humphrey LS, Borkon AM, et al. Value of intraoperative left ventricular microbubbles detected by transesophageal two-dimensional echocardiography in predicting neurologic outcome after cardiac operations. *Am J Cardiol* 1985;56:773–775.

91. Mills NL, Ochsner JL. Massive air embolism during cardiopulmonary bypass. Causes, prevention, and management. *J Thorac Cardiovasc Surg* 1980;80: 708–717.

92. Spampinato N, Stassano P, Gagliardi C, et al. Massive air embolism during cardiopulmonary bypass: successful treatment with immediate hypothermia and circulatory support. *Ann Thorac Surg* 1981;32:602–603.

93. Ziser A, Adir Y, Lavon H, et al. Hyperbaric oxygen therapy for massive arterial air embolism during cardiac operations. *J Thorac Cardiovasc Surg* 1999;117:818–821.

94. Kerber RE, Carter J, Klein S, et al. Open chest defibrillation during cardiac surgery: energy and current requirement. *Am J Cardiol* 1980;46:393–396.

95. Fall SM, Burton NA, Graeber GM, et al. Prevention of ventricular fibrillation after myocardial revascularization. *Ann Thorac Surg* 1987;43:182–184.

96. Butler J, Harriss DR, Sinclair M, et al. Amiodarone prophylaxis for tachycardias after coronary artery surgery: a randomized, double-blind, placebo controlled study. *Br Heart J* 1993;70:56–60.

97. Solomon AJ, Greenberg MD, Kilborn MJ, et al. Amiodarone versus a beta-blocker to prevent atrial fibrillation after cardiovascular surgery. *Am Heart J* 2001;142:811–815.

98. Curtis J, Walls J, Boley T, et al. Influence of atrioventricular synchrony on hemodynamics in patients with normal and low ejection fractions following open heart surgery. *Am Surg* 1986;52:93–96.

99. Hartzler GO, Maloney JD, Curtis JJ, et al. Hemodynamic benefits of atrioventricular sequential pacing after cardiac surgery. *Am J Cardiol* 1977;40: 232–236.

100. Yiu P, Tansley P, Pepper JR. Improved reliability of post-operative pacing by use of bipolar temporary pacing leads. *Cardiovasc Surg* 2001;9:591–595.

101. Waldo AL, Henthorn RW, Plumb VJ. Temporary epicardial wire electrodes in the diagnosis and treatment of arrhythmias after open heart surgery. *Am J Surg* 1984;148:275–283.

102. Wigneswaran WT, Jamieson MP. Temporary pacing leads in cardiac surgery. A comparison of multifilament braided electrodes and localized solitary stainless steel electrodes. *J Cardiovasc Surg (Torino)* 1986;27:609–612.

103. Kallis P, Batrick N, Bindi F, et al. Pacing thresholds of temporary epicardial electrodes: variation with electrode type, time, and epicardial position. *Ann Thorac Surg* 1994;57:623–626.

104. Ochiai Y, Morita S, Tanoue Y, et al. Use of transesophageal echocardiography for postoperative evaluation of right ventricular function. *Ann Thorac Surg* 1999;67:146–153.

105. Douglas PS, Edmunds LH, St. John Sutton M, et al. Unreliability of hemodynamic indexes of left ventricular size during cardiac surgery. *Ann Thorac Surg* 1987;44:31–34.

106. Al-Tabbaa A, Gonzalez RM, Lee D. The role of state-of the-art echocardiography in the assessment of myocardial injury during and following cardiac surgery. *Ann Thorac Surg* 2001;72:S2214–S2219.

107. Vlahakes GJ. Right ventricular failure following cardiac surgery. *Coronary Artery Disease* 2005;16:27–30.

108. Edmunds LH Jr. Inflammatory response to cardiopulmonary bypass. *Ann Thorac Surg* 1998;66:S12–S16.

109. Boyle EM Jr, Morgan EN, Kovacich JC, et al. Microvascular response to cardiopulmonary bypass. *J Cardiothorac Vasc Anesth* 1999;4(suppl 1):30–37.

110. Laffey JG, Boylan JF, Cheng DCH. The systemic inflammatory response to cardiac surgery. *Anesthesiology* 2002;97:215–252.

111. Heames RM, Gill RS, Ohri SK, et al. Off-pump coronary artery surgery. *Anaesthesia* 2002;57:676–685.

112. Mack MJ. Coronary surgery: off-pump and port access (review). *Surg Clin North Am* 2000;80:1575–1591.

113. Ascione R, Caputo M, Angelini GD. Off-pump coronary artery bypass grafting: not a flash in the pan. *Ann Thorac Surg* 2003;75:306–313.

114. Plomondon ME, Cleveland JC Jr, Ludwig ST, et al. Off-pump coronary artery bypass is associated with improved risk-adjusted outcomes. *Ann Thorac Surg* 2001;72:114–119.

115. Puskas JD, Thourani VH, Marshall JJ, et al. Clinical outcomes, angiographic patency, and resource utilization in 200 consecutive off-pump coronary bypass patients. *Ann Thorac Surg* 2001;71:1477–1483.

116. Kshettry VR, Flavin TF, Emery RW, et al. Does multivessel, off-pump coronary bypass reduce postoperative morbidity? *Ann Thorac Surg* 2000;69: 1725–1731.

117. Bull DA, Neumayer LA, Stringham JC, et al. Coronary bypass grafting with cardiopulmonary bypass versus off-pump bypass grafting: does eliminating the pump reduce morbidity and cost? *Ann Thorac Surg* 2001;71:170–175.

118. Van Dijk D, Nierich AP, Jansen EWL, et al. Early outcome after off-pump versus on-pump coronary bypass surgery: results from a randomized study. *Circulation* 2001;104:1761–1766.

119. Sellke FW, DiMaio JM, Caplan LR, et al. Comparing on-pump and off-pump coronary bypass grafting. Numerous studies but few conclusions. *Circulation* 2005;111:2858–2864.

120. Arom KV, Flavin TF, Emery RW, et al. Safety and efficacy of off-pump coronary bypass grafting. *Ann Thorac Surg* 2000;69:704–710.

121. Sabik JF, Gillinov AM, Blackstone EH, et al. Does off-pump coronary surgery reduce morbidity and mortality? *J Thorac Cardiovasc Surg* 2002;124: 698–707.

122. Zhao DX, Leacche M, Balaguer JM, et al. Routine intraoperative completion angiography after coronary bypass grafting and 1-stop hybrid revascularization results from a fully-integrated hybrid catheterization laboratory/operating room. *J Am Coll Cardiol* 2009;53:232–241.

123. Tokuda Y, Song M-H, Oshima H, et al. Predicting midterm coronary bypass graft failure by intraoperative transit time flow measurement. *Ann Thorac Surg* 2008;86:532–536.

124. Gallo JI, Artinano E, Duran CMG. Clinical experience with glutaraldehyde-preserved heterologous pericardium for the closure of the pericardium after open heart surgery. *Thorac Cardiovasc Surg* 1982;30:306–309.

125. Opie JC, Larrieu AJ, Cornell IS. Pericardial substitutes: delayed reexploration and findings. *Ann Thorac Surg* 1987;43:383–385.

126. Laks H, Hammond G, Geha AS. Use of silicone rubber as a pericardial substitute to facilitate reoperation in cardiac surgery. *J Thorac Cardiovasc Surg* 1981;82:88–92.

127. Minale C, Hollweg G, Nikol S, et al. Closure of the pericardium using expanded polytetrafluoroethylene GORE-TEX surgical membrane: clinical experience. *Thorac Cardiovasc Surg* 1987;35: 312–315.

128. Mills SA. Complications associated with the use of heterologous bovine pericardium for pericardial closure. *J Thorac Cardiovasc Surg* 1986;92:446–454.

129. Skinner JR, Kim H, Toon RS, et al. Inflammatory epicardial reaction to processed bovine pericardium: case report. *J Thorac Cardiovasc Surg* 1984;88: 789–791.

130. Labitzke R, Schramm G, Witzel U, et al. "Sleeve-rope closure" of the median sternotomy after open heart operations. *Thorac Cardiovasc Surg* 1983;31: 127–128.

131. Robicsek F, Daugherty HK, Cook JW. The prevention and treatment of sternum separation following open-heart surgery. *J Thorac Cardiovasc Surg* 1977;73:267–268.

132. Sanfelippo PM, Danielson GK. Complications associated with median sternotomy. *J Thorac Cardiovasc Surg* 1972;63:419–423.

133. Losanoff JE, Richman BW, Jones JW. Disruption and infection of median sternotomy: a comprehensive review. *Eur J Cardiothorac Surg* 2002;21:831–839.

134. Davidson BR, Bailey JS. Incisional hernia following median sternotomy incisions: their incidence and aetiology. *Br J Surg* 1986;73:995–996.

135. Anderson CA, Filsoufi F, Aklog L, et al. Liberal use of delayed sternal closure for postcardiotomy hemodynamic instability. *Ann Thorac Surg* 2002;73:1484–1488.

136. Insel J, Weissman C, Kemper M, et al. Cardiovascular changes during transport of critically ill and postoperative patients. *Crit Care Med* 1986;14:539–542.

3 Postoperative Management

Postoperative care of the cardiac surgical patient begins at the time of transfer from the operating room to the intensive care unit (ICU). This is a hazardous period that requires the strict attention of both the anesthesiologist and the surgeon. Electrocardiogram (ECG) and arterial pressure monitoring by a portable, battery-powered unit is essential during the transfer, and basic resuscitation medications (such as epinephrine) should be readily available for quick administration en route to the ICU, if required. A portable defibrillator also accompanies the patient.

On arrival in the ICU, pressure monitoring lines and ECG leads are transferred to the bedside monitor without delay. Routine monitoring includes ECG, continuous arterial blood pressure, central venous pressure, pulmonary artery (PA) pressure and temperature (if a PA catheter is present), and arterial hemoglobin oxygen saturation using a cutaneous pulse oximeter sensor. The external pacemaker, having been attached to the patient's temporary pacing wires in the operating room, is checked to make sure that it is turned on and the settings are appropriate (most often a "back-up" demand ventricular pacing rate appropriate for the patient's age). A verbal report of the patient's condition is given to the primary nurse by the anesthesiologist. This includes a description of the procedure performed, any problems encountered including difficulties with intubation, details regarding the filling (pulmonary capillary wedge or PA diastolic) pressure at which the patient's heart appears to function best, and any ongoing drug infusions. Blood samples are sent for arterial blood gas analysis, hemoglobin level, and sodium and potassium concentrations. Routine measurement of platelet count and other clotting studies are not necessary for the patient who is not bleeding excessively.

The heart is auscultated to determine the presence or absence of murmurs and the loudness of the heart sounds to provide a baseline for later reference. For example, the later development of a murmur may indicate detachment of a prosthetic valve or patch, and, similarly, muffled heart sounds later on may suggest cardiac tamponade. The chest is auscultated to determine that there are adequate breath sounds bilaterally. If not already present, an oro- or nasogastric tube may be inserted depending on the preference of the surgeon or the presence of abdominal distension. A chest x-ray is usually obtained but may not be necessary for the stable patient (1). This provides verification of the

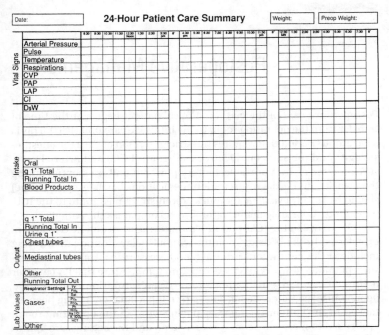

FIGURE 3.1 Intensive care unit flow sheet for recording patient data. CI, cardiac index; CVP, central venous pressure; LAP, left atrial pressure; PAP, pulmonary arterial pressure.

position of the endotracheal tube, nasogastric tube, chest tubes, and monitoring cannulas; establishes a baseline measurement of the mediastinal silhouette; and rules out pneumothorax, hemothorax, or atelectasis. If a PA catheter is present, baseline determinations of the patient's thermodilution cardiac output are obtained early after arrival in the ICU.

Vital signs, fluid input and output, and hemodynamic data are recorded at regular intervals on a standardized flow sheet as shown in Fig. 3.1. The importance of a permanent staff of nurses trained in cardiac surgery care cannot be overemphasized. These nurses can accurately record measurements, recognize ECG abnormalities, perform physical assessment of the patient, titrate medications, and initiate treatment for problems before they become major ones. Suggestions or concerns raised by an experienced cardiac surgery nurse should not be dismissed lightly by the physicians participating in the care of the postoperative patient.

Preprinted postoperative order sheets or computer templates are used. These not only allow for individualization in differing circumstances but also contain the common orders that are needed for most patients. This increases efficiency and helps prevent the omission of important directives. Likewise, when the patient is ready to be transferred out of the ICU, preprinted transfer orders or computer templates are again employed. Protocols for the management of specific problems (such as low cardiac output, excessive bleeding, or atrial fibrillation) that have been developed by multidisciplinary consensus are employed by most cardiac surgery programs and are very useful for patient management.

MANAGEMENT OF THE HEMODYNAMIC STATE

Evaluation and Monitoring of Cardiovascular Function

Assessment of the patient's cardiovascular status after cardiac surgery begins with physical examination. The patient with satisfactory cardiac output and blood pressure typically is alert (if not anesthetized), warm to the touch, and has palpable pedal pulses (in the absence of lower extremity obstructive vascular disease); whereas the patient with inadequate cardiac output and blood pressure typically may be agitated or lethargic, have cool skin and slow capillary refill, and may not have palpable pedal pulses. The patient with cardiac failure, unless hypovolemic, often has jugular venous distention, but more subtle and chronic signs of heart failure, such as a third heart sound or pulmonary crackles, may be difficult to discern in the noisy ICU environment. The assessment can be confounded by the effects of hypothermia (causing peripheral vasoconstriction and cool extremities) and anesthetic agents (causing unresponsiveness). Congestive heart failure in infants is not manifested by peripheral edema or orthopnea as it is in adults. One must look instead for hepatomegaly, facial puffiness, unexplained tachycardia, weight gain, cardiac enlargement, or tachypnea.

Other parameters such as hourly urine output are taken into account but can be misleading early after open heart surgery. Patients usually exhibit a relative diuresis early after surgery due to the effects of hemodilution and osmotic agents that may have been administered during cardiopulmonary bypass (CPB). Because of these factors, even patients with poor cardiovascular performance early after surgery may continue to produce significant amounts of urine for several hours after the operation. Later, when the effects of CPB have cleared, urine output becomes a more sensitive measure of cardiac output and blood pressure: a low urine output (30 to 50 mL per hour in adults or 0.5 mL per hour in infants) indicates possible inadequate hemodynamic performance and requires prompt investigation and treatment.

Invasive measurements provide important complementary information to these noninvasive observations (2). It must be remembered, however, that all catheters, cannulas, monitors, and tracings may be inaccurate, misread, or mislabeled. *Proper management of the cardiac surgery patient never relies on a single "number" to dictate the direction of therapy, but rather takes into account all of the noninvasive and invasive information that is available.*

Arterial pressure is monitored continuously, usually via a cannula in the patient's radial artery. Although systolic arterial pressure reflects the systolic pressure within the left ventricle (in the absence of obstructive lesions such as aortic stenosis), arterial blood pressure is not a sensitive measure of overall hemodynamic status. The ability of the systemic circulation to vasoconstrict and maintain a relatively normal blood pressure, even in the presence of very poor cardiac function, makes this measure of hemodynamic function often the "last to fall" before total cardiovascular collapse.

Flow-directed PA catheters are utilized routinely for monitoring adult patients undergoing cardiac surgery at many, but not all, hospitals or only in selected patients at other institutions. These catheters provide continuous measurement of the PA systolic, diastolic, and mean pressures; allow for thermodilution measurements of the right heart cardiac output. They also provide access for blood sampling from the PA (mixed venous blood).

The concepts of *preload* and *afterload* are important in the care of cardiac surgery patients. For the ventricle to produce an adequate output, it first must be adequately filled. Technically, the volume of blood within the ventricle at the end of diastole is the best measure of ventricular filling and best reflects the preload of the heart, but this is difficult to measure routinely. The left ventricular end-diastolic pressure (LVEDP) reflects the ventricular volume (ignoring the effects of compliance). However, to measure the LVEDP, a catheter must be placed within the left ventricle, which is impractical. The mean left atrial pressure is a good estimate of LVEDP. Although occasionally used in infants and small children, left atrial catheters are very infrequently used in adults. Safer and more convenient is the pulmonary capillary wedge pressure (PCWP), which is obtained at the end of the PA catheter when the vessel is occluded (or "wedged") by temporary inflation of a balloon positioned at the end of the catheter. The PCWP closely approximates LVEDP in patients with normal hearts and lungs, although it tends to be lower than the LVEDP in many patients with cardiac disease (3). Inflation of the balloon to measure PCWP has a small risk of injury to the PA branch, especially in patients with pulmonary hypertension. For that reason, many hospitals rely on the PA diastolic pressure as a reasonably good approximation of the PCWP as this does not require balloon inflation.

Thermodilution cardiac output determination is based on the principle of temperature dilution. The PA catheter has three lumens: one proximally opening into the right atrium, the second at the catheter tip for pressure measurements, and the third for filling the balloon. The catheter and the associated computer derive the cardiac output by analysis of the decrement in temperature in the PA produced by the dilution of a bolus of cold saline injected into the right atrial port; the temperature sensor is at the distal tip of the catheter. Thermodilution measurements of right heart cardiac output (and, normalized to body surface area, the cardiac index) provide generally reliable and useful information regarding the hemodynamic state of the patient, since the left ventricular output is usually identical. The computed cardiac output value can, however, be erroneous due to the improper injection rate or injectate volume of saline, incorrect entry of the patient's weight or height into the computer, or the presence of a left-to-right shunt such as a postinfarction ventricular septal defect. In the latter situation, the computer-derived right heart cardiac output will provide a falsely elevated determination of the left ventricular output. Severe tricuspid valve insufficiency may make the cardiac output determination less accurate by producing artifacts in the thermodilution curve. In addition, in patients of short stature, the central venous injection port on the PA catheter may actually lie within the venous insertion sheath, resulting in loss of injectate.

PA catheters are useful, but not required, for the management of heart surgery patients, particularly those with impaired ventricular function (4,5). Complications related to PA catheters occur in 0.1% to 0.5% of patients. Risks of using the catheter include ventricular arrhythmias, right ventricular perforation, knotting of the catheter, and PA rupture (6,7). Complete heart block can occur during PA catheter insertion or removal in patients with left bundle branch block. Presence of PA rupture should be suspected in any patient with a PA catheter who experiences hemoptysis. Most commonly, the right PA or its branch is the bleeding source. The presentation may be a small "herald" bleed, delayed recurrent hemorrhage, or exsanguination (8). Constant awareness of this rare but catastrophic complication is essential. Management of catheter-induced PA perforation is individualized and involves removal of the catheter, establishment of adequate ventilation, and evaluation and intervention to achieve control of the bleeding (9,10). Depending on the amount of bleeding and other circumstances, management options include bronchoscopy, intrabronchial tamponade with a balloon catheter to protect the remaining airway, early pulmonary arteriography with embolization occlusion of the bleeding vessel, and emergency lung resection.

By measuring the arterial pressure, central venous pressure, and cardiac output, it is possible to calculate the systemic vascular resistance (SVR; Table 3.1). This parameter is also referred to as *afterload*; high afterload indicates vasoconstriction, whereas low afterload indicates

TABLE 3.1	Hemodynamic Parameters	
Parameter	**Formula**	**Normal Values**
Mean arterial blood pressure (MAP)	[SBP + (2 × DBP)]/3	60–105 mm Hg
Cardiac output (CO)	SV × HR	4–8 L/min
Cardiac index (CI)	CO/BSA	2.5–4.0 L/min/m^2
Stroke volume (SV)	CO/HR × 1,000	60–100 mL/beat
Systemic vascular resistance (SVR)	(MAP – RAP or CVP)/CO × 80	800–1,400 dyne-sec/m^5
Pulmonary vascular resistance (PVR)	(PAP$_m$ – PCWP)/CO × 80	100–150 dyne-sec/m^5
Left ventricular stroke work (LVSW)	SV/(MAP – PCWP) × 0.0136	60–80 g-m/beat

BSA, body surface area; CVP, central venous pressure; DBP, diastolic blood pressure; HR, heart rate; PAP$_m$, pulmonary artery pressure (mean); PCWP, pulmonary capillary wedge pressure; RAP, right atrial pressure; SBP, systolic blood pressure; SV, stroke volume.

vasodilatation. The magnitude of afterload is based on arterial pressure and cardiac output. A high calculated SVR indicates a high resistance to the ejection of blood from the left ventricle or a state of low cardiac output with compensatory vascular constriction to maintain the blood pressure. Low afterload is a state of reduced vascular tone (vasodilation) that may be associated with low blood pressure. Pharmacologic management of the SVR is an important aspect of the management of altered hemodynamic states such as low cardiac output. It must be realized, however, that the SVR is derived from three measurements (mean aortic pressure, right atrial pressure, and cardiac output), each of which has potential sources of error and degrees of inexactness. Thus, derived vascular resistance should be considered an estimate, but not an accurate determination, of the state of constriction of the circulation. Likewise, pulmonary vascular resistance (PVR) may be derived as shown in Table 3.1.

Oxygen saturation of the PA mixed venous blood (Svo$_2$) is indicative of both oxygen delivery (cardiac output, arterial saturation, hemoglobin level) and oxygen consumption. PA catheters that have a built-in oxygen saturation sensor at the distal tip can continuously measure the Svo$_2$, which is displayed on a bedside monitor. The normal Svo$_2$ is approximately 80%. Factors that can lead to a decrease in the Svo$_2$ include decreased cardiac output, hypoxia, anemia, and patient shivering. Being a continuously monitored parameter, the Svo$_2$ may provide an early indication of significant hemodynamic alterations (11). But, being somewhat nonspecific and requiring a more expensive central catheter, the technique is not universally applied in adult cardiac surgery patients. The use of Svo_2 measurement in congenital heart surgery is discussed in Chapter 7.

In some patients, at the time of surgery, a small catheter may be introduced into the left atrium and brought out through the chest wall to a transducer for pressure monitoring. These catheters are particularly useful for infants, who are too small for commercially available balloon-tipped PA catheters. The left atrial catheter provides for direct continuous measurement of the filling pressure of the left ventricle. Because they are a direct link between the inside of the left heart and the outside of the patient, extreme care must be taken to avoid air or other embolism.

Thermodilution determination of cardiac output is usually made every 2 to 4 hours during the first 12 to 24 hours after surgery and more frequently if low cardiac output or other problems are present. Alternatively, there are commercially available systems that provide continuous measurement of the patient's cardiac output. In this manner, the effectiveness of therapeutic interventions such as inotropic drug therapy may be determined. For most patients who undergo uncomplicated cardiac surgery, intensive hemodynamic monitoring is employed for 12 to 24 hours after operation. If, on the day after surgery, the patient is stable with satisfactory hemodynamic parameters, the PA or left atrial catheter is removed to minimize the risks of catheter sepsis and emboli. In a patient with a left atrial line, the chest tubes remain in place until after the line is removed. The left atrial catheter should not be withdrawn until confirmation of normal coagulation status has been obtained to avoid bleeding from the insertion site. The radial artery cannula may be left in place longer (usually until the time of transfer from the ICU) to provide access for arterial blood sampling.

Management of the Cardiac Output

Cardiac surgery is often associated with some degree of postoperative ventricular dysfunction. Low cardiac output (defined as a cardiac index of <2.0 L/min/M^2) may result from one or a combination of the following factors: decreased myocardial contractility (of left, right, or both ventricles), abnormal heart rhythm, inadequate preload, or excessive afterload. Low cardiac output results in poor systemic perfusion and, if severe enough, ischemia of vital organs. If not successfully treated, the predictable complications include renal, hepatic, and neurologic dysfunction, with worsening cardiac failure and eventual death. Despite careful preoperative evaluation, perfect repair of the cardiac lesion, and satisfactory intraoperative myocardial preservation, low cardiac output still may follow cardiac surgery. Early recognition of the low output state and appropriate management can lead to reversal of the situation and survival of the patient. Management of postoperative low cardiac output is detailed in Chapter 4.

Management of the Blood Pressure

Generally, it is desirable to maintain the adult patient's systolic blood pressure at 100 to 120 mm Hg (mean arterial pressure, 60 to 70 mm Hg), although elderly patients with long-standing hypertension and inelastic arteries may require a higher blood pressure to adequately perfuse end organs.

Postoperative Hypotension

Hypotension in the early period after cardiac surgery may be due to re-duced cardiac output (due to poor ventricular function or inadequate preload) or to low vascular tone (i.e., low afterload). While hypotension due to reduced cardiac output is usually associated with elevation of the SVR, hypotension due to low afterload is characterized by normal or elevated cardiac output and low SVR.

Hypotension secondary to low intravascular volume (preload) sta-tus, as measured by the central venous pressure, PCWP or diastolic pressure, or left atrial pressure, usually responds to volume infusion. The choice of fluids to achieve this includes crystalloid such as normal saline or colloid such as albumin (most often 5%) or hydroxyethyl starch preparations (hetastarch, pentastarch). Further discussion re-garding choice of fluid for volume infusion follows in the section "Post-operative Fluid Management."

Patients with mild to moderate hypotension with low SVR (low af-terload) may respond well to dopamine infusion (2.5 to 10.0 μg/kg per minute) although tachycardia often limits the usefulness of this drug. Significant hypotension (mean arterial pressure <60 mm Hg) is usually best treated with an α-adrenergic agonist agent such as phenylephrine or with norepinephrine, which has both α- and β-agonist actions. In fact, for the patient with normal or high cardiac output but mild hy-potension and moderately low SVR, it is common to use neosynephrine infusion to "tighten up" the patient's SVR. This will cause the blood pressure to rise and helps to avoid the administration of large vol-umes of fluid leading to weight gain and contributing to pulmonary complications.

Occasional patients (perhaps 10%) will experience severe hypoten-sion with low SVR (<1,200 dynes·second/cm^5) and normal or high car-diac output. This state of *vasodilatory or vasoplegic shock* may be related to CPB-induced systemic inflammatory response and is more common in patients treated with angiotensin-converting enzyme (ACE) inhibitors, β-blockers, amiodarone, and/or phosphodiesterase III inhibitors (12,13).

In this situation, the patient's blood pressure response to neosynephrine or norepinephrine may be inadequate and maintenance of the blood pressure may become a serious problem. Vasodilatory shock may be related to increased bradykinin and decreased plasma vasopressin levels (14,15). Treatment of patients in this setting with continuous arginine vasopressin infusion usually results in successful elevation of the blood pressure and organ perfusion (16–18). Administered through a central venous catheter, vasopressin is started at 0.04 U per minute (adult dose) and titrated upward to achieve a mean arterial blood pressure of 60 to 70 mm Hg (19). Administration of methylene blue (2 mg/kg) has also been reported to be effective treatment for vasoplegic shock, although experience is limited (20).

Postoperative Hypertension

Hypertension after cardiac surgery is less common today than previously, likely due to better preoperative management of hypertension and the preoperative administration of β-blocker drugs. Emergence from anesthesia, pain, irritation from the endotracheal tube, and disorientation may all contribute to an adrenergically mediated increase in peripheral vascular resistance and tachycardia that result in elevation of the blood pressure. Early postoperative hypertension is associated with increased myocardial oxygen consumption, bleeding, and the potential disruption of suture lines; it may also contribute to neurologic injury. For adults, efforts to lower the blood pressure should be undertaken whenever the mean arterial pressure exceeds 90 to 100 mm Hg. In infants and children, postoperative hypertension is treated at correspondingly lower levels.

Hypertension occurring early after heart surgery is treated with short-acting drugs that are administered by continuous infusion (21,22). A variety of drugs are available for this purpose (Table 3.2). The most popular drug, particularly for adults with coronary artery disease, is *nitroglycerin*. Nitroglycerin acts to dilate preferentially the venous capacitance vessels at low doses, affecting the resistance arteries only at higher doses. Although heart rate may increase somewhat, arterial impedance (afterload) is reduced. This results in favorable effects on myocardial metabolism. Nitroglycerin reduces the propensity of the coronary arteries to vasoconstriction (spasm) and results in improved internal mammary and radial artery flow rates (23). Nitroglycerin infusion in adults is begun at 10 to 20 μg per minute and the rate of infusion is increased by 5 to 10 μg per minute every 5 minutes (up to 200 μg per minute) until the desired reduction in blood pressure is reached. Patients with low filling pressures may be particularly sensitive to nitroglycerin's hypotensive effect. Nitroglycerin is rapid in onset and its

TABLE 3.2	Drugs for the Acute Treatment of Early Postoperative Hypertension (Adult Intravenous Doses)	
Drug	**Intravenous Dose**	**Comment**
Nitroglycerin	20–300 μg/min or 0.1–5.0 μg/kg/min	Not as effective as nitroprusside, but better for coronary flow and radial artery spasm
Nitroprusside	0.10–10.0 μg/kg/min	Limit duration of use due to toxicity, especially if renal insufficiency is present
Esmolol	Load with 500 μg/kg, then 50- to 150-μg/kg/min infusion	Rapid onset and short duration of effect; easy to titrate for effect. Use with caution in presence of poor left ventricular function or bradycardia
Fenoldopam	Start with 0.025–0.3 μg/kg/min; max 1.6 μg/kg/min	For short-term use; may be useful for patient with renal insufficiency; caution in patients with glaucoma
Labetalol	Load with 5–40 mg over 2 min, then 1- to 3-mg/min infusion	Longer acting than esmolol; causes vasodilation in addition to β-blockade; do not use if ventricular function is poor
Nicardipine	2.5- to 15-mg/h infusion (adult)	Caution if cardiac conduction impaired; relatively long half-life makes titration more difficult
Clevidipine	Start at 1–2 mg/h; titrate to desired effect; usual dose 4–6 mg/h (adult)	Metabolism not affected by renal or hepatic function
Enalaprilat	0.625–2.50 mg by slow infusion (>5 min); repeat every 6 h (adult)	May cause renal insufficiency in patients with renal artery stenosis

Note: For all the above drugs given intravenously, continuous blood pressure monitoring is recommended, and the drug dose should be carefully titrated to the desired result to avoid hypotension.

effect resolves quickly when the drug is discontinued. Continuous measurement of the blood pressure is required when nitroglycerin is being used for blood pressure control. Side effects include headache, flushing, and tachyarrhythmias.

While nitroglycerin has advantages, it is often not sufficiently effective in controlling postoperative hypertension and may fail to provide adequate blood pressure control in at least 15% of patients (24). *Nitroprusside* is a highly effective agent that acts by dilating both the arterial and venous capacitance vessels. Treatment is begun at 0.1 μg/kg per minute and titrated upward until the desired reduction in blood pressure is achieved. The maximum recommended dose is 2 μg/kg per minute. Excessively lowering the blood pressure with nitroprusside in coronary bypass patients may be deleterious for the myocardial oxygen supply–demand relationship, may cause intracoronary steal of blood away from ischemic areas, and may have detrimental effects on internal mammary artery bypass graft flow. Tachycardia is common. The use of nitroprusside should be limited to 12 hours or less, and to even shorter periods of time in patients with renal insufficiency to avoid cyanogen (cyanide radical) accumulation. Cyanogen toxicity is characterized by metabolic acidosis, drug tachyphylaxis, coma, absent reflexes, dilated pupils, and pink skin color. In general, nitroprusside should be used only when necessary and for as short a duration as possible (21).

Alternatives to nitroprusside include β-blockers, ACE inhibitors, and calcium channel blocking (CCB) drugs. Short-acting β-blockers, namely *esmolol* and *labetalol*, are effective, especially for patients with both hypertension and tachycardia. Esmolol is a fast-acting β1-receptor blocking agent that has a very short half-life (9 minutes), allowing for rapid control of the blood pressure with rapid reversal of its effect when discontinued (25,26). As a specific β1-receptor blocker, it inhibits the cardiac β-receptors (cardioselective) while having little effect on bronchial and vascular smooth muscle. Esmolol reduces the heart rate, a useful property for patients with coronary insufficiency. For adults, administration is begun with a loading dose of 0.5 to 1.0 mg/kg over 1 minute, followed by a maintenance dose of 25 to 300 µg/kg per minute. Effectiveness of esmolol in postoperative pediatric heart surgery patients has also been described (27). The patient's blood pressure and heart rate must be monitored closely to avoid overshooting the desired result. *Labetalol* has both β-receptor and α-receptor blocking properties. When used for postoperative hypertension control, the drug exerts moderate negative inotropic and chronotropic properties resulting in blood pressure reduction without reflexive vasoconstriction (28). Cerebral, renal, and coronary artery blood flow are maintained. It should, however, be used with caution in patients with poor ventricular function. β-Blocker drugs should be used with care in patients with bradycardia, conduction abnormalities, congenital heart defects with right-to-left shunting, reactive airway disease, diabetes, and peripheral vascular disease. In our practices we find esmolol to most often be appropriate for younger adult patients with postoperative hypertension and tachycardia and relatively normal left ventricular function. Labetalol is quite useful for perioperative management of patients with aortic dissection and following adult aortic coarctation repair.

ACE inhibitors cause reduced SVR with generally little effect on heart rate. Patients with congestive heart failure who are treated with ACE inhibitors experience increased cardiac output and decreased PCWP. Thus, the postoperative use of the ACE inhibitors may be of value, particularly for the hypertensive patient with impaired ventricular function. For treatment during the early postoperative period, the intravenous (IV) form of enalapril, *enalaprilat*, may be useful (29). The initial adult dose is 0.625 to 1.25 mg infused over 5 minutes, with further doses (up to 5.0 mg) every 6 hours as indicated. The use of enalaprilat in this setting results in improved cardiac output in conjunction with reduced blood pressure. When the patient is able to take oral medications, conversion to oral enalapril or another ACE inhibitor may be accomplished. When administering ACE inhibitors to patients with renal insufficiency, the serum creatinine level should be closely followed.

CCB drugs block transmembrane flow of calcium, resulting in peripheral vascular and coronary artery dilation, reduced myocardial contractility, and lower blood pressure (30). *Nicardipine* has been demonstrated to be effective for the treatment of postoperative hypertension when used as continuous, titratable infusion (31–33). The ultra–short-acting dihydropyridine CCB *clevidipine* has also been found to be safe and effective for rapid treatment of acute hypertension after cardiac surgery (34,35). The CCB *nifedipine* is not recommended for the urgent or emergency treatment of hypertension (21).

Hydralazine is also useful for the acute treatment of hypertension, especially in patients with heart failure. The initial adult dose is 5 to 10 mg IV every 20 minutes until the goal blood pressure is reached or a maximum dose of 40 mg has been administered. The duration of action of hydralazine is, however, prolonged (up to 10 hours) and shorter acting drugs are generally preferred for the treatment of acute postoperative hypertension.

Fenoldopam is a unique drug with selective dopamine-1 receptor agonist properties, making it useful for the treatment of hypertension, particularly in patients with renal impairment (36). When given intravenously, fenoldopam has a moderately rapid onset of action (5 to 15 minutes). The usual starting dose is 0.1 μg/kg per minute with the drug dose increased by 0.05 to 0.1 μg/kg per minute increments until the desired blood pressure (or maximum dose of 1.6 μg/kg per minute is reached. Reported clinical experience with fenoldopam in heart surgery has been favorable and may be particularly valuable in postoperative patients with hypertension and renal insufficiency (37–39).

PULMONARY CARE

General anesthesia, inhalation anesthetic agents, and CPB impair lung function. Contributing factors include pulmonary sequestration of activated leukocytes and platelets in pulmonary capillaries, complement activation, microemboli (gas or tissue debris), increased capillary permeability, and alveolar hypoperfusion (40,41). Furthermore, a significant proportion of cardiac surgery patients have pre-existing pulmonary dysfunction as either the result of their cardiac condition or smoking-induced emphysema. Postoperative respiratory failure occurs in about 10% of patients undergoing cardiac surgery and is associated with increased hospital and long-term mortality (42). Optimal perioperative management of the pulmonary system is an important aspect of successful care of cardiac surgery patients.

Identification of patients with compromised pulmonary function before surgery can assist in the management of the patient postoperatively by setting postoperative expectations. Note should be made of a history of smoking, frequent respiratory infections, episodes of wheezing, chronic sputum production, recent respiratory tract infections, and previous cardiac surgery in which damage to a phrenic nerve might have occurred. Long-term preoperative amiodarone treatment may be associated with an increased incidence of postoperative adult pulmonary insufficiency (43,44). For patients with known pulmonary disease or positive risk factors in their history, preoperative pulmonary function tests and room air arterial blood gas determinations will quantify abnormalities of ventilation and gas exchange and provide baseline information for postoperative comparison. Independent variables associated with the need for prolonged postoperative ventilation include advanced age, forced expiratory volume in one second (FEV_1 <70% of predicted), elevated serum creatinine level, ejection fraction <30%, recent myocardial infarction, emergency surgery, mitral valve procedures, and the use of CPB. Using these preoperative factors, a "prolonged ventilation score" may be derived to predict an individual patient's risk (45).

All patients are instructed preoperatively in the use of an incentive spirometer (Fig. 3.2). Patients with chronic obstructive pulmonary disease should have their medications optimized prior to undergoing operation (46). Patients who smoke should be encouraged to stop before surgery, although the benefit of doing so is most apparent if the patient quits at least 2 months preoperatively.

Some patients, usually younger ones with little or no pulmonary disease who have undergone an uncomplicated cardiac repair, are sometimes extubated in the operating room before transfer to the ICU or soon after arrival in the ICU. However, most cardiac surgery patients are transported to the ICU with the endotracheal tube in place, still receiving mechanical ventilation. Expeditious weaning of the patient from the ventilator with early extubation, often within a few hours of ICU arrival, has been demonstrated to be safe and advantageous. This is the goal in nearly all patients (both adult and pediatric) who have undergone uncomplicated operations (47–52). Exceptions to a "fast track" toward early extubation include patients with low cardiac output or hemodynamic instability, patients with an intra-aortic balloon pump in place, patients with an apparent neurologic deficit, and those who are bleeding excessively.

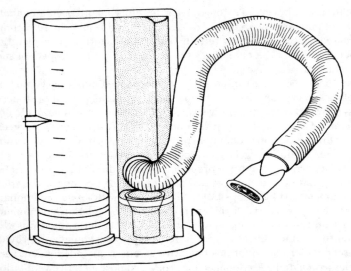

FIGURE 3.2 Disposable incentive spirometer. The patient inhales deeply through the mouthpiece. The float on the left rises according to the inspiratory flow rate.

Mechanical Ventilators

Mechanical ventilators provide positive pressure within the airways causing inspiration; expiration follows as a passive process. Control of ventilation may be based on volume (where the ventilator delivers a set volume of gas, no matter what the pressure is required to achieve that set volume) or based on pressure (where the ventilator delivers gas until a desired airway pressure is achieved with the variable being the delivered tidal volume). Most ventilators in use today have the capability of either volume- or pressure-control modes. For adults, the volume-control mode is used most frequently and for infants the pressure-control mode is most common. When using the volume-control mode, the operator sets the tidal volume, respiratory rate, and inspiratory gas flow or inspiratory time, and positive end-expiratory pressure (PEEP). For pressure control, the settings are the ventilator rate, the inspiratory time, the desired peak airway pressure, and PEEP.

For an adult patient, typical initial postoperative ventilator settings are: tidal volume 6 to 8 mL/kg, rate 10 to 12 per minute and fractional inspired oxygen (FIO_2) 50% using the continuous mandatory ventilation mode. A PEEP level of 5 cm is ordered. Minute ventilation equals the tidal volume multiplied by the respiratory rate, thus this provides a set minute ventilation of 60 to 96 mL/kg per minute. Since the normal ratio of dead space (airways and nonperfused alveoli) to tidal volume is 0.33, the alveolar ventilation will be about 40 to 64 mL/kg per minute or about 2.4 to 3.8 L per minute, which is a ventilation volume usually sufficient to remove metabolically produced carbon dioxide. For the patient with normal lungs, the inspiratory flow rate or inspiratory time is adjusted so that the ratio of inspiration time to expiration time (I/E ratio) is about 1:3. If the patient is experiencing high airway pressures (above 35 cm H_2O), the flow rate is decreased so that the I/E ratio is decreased. Alternatively, the tidal volume may be decreased resulting in decreased plateau pressure (the airway pressure during a 1- to 2-second inspiratory pause), which is the major determinant of barotrauma to the lung. Ideally, the plateau pressure is kept below 30 to 32 mm cm H_2O to prevent ventilator-induced lung injury. Patients with significant chronic obstructive pulmonary disease may benefit from a combination of lower ventilator rate and longer expiratory times to prevent air trapping (53). The inspired oxygen level is titrated to maintain the arterial oxygen saturation 90% to 93%. If the F_{IO_2} requirement exceeds 60%, the PEEP level may be increased, although we generally aim to keep it below 10 cm.

Ventilators can provide various modes of ventilation (54). For the comatose, anesthetized or paralyzed patient, the *controlled* mechanical mode is used in which the ventilator simply delivers breaths at set time intervals (depending on what rate has been chosen) irrespective of what the patient may do. This mode is generally used only in the operating room. As the patient awakens and begins to initiate breaths, the *assist-control* or *volume-control* mode may be used. In this mode, the set breath volume (the tidal volume) is delivered every time the patient initiates a breath. The sensitivity of the assist-control mode is adjusted so as to prevent over- or underventilation and a back-up (control) rate is specified to provide a minimum number of breaths per minute if the patient is not initiating respiration. This allows the patient to adjust his or her breathing rate to provide for normocapnia. Alternatively, the *synchronized intermittent mandatory* ventilation (SIMV) mode may be used. In this mode, the patient receives a set number of breaths per minute but may take self-initiated breaths in-between those delivered by the ventilator. The tidal volume of these patient-initiated breaths is dependent upon the amount of pressure support applied, patient strength and effort, and chest compliance. The SIMV mode detects when the patient takes his own breath and avoids "stacking" a delivered breath on top of a spontaneous one to allow for better patient–ventilator synchrony. It is common to add some level of *pressure support* to the SIMV mode. This provides a constant small (5 to 10 cm H_2O) degree of inspiratory pressure with patient-initiated breaths so as to overcome the endotracheal tube and ventilator tubing resistance. To avoid hypoventilation with SIMV mode, the *mandatory minute ventilation* mode can be utilized. This mode monitors the patient's minute ventilation. If the patient is not breathing spontaneously at a sufficient rate to ensure that a preset minute ventilation is reached, the ventilator will deliver breaths at the preset tidal volume so as to make up the difference between the patient's efforts and the preset required minute ventilation. If, however, the patient breathes at a rate and tidal volume equal to, or in excess of, the preset minute ventilation, the ventilator will not deliver additional breaths to the patient.

PEEP increases the patient's functional residual capacity. This form of pressure support maintains some degree of lung inflation at all times. By decreasing the amount of atelectasis present, arterial oxygenation is increased for the same level of inspired oxygen. PEEP is therefore quite useful for the treatment of respiratory failure characterized by impaired gas exchange; however, high levels of PEEP (above 10 cm H_2O) may reduce the patient's preload and hence, cardiac output, which can limit its usefulness in some cardiac surgery patients. This may be particularly true in patients with right heart failure or after the Fontan procedure where PEEP may increase transpulmonary pressure. It can be valuable to determine the optimum PEEP curve for these patients. To construct this relationship, cardiac output determinations are made at representative levels of PEEP (e.g., 4, 8, 12, and 16 mm Hg), and the PEEP that provides improvement in oxygenation without lowering the cardiac output significantly is chosen for use.

Large tidal volumes, particularly in conjunction with high levels of PEEP, may result in overinflation of nondependent lung segments and alveolar injury. In fact, high pressures may be more damaging than high-inspired oxygen concentrations. Reduced peak inspiratory pressures may be achieved by smaller tidal volume settings. However, this may result in hypercarbia and decreased volume of aerated lung with subsequent intrapulmonary shunting caused by the reduction in minute ventilation. Thus, efforts are made to achieve a balance between pressure management, inspired oxygen concentration, and carbon dioxide removal (55).

It is recommended that the peak airway pressure be maintained at <40 cm H_2O. A sudden increase in peak inspiratory pressures may be indicative of bronchospasm, mucous plugging of a major bronchus, pneumothorax, hemothorax, obstruction of the endotracheal tube, or compression of the ventilator circuit tubing. The sudden onset of high inspiratory pressures should be evaluated by suctioning the patient, chest auscultation, obtaining a chest x-ray, and careful examination of the endotracheal tube and ventilator circuit tubing.

Use of Arterial Blood Gas Determination

Analysis of the arterial blood gases provides valuable information regarding gas exchange and the patient's acid–base status. Elevation of the partial pressure of carbon dioxide (Pco_2) indicates inadequate ventilation. If severe, the patient may require intubation and mechanical ventilation. If already on the ventilator, the hypercarbic patient is most likely in need of a higher minute volume. A diminished partial pressure of oxygen (Po_2) may be caused by a ventilation–perfusion imbalance secondary to atelectasis, pneumonia, congestive heart failure, or by an unrecognized, right-to-left cardiac shunt. When lung disease is present, increasing the inspired oxygen concentration (Fio_2) will usually increase the Po_2. When the Po_2 increases little in the presence of a high Fio_2 there may be a fixed anatomic intracardiac right-to-left shunt or an intrapulmonary shunt. In this situation, echocardiography may be performed to rule out an intracardiac shunt.

The base deficit (calculated from the pH and Pco_2) is usually provided as a part of the blood gas determination results. From this, the amount of sodium bicarbonate necessary to correct any metabolic acidosis can be calculated.

Weaning Ventilator Support

It is the goal to remove all patients from mechanical ventilation as soon as it is safe to do so. Early extubation is safe and advantageous for the patient and cost-effective for the hospital. An important factor in the development of early extubation protocols has been the application of intraoperative anesthetic techniques that reduce narcotic administration with concomitant use of inhalational anesthetic agent (56). This allows for the earlier attainment of consciousness, spontaneous breathing, and early weaning from the ventilator. Patient characteristics favorable for early extubation are shown in Table 3.3.

As the patient emerges from anesthesia, narcotic administration is limited to that which is necessary to keep the patient comfortable but

---

TABLE 3.3	Patient Characteristics for Early Extubation

- Uncomplicated operation with CPB time of <2.5 h
- Awake, alert, neurologically intact patient
- Adequate urine output
- No significant arrhythmias
- Hemodynamically stable
- IABP support not required
- Fully rewarmed
- Not bleeding excessively (<150 mL over 2 h)
- Satisfactory chest x-ray appearance

CPB, cardiopulmonary bypass; IABP, intra-aortic balloon pump.

not overly sedated. As the patient begins to initiate more spontaneous breaths and is responding to verbal commands, the ventilator mode is changed to pressure support. For this, the patient is placed on pressure support at 5 cm and allowed to breath on his or her own. The pressure support lessens the work of breathing but does not provide excessive assistance. Alternatively, the patient may be placed on a T tube and allowed to breathe on his own through the endotracheal tube but without mechanical assistance. After breathing 40% inspired oxygen concentration (either on pressure support or on a T tube) for 30 minutes or so, simple spirometric measurements are made (tidal volume, inspiratory force, minute ventilation) and the arterial blood gases are checked. If the pH is ≥ 7.31, the partial pressure of carbon dioxide, arterial ($Paco_2$) ≤ 45 mm Hg, and oxygen saturation as measured by pulse oximetry (Spo_2) $>93\%$, the endotracheal tube is removed. Alternatively, respiratory mechanics may be measured with the criteria for extubation being shown in Table 3.4. If the patient does not meet these criteria, the previous ventilator settings are resumed and the patient is re-evaluated in 1 to 2 hours.

The *Rapid-Shallow-Breathing Index* is a potentially useful tool for predicting successful extubation. During a trial of spontaneous breathing, measurements of the breathing rate (f, in breaths per minute) and the tidal volume (TV, in liters) are made. If the index, f/TV, is <105, successful extubation is likely. Serial measurements over several hours increase the ability of the index to predict successful weaning from the ventilator (57).

After extubation, humidified oxygen is delivered to the patient by face mask or nasal prongs (which are more comfortable). The inspired oxygen concentration is decreased gradually over 24 to 36 hours while continuing

---

TABLE 3.4	Criteria for Extubation

- Hemodynamic stability (cardiac index $>$ 2.0 L/min/m^2)
- No more than modest amount of inotropic drug support (i.e., <5 μg/kg/min dobutamine)
- Stable heart rhythm, lack of significant tachycardia
- Conscious, alert, follows commands
- Not bleeding excessively
- Measured on ventilator
  Minute ventilation $<$ 10–15 L/min
  Maximum inspiratory force $>$ –20 cm H_2O
- Successful spontaneous breathing trial with
  Respiratory rate $<$ 25 breaths per minute
  Tidal volume $>$ 3 mL/kg
  Vital capacity $>$ 10 mL/kg
  P_aO_2 $>$ 70 mm Hg on F_iO_2 40%
  P_aCO_2 $<$ 45 mm Hg

to monitor the patient's arterial oxygen saturation. The patient is usually on nasal-prong oxygen at the time of transfer from the ICU to the postoperative care ward. Over the next few days, the nasal-prong oxygen delivery rate is gradually reduced with periodic determinations of the arterial oxygen saturation by pulse oximetry, generally aiming to keep it above 92%.

Respiratory care during the early postoperative period is simple but important. At the time of surgery, the patient's chest and mediastinal tubes are connected to a commercially available three-chamber system to prevent the intrathoracic accumulation of blood and fluid (Fig. 3.3). For the intubated patient, frequent endotracheal suctioning, humidification of the inspired gases, and frequent changes of body

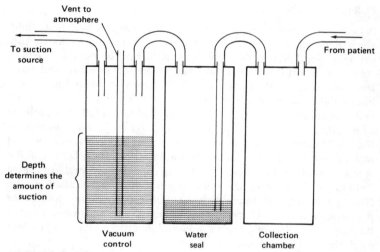

FIGURE 3.3 Principles of a chest tube suction system. The essential components of commercially available suction systems for chest tube drainage are the following: **(A)** A fluid collection chamber (*right*) in which the fluid or blood draining from the chest may be collected sterilely, measured accurately, and (in some systems) detached for connection to an intravenous line, so that the shed blood can be reinfused into the patient. **(B)** A water seal chamber (*middle*) that functions as a one-way valve to prevent the backward flow of air into the chest and as a monitor for air leakage from the chest. Leaking air appears as bubbles from the underwater portion of the tube. The water level in this chamber is usually set at 2 cm. **(C)** A vacuum control chamber (*left*) in which the water level is usually set at 20 cm H_2O, the amount of negative pressure applied to the chest tubes through the other chambers. The connection to atmosphere will relieve any negative pressure in excess of this amount that is applied by the wall suction. The suction source should be adjusted to provide gentle, continuous bubbling in this chamber to ensure that the intended vacuum is being maintained. Excessive bubbling will result in a lowered water level and decreased suction.

position are important to prevent retained secretions and atelectasis. After extubation, the patient is encouraged to sit up, dangle his or her legs, and to use the incentive spirometer. The incentive spirometer is a very effective method for preventing postoperative atelectasis (58). Early ambulation is encouraged and the level of exertion is increased incrementally after the patient's chest tubes are removed.

Most patients are extubated within 6 hours of surgery. Some, for a variety of reasons, may be difficult to wean from the ventilator. Management of these patients is discussed in Chapter 4.

FLUIDS AND ELECTROLYTES

Postoperative Fluid Management

Patients who undergo cardiac surgery invariably gain total body fluid. For patients undergoing surgery with CPB, this gain in predominantly extravascular fluid occurs as the result of the bypass circuit prime fluid volume, hemodilution with loss of plasma oncotic pressure, and capillary leakage during the period of CPB. The degree of hemodilution and interstitial tissue edema is proportional to the length of time on CPB and is proportionally greater in very small children (59). For patients who undergo surgery without the use of CPB ("off pump") intraoperative fluid loading is often necessary to prevent hypotension associated with manipulation of the beating heart. Because of these factors, at the completion of surgery, most patients are considerably fluid in positive fluid balance. Initial fluid orders should specify a low infusion rate: 50 mL per hour for adults and one half of the usual maintenance rate for pediatric patients. A 5% dextrose-containing solution is used. Further fluid and electrolyte administration is tailored to the individual patient on the basis of hemodynamic criteria.

Despite an increase in total body fluid of up to 20% to 30%, the intravascular volume status of the patient during the early postoperative period is dynamic, and volume administration may be required to maintain adequate filling (ventricular preload) of the heart. The effects of hemodilution, capillary leak with redistribution of fluid, vasodilation, and other factors may result in low preload despite the gain in total body fluid. Monitoring the heart rate, arterial pressure, cardiac output, central venous pressure, PA pressure, left atrial pressure (if available), and urine output provides information to allow one to adjust colloid or crystalloid administration to the patient appropriate to the circumstances. When arterial pressure, filling pressures, and urine output are low, a trial of volume infusion should be given. Intravascular depletion also usually causes tachycardia, but this response may be blunted in patients who received β-adrenergic antagonists preoperatively.

For volume loading, the use of normal saline, 5% albumin, or hydroxyethyl starch preparations is customary. Considerable debate has been held regarding the relative efficacy and safety of these choices (60,61). Hetastarch interferes with platelet function and, in large doses, may cause transient prolongation of the prothrombin, partial thromboplastin, and bleeding times. Its use in CPB patients is associated with impaired blood coagulation and postoperative bleeding as compared to the patients who receive albumin (62–64). Albumin, being a pooled plasma product does carry a very small risk of transmitted infection. In our practices, we generally prefer the use of normal saline alternating with 5% albumin (each as 250 or 500 mL boluses for adults) for fluid administration when given for the purpose of increasing the patient's preload. The administration of blood products such as plasma or red blood cells (RBCs) for the purpose of volume expansion is not appropriate.

For the patient with low preload but adequate systemic blood pressure, heart rate, and cardiac output, volume loading is not indicated. For the adult patient with low preload, hypotension, and low cardiac output (with or without tachycardia), a bolus of 250 to 500 mL of fluid is given over 10 minutes with monitoring of the patient's hemodynamic parameters. If the filling pressure (central venous, PA diastolic, or left atrial) quickly rises above 15 mm Hg, the bolus infusion should be slowed and the situation reassessed. For infants, the usual trial fluid bolus is 5 to 10 mL/kg. If hypotension and low preload persist, the fluid bolus should be repeated. Generally, 6 to 12 hours after surgery, the patient's volume status stabilizes and further boluses of volume- expanding solutions are not required.

Beginning the first day after surgery, to reduce interstitial edema, patients with an uncomplicated postoperative course are usually fluid-restricted to approximately 50% of normal requirements. IV fluid administration is minimized, and the patient is allowed to take small amounts of fluid by mouth. Diuretic therapy is usually employed to return the patient to their preoperative weight. This is accomplished gradually, over 3 to 4 days following surgery. Depending on how much water weight the patient has gained, furosemide is administered either intravenously or orally, usually every 8 hours for 24 to 48 hours. Daily weights are measured and the dose is adjusted accordingly. Frequent potassium level determinations and supplementation as needed is important. Severely fluid-overloaded patients, especially if renal and/or respiratory insufficiency is present, may benefit from continuous furosemide infusion (65,66). This is accomplished with a loading dose of 0.5 mg/kg followed by 0.125 to 0.5 mg/kg per hour. For adults, the typical infusion rate is 5 to 40 mg per hour. The rate of furosemide infusion is adjusted according to the urine output response. For adults who are considerably above their preoperative weight, the urine output goal is

100 to 150 mL per hour. As the patient's weight approaches the preoperative level, the furosemide infusion is slowed and then discontinued.

Potassium

Hypokalemia is the most common electrolyte abnormality encountered in hospitalized patients (67). Patients on long-term preoperative diuretic therapy frequently have decreased preoperative total body potassium stores even though their serum potassium levels may be within the normal range. When CPB is utilized, a high rate of intraoperative urine output is common, with concomitant potassium loss. This effect usually continues for several hours after the operation and will be exacerbated in hyperglycemic patients. The associated potassium loss can be considerable and may result in severe hypokalemia.

Postoperative hypokalemia may be associated with nonsustained ventricular tachycardia and, perhaps, atrial fibrillation (68,69). Severe hypokalemia causes muscular weakness, metabolic alkalosis, arrhythmias, ECG changes (T-wave flattening and inversion, U-wave prominence, and ST-segment depression), and increased susceptibility to digoxin toxicity. Depletion of serum potassium levels can occur quickly; therefore, frequent potassium level determinations and replacement as required are indicated. For an adult, a decrease of 1 mEq/L in the serum potassium level represents a total body deficiency of at least 100 mEq. Thus, large amounts of potassium supplementation may be required for the severely depleted patient. When possible, oral administration is preferred (20 to 40 mEq two to three times per day for adults). For adults, IV potassium is administered at a rate of 10 to 20 mEq per hour. This should be mixed in 100 mL of 5% dextrose and given through a central vein catheter to prevent vein irritation. The rate of infusion must be controlled by an infusion pump to prevent inadvertent rapid delivery, which can result in serious arrhythmias. For infants, potassium chloride may be given through a central line in doses up to 0.5 mEq/kg per hour mixed in 3 to mL/kg of 5% dextrose. The serum potassium level should be maintained between 4.0 and 5.0 mEq/L.

If the patient is receiving potassium-sparing diuretics such as triamterene or spironolactone, a regularly scheduled dose of potassium generally *should not* be given because dangerous hyperkalemia may result. Individually ordered doses may be needed, but patients receiving potassium supplementation in addition to a potassium-sparing diuretic should have frequent potassium level determinations.

Although uncommon, hyperkalemia may occur after cardiac surgery, most frequently in patients with impaired renal function. The combination of pre-existing renal insufficiency, large doses of hyperkalemic cardioplegia solution infusion, red cell damage during CPB, and (when low cardiac output is present) hypoperfusion of tissues with release of intracellular potassium can quickly result in dangerous hyperkalemia in the early postoperative period. Use of hemofiltration during operation can help lessen this problem. One maneuver useful for the patient with hyperkalemia and relatively normal renal function is to administer a moderate dose of furosemide (40 mg IV for the adult) and to replace the resultant urine output with a crystalloid, potassium-free solution. Severe hyperkalemia (above 6.5 mEq/L) may cause weakness, paresthesia, and ECG changes (peaked T waves, atrioventricular block, and widened QRS complex) and may lead to arrhythmic death of the patient. Specific treatment is begun when the serum potassium level exceeds 6.5 mEq/L, even in the absence of ECG changes (70). If ECG changes are present, calcium gluconate should be administered (10 mL of 10% solution IV over 3 to 5 minutes); however, calcium reversal of the cardiac effects of hyperkalemia will be short-lived (30 to 60 minutes). Glucose (50 mL of 50% dextrose solution) with insulin (10 units of regular insulin added to the solution) may be administered over 10 minutes to drive serum potassium into the intracellular space. Definitive removal of excess potassium from the body requires the use of the cation-exchange resin sodium polystyrene sulfonate (20 to 60 g mixed with 70% sorbitol to prevent constipation) given orally or rectally. Dialysis or venovenous hemofiltration will likely be needed to treat hyperkalemia associated with severe renal failure.

Sodium

Cardiac surgery using CPB causes a significant increase in the patient's total body fluid volume, which is often associated with a moderate reduction in the serum sodium concentration. In this setting, hyponatremia is nearly always dilutional, the result of excess free water rather than a deficit in total body sodium. Loss of the accumulated extra free water over the first few days after surgery, often assisted by the administration of diuretic agents, results in normalization of the sodium level. Thus, treatment of asymptomatic hyponatremia in the early postoperative period by administration of sodium-containing solutions is usually not necessary. The fundamental disorder is water overload and hemodilution, not sodium deficiency; therefore, mild to moderate fluid restriction is in order. If the hyponatremia is symptomatic and/or severe, with the serum sodium level <120 mEq/L, administration of 3% saline may be indicated (71).

Serious hypernatremia (serum sodium level above 160 mEq/L) is rare and is usually the result of excessive diuretic treatment and dehydration. Generally, the patient's serum blood urea nitrogen and creatinine levels will also be elevated. Less frequent causes include excessive sodium administration (often in the form of sodium bicarbonate used to treat acidosis) and diabetes insipidus. Symptoms of severe hypernatremia include restlessness, irritability, ataxia, and seizures. Treatment is the cautious administration of free water at a rate that does not correct the serum sodium level faster than 0.7 mEq/L per hour (72).

Calcium

Ionized (and total) serum calcium levels decrease modestly during CPB and, if untreated, remain below normal during the early postoperative period largely due to hemodilution. There is no adverse consequence of mild hypokalemia; myocardial performance is not impaired. The calcium level usually returns to normal during the first 24 hours after operation (73). The normal total plasma serum calcium level is approximately 9.0 to 10.5 mg/dL (2.2 to 2.6 mmol/L), with the physiologically active ionized fraction being about 1.1 to 1.3 mmol/L (4.5 to 5.6 mg/dL). While citrate-anticoagulated banked blood will briefly reduce the serum calcium concentration, this effect is very transient, as the citrate is cleared quickly, and for significant hypocalcemia to result, an extremely fast rate of blood infusion (more than 1 unit every 5 minutes for an adult) is required. Thus, the administration of calcium with red cell transfusions is not recommended, even during massive transfusion, and may actually be harmful (74). Neonates may be more sensitive to the effects of citrated blood transfusion (due to liver immaturity) but calcium administration should be guided by measurement of the ionized calcium level.

In general, asymptomatic hypocalcemia does not warrant treatment. In fact, calcium administered to the recently ischemic myocardium may be injurious to the muscle and may contribute to myocardial dysfunction and other complications (75–77). In addition, calcium may interfere with exogenously administrated catecholamine such as epinephrine and dobutamine (78). Calcium administration is not generally recommended unless specifically indicated for symptomatic, documented hypocalcemia.

Symptoms of hypocalcemia may develop when the ionized calcium level falls below 2.5 mg/dL. Manifestations of hypocalcemia include low cardiac output, hypotension, arrhythmias, and ECG abnormalities (prolongation of QT and ST segments and T-wave inversion). Noncardiac effects of hypocalcemia include weakness, tetany, seizures, apnea, paresthesias, laryngospasm, and psychosis. When administered, calcium should be given intravenously. Initially, for adults, a bolus of 100 to 200 mg of elemental calcium (10 to 20 mL of 10% calcium gluconate or 4 to 8 mL of 10% calcium chloride) is given, followed by infusion of 1 to 2 mg/kg per hour. The calcium chloride form is more effective in raising the ionized serum calcium level quickly. Administration through a central line is mandatory because calcium solutions are irritating to peripheral veins and extravasated calcium chloride causes tissue necrosis. Attention should also be paid to the serum magnesium, potassium and pH. Hypomagnesemia will make it more difficult to correct hypocalcemia (67).

Severe, symptomatic hypocalcemia tends to occur most often in newborn infants undergoing operation, likely as a result of inadequate calcium stores and immature parathyroid glands. In the infant, significant hypocalcemia may be manifested by twitching, jitteriness, and seizures. Treatment is by *slow, central venous* catheter injection of 10% calcium gluconate, 10 to 20 mg/kg, or 10% calcium chloride, 5 mg/kg.

Magnesium

Magnesium is an important intracellular element. Less than 1% of the total body magnesium content is present in the blood. The normal adult magnesium concentration is 1.7 to 2.3 mg/dL but the blood level may not accurately reflect intracellular stores. Normal levels may be lower in neonates and higher in infants, and preoperative hypomagnesemia is frequent in patients undergoing surgery for congenital heart disease (79).

Magnesium is important in the regulation of many cellular functions including calcium and potassium fluxes, smooth muscle tone, coronary vascular reactivity, and nitric oxide synthesis. A decrease in the patient's serum magnesium level, largely due to hemodilution, often occurs after cardiac surgery using CPB with gradual return to normal in a few days (80). Magnesium administration to the cardiac surgery patient may enhance hemodynamic performance, especially for the magnesium-deficit patient and appears to reduce the incidence of postoperative atrial fibrillation (81–83). The exact role of magnesium supplementation to the cardiac surgery patient is unclear but administration appears to be safe; in our practices it is common to administer 2 g (adult dose) of magnesium sulfate intravenously to the patient just prior to weaning the patient from CPB. In addition, hypomagnesemia may be a contributor to the development of hypokalemia; both should be corrected when hypokalemia is present.

ACID–BASE BALANCE

Measurement of the arterial blood gases will determine the diagnosis of acidemia or alkalemia although compensatory changes will occur so as to reduce the changes in the ratio of bicarbonate (HCO_3) to carbon dioxide (PCO_2), thereby reducing the magnitude of the pH disturbance. Table 3.5 outlines the basic acid–base disturbances.

| TABLE 3.5 | Acid–Base Disturbances |

		Primary		Secondary Response	
Disorder	pH	HCO_3	Pco_2	HCO_3	Pco_2
Metabolic acidosis	↓	↓			↓
Metabolic alkalosis	↑	↑			↑
Respiratory acidosis	↓		↑	↑	
Respiratory alkalosis	↑		↓	↓	

From Wait RB, Kahng Ku, Dresner LS. Fluids and electrolytes and acid base balance. In: Greenfield LJ, Mulholland MW, Oldham KT, et al., eds. *Surgery: scientific principles and practice,* 2nd ed. New York: Lippincott-Raven Publishers, 1997: 261.

Acidosis

Metabolic acidosis most often occurs when endogenous acid production exceeds bicarbonate content and production. In cardiac surgery patients, this is most often the result of low cardiac output and tissue hypoperfusion with lactate release from tissues secondary to anaerobic metabolism. Impaired renal perfusion, low filling pressures, high doses of administered catecholamines, and the presence of hyperglycemia may also contribute to the accumulation of acid. Pre-existing renal dysfunction and/or treatment with the oral hypoglycemic drug metformin may predispose the patient to postoperative metabolic acidosis. Severe postoperative metabolic acidosis may be the result of unsuspected gut ischemia or infarction or an ischemic limb.

Hyperventilation, the respiratory response to the decreased pH, cannot be relied on as compensation for metabolic acidosis as full compensation requires 12 to 24 hours. More importantly, respiratory compensation for metabolic acidosis does not correct the underlying cause of the acidosis. Metabolic acidosis results in reduced myocardial contractility, increased PVR, peripheral arteriolar dilatation, central venous constriction, and reduced responsiveness to administered adrenergic agents such as epinephrine. Other, less common causes of metabolic acidosis in cardiac surgery patients include uremic acidosis due to acute or chronic renal failure and ketoacidosis secondary to insulin deficiency.

The important principle regarding the treatment of metabolic acidosis is to correct the underlying cause. For patients with lactic acidosis due to tissue hypoxia, this requires optimization of cardiac output (both myocardial function and volume status) and oxygenation. If gut ischemia is suspected, abdominal computed tomography scan or colonoscopy may be indicated. Efforts to correct the pH by the administration of alkali without correction of the underlying cause of the acidosis are generally not successful. When used to treat acidemia, the alkali of choice is IV sodium bicarbonate. Bicarbonate administration is generally not, however, indicated unless the pH is below 7.2 and rapid bolus infusion should be avoided, especially in infants. Using the base deficit determined from the arterial blood gas result, the amount of sodium bicarbonate to administer may be estimated by this formula:

$$NaHCO_3 \text{ (mEq)} = 0.3 \times \text{body weight (kg)} \times \text{base deficit (mEq/L)}$$

To avoid overcorrection, the initial dose should be *one half* of this calculated dose. For example, a 70-kg patient with a base deficit of -5 would be calculated to receive 105 mEq of sodium bicarbonate; since each ampoule contains 44.6 mEq, we would begin by giving the patient a single ampoule and then recheck the arterial blood gases in 20 minutes.

It is important to be aware of the patient's current serum potassium level before administering bicarbonate. If the patient is significantly hypokalemic (below 3.5 mEq/L), the rapid administration of bicarbonate can further reduce the serum potassium level, potentially resulting in serious arrhythmias. Potassium administration prior to treating the patient with sodium bicarbonate is indicated in this situation.

Overcorrection of metabolic acidosis by excessive administration of bicarbonate should be avoided, as the resultant "overshoot" alkalosis may be detrimental to cardiac function, predispose to arrhythmias, result in increased CO_2 production, and impair oxygen delivery to the tissues by increasing hemoglobin's affinity for oxygen. Rapid correction of extracellular acidosis may actually cause worsening of intracellular acidosis (84). Because of the potential detrimental effects of administered bicarbonate, any respiratory component to the acidosis should be corrected first to lessen the need for bicarbonate. Furthermore, sodium bicarbonate administration can lead to hypernatremia and volume overload, especially in infants. *Tromethamine* (THAM) can be substituted for sodium bicarbonate, especially when the serum sodium level is above 155 mEq/L. It is an effective buffer and is sodium free but may have serious side effects (85). We rarely use it.

Respiratory acidosis is due to carbon dioxide accumulation as the result of inadequate ventilation. Acutely, a small compensatory increase in the plasma bicarbonate will occur but this does not become significant unless the hypercapnia is sustained for days. Hypercarbia is associated with increased in PVR, which may result in impairment of right ventricular function (86,87). As the P_{CO_2} rises, a decrease in the P_{O_2} level may occur with hypoxia resulting that may become the principal threat to life in this situation. Respiratory acidosis in the early postoperative patient who is on a mechanical ventilator is usually simple to correct: increasing the minute ventilation by increasing the ventilator rate or delivered volume will lead toward normalization of the Pco_2 and arterial pH. A portable chest x-ray will help rule out mechanical causes of compromised ventilation such as pneumothorax or large pleural effusion, which can be easily corrected. If conservative measures fail to provide adequate ventilation and carbon dioxide excretion, intubation and mechanical ventilation are required and should not be delayed.

Mixed metabolic and respiratory acidosis may occur in postoperative patients, especially in the setting of low cardiac output and/or renal insufficiency (metabolic causes) and chronic obstructive pulmonary disease and/or pulmonary edema (respiratory causes). Severe acidemia necessitating immediate therapy may result.

Alkalosis

Alkalosis (blood pH >7.60) results in arteriolar constriction with the potential for reduced myocardial and cerebral perfusion, hypocalcemia, neurologic abnormalities, cardiac arrhythmias, depressed respiration with hypercapnia and hypoxemia, and difficulty weaning from mechanical ventilatory support (88).

A mild degree of *metabolic alkalosis* may develop during the first few days after uncomplicated cardiac surgery, usually the result of diuretic therapy without sufficient potassium and chloride replacement. The alkalosis is characterized by an elevated arterial bicarbonate concentration and can be induced by hypokalemia, excessive losses of gastric juice with chloride depletion, or hypovolemia (since renal retention of sodium prevails over correction of alkalosis). Some degree of respiratory compensation for metabolic alkalosis can occur in the patient who is not being ventilated mechanically. Severe hypoventilation will not usually develop because this response is limited by the hypoxic respiratory drive. The tendency to retain CO_2 to compensate for significant metabolic alkalosis may hamper efforts to wean the patient with respiratory compromise from mechanical ventilation.

Hypokalemia-induced alkalosis will be reversed by the administration of potassium chloride with the goal of raising the serum potassium level above 4.5 mEq/dL. A mildly low serum potassium level (e.g., 3.5 mEq/dL) indicates a severe total body depletion of potassium, and significant amounts of potassium chloride may be needed to restore the total body reserves. In fact, patients on chronic diuretics or who are chronically overventilated may have a profound intracellular potassium deficit with a low-normal serum potassium level and significant metabolic alkalosis.

For metabolic acidosis that is not associated with significant hypokalemia, the administration of dilute hydrochloric acid (0.15 N HCl at 0.2 mEq/kg per hour IV for 12 hours via a central line) may be effective.

During the early period after cardiac surgery, *respiratory alkalosis* is most often secondary to ventilator-induced hyperventilation. Typically, the arterial blood gases will exhibit a low Pco_2 and a decreased bicarbonate concentration. For the patient still on mechanical ventilation, this is easily corrected by decreasing the patient's minute ventilation.

USE OF BLOOD PRODUCTS IN THE PERIOPERATIVE PERIOD

Cardiac surgery results in bleeding. Preoperative treatment with platelet inhibiting and antithrombotic drugs, tissue injury, multiple suture lines, the use of CPB, heparin administration, and the dilution of platelets and serum clotting factors all contribute to significant operative blood loss, postoperative bleeding, and postoperative anemia. Therefore, an important part of the management of the patient undergoing cardiac surgery involves the rational use of blood products.

The Risks of Blood Transfusion

Although blood is safer than it ever has been, risks associated with blood product transfusion still exist and are a major concern of patients undergoing cardiac surgery (Table 3.6). Risks associated with blood product transfusion include the transmission of viruses, bacterial infection (more common in platelet transfusions), acute hemolytic reaction, delayed hemolytic reaction, and transfusion related lung injury (89,90). In addition to these direct risks, RBC transfusions are associated with an increased incidence of postoperative bacterial infections such as wound infection and pneumonia (91–93). This may be due to a nonspecific immunosuppressive effect, perhaps related to transfused leukocytes that are present in the standard RBC preparation. The use of leukocyte-reduced RBCs has become standard at some, but not all, hospitals (94). Other risks of blood product transfusion to patients undergoing cardiac surgery include increased short- and long-term mortality, renal failure, longer ventilator time, atrial fibrillation, and increased length of stays in the ICU and hospital (89,95–98). The transfusion of blood products to cardiac surgery patients is clearly disadvantageous and should be avoided as is safely possible.

It is standard practice for the treating physician to discuss the indications for, and potential complications of, blood product transfusion with all cardiac surgery patients. Written permission for transfusions is obtained, usually at the time of obtaining consent for the operation.

Indications for Transfusion

Recognizing the risks, costs, and supply limitations associated with blood product transfusion, cardiac surgery programs, hospitals, and

TABLE 3.6	Risks of Blood Transfusion
Type	**Occurrence in Red Blood Cell Units Transfused**
Infections	
Human immunodeficiency virus	1 in 1.4–2.4 × 10⁶
Hepatitis B	1 in 58,000–149,000
Hepatitis C	1 in 872,000–1.7 × 10⁶
Bacterial infection	1 in 2,000
Immunologic Reactions	
Febrile nonhemolytic transfusion reactions	1 in 100
Anaphylactic transfusion reactions ABO mismatch	1 in 20,000–50,000
Hemolysis	1 in 60,000
Death	1 in 600,000
Leukocyte-related target organ injury	1 in 20 to 1 in 50
Transfusion-related acute lung injury	1 in 2000
Posttransfusion purpura	Rare
Transfusion Services Error	
Donor screening error (malaria, Trypanosoma cruzi babesioses, Creutzfeld-Jakob disease)	1 in 4 × 10⁶
Transfusion services error	1 in 14,000

From Ferraris VA, et al. Perioperative blood transfusion and conservation in cardiac surgery: STS and SCA practice guideline. *Ann Thorac Surg* 2007;83:S30, with permission.

professional society task forces have developed guidelines for the transfusion of blood products (89,99). Adherence to these guidelines is overseen by a hospital Blood Transfusion Committee, and unnecessary transfusions are reviewed with the ordering clinician. Transfusion guidelines are, however, not absolute. Deviations from the guidelines are necessary to take into account individual patient characteristics (including age and coexisting diseases) but written justification in the patient's medical record for "out of protocol" transfusions is recommended. The goal of these measures is to reduce unnecessary blood product transfusions thereby decreasing the incidence of transmission of blood-borne infections, reducing the impact of transfusion-related immunosuppression, and helping to maintain the supply of blood products. Table 3.7 lists suggested transfusion guidelines.

Thrombocytopenia is very common following cardiac surgery. Nearly all patients will experience a 30% to 60% reduction in their

TABLE 3.7 Blood Product Transfusion Guidelines in Postoperative Cardiac Surgery Patients

Red Blood Cells

If hemoglobin level is <7.0 g/dL:
Most patients will require transfusion, although young healthy patients may tolerate

If hemoglobin level is 7–8 g/dL:
Most stable patients will tolerate without difficulty, but consider transfusion if:
- Ongoing bleeding is present
- Cardiovascular instability is present
- Patient is symptomatic (syncope, dyspnea, angina)
- Cardiovascular instability is present
- Age > 70 yr

If hemoglobin level is ≥9 g/dL:
Most patients will *not* require transfusion; should be performed only if clear-cut symptoms are present or if patient is bleeding severely. At most hospitals, transfusions for hemoglobin > 9 g/dL are reviewed for appropriateness.

In general, for an adult, 1 U of packed red blood cells will raise the hemoglobin by 3 g/dL.

Platelets

If platelet count is <50,000/mm³:
Consider transfusion, even if not bleeding, if patient is within 24 h of surgery

If platelet count is ≥50,000/mm³:
If bleeding, transfusion indicated, especially if patient recently received platelet inhibitor
If *not* bleeding, transfusion not usually indicated

If platelet count is >100,000/mm³:
If bleeding and platelet dysfunction are suspected due to recent cardiopulmonary bypass or platelet inhibitor drugs, transfusion may be indicated

Note: If heparin-induced thrombocytopenia is suspected, platelet transfusion is not indicated (see text). In general, for an adult, 1 platelet apheresis unit will increase the platelet count by 30,000–40,000/mm³.

Fresh Frozen Plasma

If prothrombin time is ≥16 sec (or INR ≥ 1.5):
If patient bleeding, transfusion indicated
If patient *not* bleeding, transfusion not usually indicated

If prothrombin time is <16 sec (or INR < 1.5):
Transfusion *not* indicated

Cryoprecipitate

If fibrinogen level is <100 mg/dL:
If patient bleeding, transfusion indicated
If patient *not* bleeding, transfusion not indicated

If fibrinogen level is >100 mg/dL:
Transfusion *not* indicated

In general, for an adult, 6 U of cryoprecipitate will increase the fibrinogen level 100–150 mg/dL.

INR, international normalized ratio.
Note: These are only guidelines; transfusion protocols vary among hospitals. Specific patient circumstances may require deviations. Written documentation in the patient's medical record regarding out-of-protocol transfusions is usually required.

platelet count on the first postoperative day, largely due to hemodilution and consumption during CPB. If the patient is not bleeding, there is no need to transfuse platelets. If the platelet count is $<100,000/mm^3$, it should be repeated within 24 hours. If the platelet count is severely depressed, or if it continues to fall, or if it rises and then falls, the possible presence of *heparin-induced thrombocytopenia* (HIT) should be entertained. This serious immune-mediated prothrombotic condition results in thrombocytopenia, the potential for venous and/or arterial thrombosis and thromboembolism, renal failure, and death (100). Administration of heparin in this setting may precipitate life-threatening clot formation. The diagnosis of HIT may be difficult to make and is based on the presence of thrombocytopenia (usually a $>50\%$ reduction from baseline), blood assay tests, and the presence of thrombosis, either arterial or venous. The two assays used to aid in the diagnosis of HIT are the serotonin release assay (which is relatively specific but not particularly sensitive) and the enzyme-linked immunosorbent assay (ELISA) (which is more sensitive but less specific). A negative ELISA makes the diagnosis of HIT unlikely (101). If the presence of HIT is suspected, all heparin should be discontinued (including that used to flush catheters). If strongly suspected or proven by assay testing and/or clinical picture, anticoagulation with a nonheparin agent (such as argatroban, lepirudin, or bivalirudin) should be instituted. Platelet transfusion, despite rather severe thrombocytopenia, is not routinely indicated because bleeding is not usually a problem with HIT. Consultation with a hematologist is highly recommended (102,103). The possibility of HIT should always be entertained in the patient with new onset thrombocytopenia and/or unexpected thrombotic complications.

Reducing Postoperative Bleeding and Transfusions

Predicting the Need for Blood Product Transfusions

Recognition of patient and procedure characteristics that are associated with excessive postoperative bleeding allows for efforts to proactively reduce bleeding and the need for transfusion. Many studies have analyzed the preoperative patient factors associated with perioperative transfusion in cardiac surgery (89). Table 3.8 lists the more significant and common factors. Predictive formulas have been developed to assist in the preoperative identification of patients likely to require transfusions (104–106).

Preoperative Measures to Reduce Bleeding and Transfusions

Preoperative methods reported to reduce bleeding and transfusions in cardiac surgery patients include preoperative discontinuation of

| TABLE 3.8 | Risk Factors Associated with Bleeding and Transfusion |

Patient-related Variables
Age > 70 yr
Preoperative anemia
Female gender
Small body surface area
Preoperative antithrombotic therapy
  High intensity (abciximab, clopidogrel, direct thrombin inhibitors, low-molecular-weight heparin, long-acting direct thrombin inhibitors, thrombolytic therapy)
  Low intensity (aspirin, dipyridamole, eptifibatide, tirofiban)
Preoperative coagulopathy
  Hereditary coagulopathy or platelet defect (von Willebrand's disease, Hermansky–Pudlak, hemophilia A or B, clotting factor deficiencies, etc.)
  Acquired coagulopathy or platelet defect (abnormal platelet function test, chronic lymphocytic leukemia, cirrhosis, lupus anticoagulant, drug-related polycythemia vera, etc.)
Cardiogenic shock
Renal insufficiency
Insulin-dependent adult-onset diabetes mellitus
Peripheral vascular disease
Preoperative sepsis
Liver failure or hypoalbuminemia

Procedure-related Variables
Prolonged CPB time
Reoperation
Complexity of operation
Increased protamine dose after CPB
Increased cell-saving volume
Need for transfusion while on CPB

Process-related Variables
Lack of transfusion algorithm with point-of-care testing
Use of internal mammary artery
Reduced heparin dose for CPB
Low body temperature in intensive care unit

CPB, cardiopulmonary bypass.
From Ferraris VA, et al. Perioperative blood transfusion and conservation in cardiac surgery: STS and SCA practice guideline. *Ann Thorac Surg* 2007;83:S32, with permission.

antithrombotic drugs, preoperative autologous blood donation, and preoperative erythropoietin administration.

A major contributor to the need for perioperative blood product transfusion is preoperative antithrombotic drug treatment. While aspirin does contribute to increased transfusion requirements to some degree, this effect is generally not severe and preoperative aspirin treatment is generally associated with improved postoperative outcomes in coronary artery bypass graft (CABG) surgery patients (107). Therefore, we do not usually discontinue aspirin prior to CABG, especially for patients with acute coronary syndromes. Preoperative clopidogrel treatment is, however, associated with serious increases in bleeding, transfusions, the incidence of reoperation for bleeding, and other complications. Therefore, if possible, clopidogrel should be discontinued for at least 4 to 6 days prior to surgery (108–111).

Preoperative donation of packed RBCs may be useful for the individual patient to reduce the need for transfusion of donated RBCs, but this technique has limited applicability as it can only be applied to very elective patients (112–114). In most practices predonation is used infrequently, in part due to the large number of unplanned urgent and emergency operations. With this method the patient donates a unit of blood, waits 1 to 2 weeks and donates a second unit and then waits about 1 to 2 weeks before undergoing surgery. The predonated RBC units are transfused to the patient during or after surgery using usual criteria. Contraindications to predonation include anemia, unstable angina, severe aortic valve stenosis, bacteremia, uncontrolled heart failure, severe cyanosis, and pregnancy. While appealing, this technique of autologous predonation is not without risk to the patient, is not cost-effective, and considerable numbers of units of predonated RBCs are wasted (115,116). Widespread utilization has not been adopted. We no longer use this method of blood conservation except for rare special circumstances.

Recombinant erythropoietin is an effective stimulator of RBC production. Preoperative administration has been reported to be useful for patients undergoing heart surgery, particularly when used in conjunction with autologous RBC predonation (117,118). The use of erythropoietin in this setting is "off label" and safety of this blood conservation technique, particularly for patients with coronary artery disease, is not well demonstrated (119,120). Therefore, preoperative erythropoietin is not recommended, except for special circumstances in which the benefit of preoperative red cell augmentation will likely outweigh the uncertain degree of risk (such as the patient who refuses blood transfusion for religious reasons and suffers preoperative anemia).

Intraoperative Measures to Reduce Bleeding and Transfusions

For suitable CABG surgery patients, performance of the operation without the use of CPB ("off pump") is associated with reduced bleeding and transfusions (121,122). This is likely due to a reduction in postoperative platelet dysfunction and depletion with a reduction in the activation of various inflammatory mediators that is caused by the use of extracorporeal circulation. The decision regarding the use of CPB for coronary surgery is based on patient characteristics and coronary anatomy.

CPB provides whole body perfusion to replace the heart and lung functions during cardiac surgery. This extracorporeal circuit is composed of nonendothelialized tubing and oxygenator surfaces that are associated with blood activation in terms of coagulation, complement, fibrinolysis, kallikrein, leukocytes, and platelets (123). Efforts to reduce these adverse effects of CPB have included the application of bio/blood-compatible surface materials, principally through the development of heparin coating for the synthetic surfaces of the CPB circuit (124). The use of *biocompatible surfaces* for the extracorporeal circuit is associated with improved outcomes, including reduced bleeding and transfusions, and has become commonplace (125). Some surgeons have recommended the administration of reduced heparin doses in conjunction with the heparin-bonded tubing, but this reduced anticoagulation protocol has raised safety concerns and is not used by our institutions (126,127). In fact, the use of more heparin, rather than less, during CPB is likely associated with reduced consumption of coagulation factors and platelets with improved postoperative coagulation and reduced need for postoperative blood product transfusion (89).

Reducing the volume of prime solution present in the CPB circuit helps to reduce the degree of hemodilution that occurs. This may be accomplished by removing excess tubing (and the contained prime solution) at the time of cannulation. Despite this, most infants will require the addition of blood to the prime solution to prevent excessive hemodilution and profound anemia on bypass. In adults or large children the technique of *retrograde autologous priming* may be employed in which, after cannulation, the perfusionist backs blood out of the patient into the prime circuit to displace the crystalloid prime solution, thereby reducing the degree of hemodilution. In adults, typically 500 to 750 mL of prime fluid volume may be displaced by the patient's own blood. During this procedure, close cooperation with the anesthesiologist is required. The patient's blood pressure is closely observed and small bolus doses of phenylephrine may be needed to maintain the systemic arterial pressure at an acceptable level. Retrograde autologous priming is simple to do and, when performed carefully, safe. (128,129).

Intraoperative autologous donation, also known as *acute normovolemic hemodilution* involves the withdrawal of blood from the patient, storing it during the period of CPB and then returning it to the patient after protamine administration (87). Following the induction of anesthesia and placement of monitoring cannulas, the blood (5 to 10 mL/kg patient weight) may be withdrawn by the anesthesiologist via a central line and stored in anticoagulant-containing blood bags. The blood is maintained in a sterile state at room temperature. The patient's volume loss is corrected by the infusion of the appropriate amount of normal saline. After the patient is weaned from CPB and protamine is administered, the blood is reinfused. This method of intraoperative hemodilution generally results in a reduction in transfusions and theoretically preserves RBCs, platelets, and clotting factors. It cannot, however, be used in unstable or anemic patients. Extreme hemodilution (hematocrit below 18% to 20%) during CPB has been identified as a contributor to poor outcomes, including increased rates of stroke and renal failure (130,131). The practicality of removing blood from the patient just prior to CPB may therefore be limited. The reported results of this technique have been mixed (132).

During surgery, it is customary to use a *cell salvage* device that provides for suctioning of blood shed from the pericardium and thoracic cavities, washing and filtering of the blood, and then reinfusion of the washed RBCs. Clotting factors and platelets are lost by this technique but RBCs are retained. In addition, after weaning from bypass and removal of the arterial and venous cannulas from the patient, the blood remaining in the pump tubing and oxygenator is processed through the cell saver for reinfusion into the patient. The use of such cell salvage techniques is standard at most hospitals.

Drugs to Reduce Bleeding and Transfusions

During surgery, one of a number of drugs may be administered for the purpose of reducing postoperative bleeding and the need for transfusions.

Aprotinin is a naturally occurring inhibitor of the serine protease enzymes (including plasmin) that, in the past, was widely used prophylactically to reduce bleeding and transfusions in cardiac surgery. It was approved for use in CABG patients in the United States in 1993 but was withdrawn from the market in 2007 due to safety concerns (133).

Aminocaproic acid and *tranexamic acid* are lysine analogs which specifically block the lysine binding site on plasminogen thereby preventing plasminogen from converting fibrin to fibrin degradation products, thus inhibiting the process of fibrinolysis. Each is administered prophylactically during cardiac procedures using CPB. Randomized controlled trials investigating aminocaproic acid and tranexamic acid are limited in number. Aminocaproic acid is not available for use in Europe. Both drugs have been reported to reduce bleeding and transfusions in patients undergoing cardiac surgery using CPB although tranexamic acid is generally felt to be more effective (134–139). A reduction in the incidence of reoperation for postoperative bleeding has not, however, been demonstrated (89). In the United States, aminocaproic acid is commonly used during adult cardiac surgery, and studies indicate reductions in chest tube drainage although reductions in transfusions have not been consistently demonstrated. Likewise, tranexamic acid has been shown to be clinically superior to placebo in terms of reduction of blood loss, although the data regarding proportions of patients requiring transfusions are not as consistent (109,140). Neither drug should be used when there is a possibility of ongoing disseminated intravascular coagulation.

A variety of dosage regimens for aminocaproic acid and tranexamic acid have been reported with no standard protocol currently being universally preferred. Generally, for aminocaproic acid, a loading dose of 5 to 10 g is administered before CPB with further similar doses being added to the pump prime solution and given after protamine administration. In addition, a constant infusion, at 2 g per hour may be employed. Tranexamic may be administered as a loading dose of 30 mg/kg with 2 mg/kg being added to the pump prime solution and 16 mg/kg per hour infusion during CPB (133). A lower dose is used in patients with impaired renal function.

The role of antifibrinolytic therapy in surgery for congenital heart disease is undefined, as are the recommended doses of the available drugs, although efficacy of antifibrinolytic therapy is apparent (141).

Desmopressin (DDAVP; an arginine vasopressin analog) likely increases plasma levels of von Willebrand's factor and appears to be useful in reducing postoperative bleeding in patients with identified platelet dysfunction after surgery, such as von Willebrand's disease (142,143). However, routine use is not recommended (89).

Postoperative Reinfusion of Shed Mediastinal Blood

Following surgery, blood, which has been shed via the mediastinal tubes into a sterile receptacle, may be filtered and reinfused to the patient. This method of postoperative autotransfusion has produced conflicting results, with some studies showing reductions in the need for homologous transfusions but other reporting either no effect or even adverse consequences of the technique. The potential for reinfusion of lipid particles, thromboemboli, inflammatory cytokines, and other adverse components has raised concern regarding the safety of this practice. Thus, direct reinfusion of filtered shed mediastinal blood from postoperative chest tube drainage back to the patient is not recommended and we do not use this technique (89).

PAIN CONTROL

Besides the discomfort, postoperative pain can cause the patient to experience tachycardia, hypertension, splinting with resultant small tidal volumes, and ineffective cough. During the early postoperative period, patients are commonly treated with IV morphine. Adults are given 2 to

10 mg by slow IV bolus at 1 mg per minute; the infant bolus dose is 0.1 to 0.5 mg/kg at a rate of 0.1 mg per minute. Redosing every hour may be required in some patients. The main hemodynamic effect of morphine is vasodilation, thereby reducing ventricular preload and afterload with favorable effects on myocardial oxygen consumption. If the patient is hypovolemic, however, hypotension may result. Thus, morphine is given slowly with careful monitoring of the patient's arterial blood pressure and filling pressures. Small, frequent IV doses are preferable to larger, less frequent intramuscular injections during the early postoperative period because of the variability in absorption when the intramuscular route is used. For infants and children, a continuous morphine infusion may be given (0.05 to 0.1 mg/kg per hour). Patients who are allergic to morphine receive oxymorphone or hydromorphone intravenously.

In general, nonsteroidal anti-inflammatory agents, other than aspirin, are avoided in patients for postoperative pain relief in patients who have undergone CABG (144). Concern has been raised regarding this class of drugs (the cyclo-oxygenase inhibitors) due to an increased incidence of cardiovascular events associated with their use (145,146). Specifically, oral *ketorolac* is contraindicated in these patients (147). Furthermore, ketorolac is contraindicated in patients receiving aspirin, may have adverse renal and gastrointestinal effects, and may promote bleeding in the postoperative period (148).

Continuous infusion of the short-acting agent *propofol* provides the advantages of effect titration and quick reversal when the drug is discontinued. The typical propofol dose for deep sedation is 25 to 100 μg/kg per minute. Since propofol induces a state of general anesthesia, controlled ventilation of the patient is required. Propofol often causes some degree of hypotension that, at times, may become significant. If this occurs, the drug should be discontinued rather than adding a vasopressor agent to counteract the reduced blood pressure. Prolonged administration of propofol is not recommended. The drug is associated with the so-called "propofol infusion syndrome" that is characterized by lactic metabolic acidosis, cardiovascular instability, and rhabomyonecrosis (149,150). While this syndrome is rare, awareness of this possibility is important. Another agent used to provide postoperative sedation is *dexmedetomidine*, an α2 agonist (151,152). Its use may be associated with a reduced incidence of postoperative delirium.

For sedation, *midazolam* is used in small IV doses (0.01 to 0.05 mg/kg) or as a continuous infusion (0.02 to 0.1 mg/kg per hour for adults) (153). When administered to intubated neonatal patients, midazolam is may be initiated at a rate of 30 μg/kg per hour without a loading dose. In general, midazolam should be administered at the lowest possible dose that provides the desired level of sedation. Being short acting, the effect of midazolam quickly wears off when the drug is discontinued and it may be used in conjunction with the infusion of the short-acting narcotic *fentanyl*. We find this combination to be useful to provide short-acting sedation and analgesia for the intubated postoperative patient. For the less agitated patient who requires a less sedating and longer-acting anxiolytic agent, *lorazepam* is useful.

Continuous subcutaneous infusion of local anesthesia to the sternotomy wound has been shown to effectively reduce pain and the need for opioid analgesic use (154). The subcutaneous catheters (6 or 10 in) are placed parallel to the incision in surgery following closure of the skin. The small catheters are attached to a continuous infusion pump that delivers local anesthetic (e.g., bupivacaine) to the wound. After 48 hours, the catheters are easily removed.

Rarely a patient, usually with severe respiratory and/or cardiac failure, will require total immobilization with a muscle relaxant. This is usually in the setting of severe hemodynamic instability, often with an intra-aortic balloon pump in place, in a patient for whom satisfactory mechanical ventilation is difficult due to high peak airway pressures. For this purpose, vecuronium (0.08 to 1.0 mg/kg IV) is used. Since the muscle relaxing agents do not provide analgesia or amnesia, concomitant administration of other agents (such as morphine) is required.

After extubation, care must be used to avoid excess narcotic administration, which may result in respiratory depression. Conversely, insufficient pain relief will result in failure of the patient to cough and clear secretions. For adults, we generally administer hydromorphone or hydrocodone orally, or for more severe pain, oxycodone. If the patient's pain is not relieved with oral agents, small doses of IV morphine (1 to 3 mg every 2 to 3 hours as needed) may be administered with careful attention to the patient's mentation and respiratory status. In younger patients, especially males who, on occasion, have difficult-to-control postoperative pain, we have used fentanyl skin patches that deliver 12 µg per hour. As oral intake is resumed, most patients find relief with combination hydrocodone with acetaminophen or codeine with acetaminophen preparations taken orally. Another less potent, but often effective, agent is propoxyphene with acetaminophen. This drug seems to be particularly useful for older, frail patients who do not tolerate the stronger agents and suffer nausea from codeine. Commonly used analgesic agents are listed in Table 3.9.

Haloperidol is an antipsychotic agent that is of value in the treatment of adult cardiac surgery patients suffering severe acute delirium (such as may occur with alcohol withdrawal and other medical conditions). In this setting, rapid treatment of the agitated delirious patient may be required to prevent injury to the patient and to others. Haloperidol may be given orally but the IV route (1.0 to 5.0 mg IV every 2 to

| | | | TABLE | | |

TABLE 3.9 Commonly Used Pain Medications

Drug	Representative Brand Name	Pain Level Indicated For	Adult Oral Dose	Parenteral Adult Dose	Pediatric Dose
Acetaminophen	Tylenol	Mild–moderate	325–650 mg q 4–6 h; max dose 4 g/day	NA	NA
Propoxyphene	Darvocet N-100 (100 mg with acetaminophen 650 mg)	Mild–moderate	1–2 tabs q 4–6 h	NA	NA
Codeine (30 mg) and acetaminophen (300 mg)	Tylenol no. 3	Mild–moderate	1–2 tabs q 4–6 h	NA	NA
Hydrocodone (5 mg) with acetaminophen (500 mg)	Vicodin	Moderate	1–2 tabs q 4–6 h	NA	NA
Hydromorphone	Dilaudid	Moderate	2–4 mg q 4–6 h p.r.n.	1–4 mg IM/IV/SC q 4–6 h	NA
Meperidine	Demerol	Moderate–severe	150–300 mg q 3–4 h	50–150 mg IM/IV q 3–4 h	1.0–1.75 mg/kg PO/IM/IV
Oxycodone	Roxicodone	Moderate–severe	5–15 mg q 4–6 h	NA	NA
Morphine sulfate	—	Severe	30–60 mg q 4–6 h	1–10 mg IV q 1–2 h p.r.n.	0.1–0.2 mg/kg IV/IM q 2–4 h
Oxymorphone	Numorphan	Severe	NA	0.5–1.5 mg q 1–3 h p.r.n.	NA
Fentanyl	Sublimaze	Severe	NA	12.5–50 μg q 1–2 h p.r.n. or 0.5 to 1.5-μg/kg/h infusion	0.5–2.0 μg/kg q 1–4 h p.r.n. or 0.5 to 1.0-μg/kg/h infusion

IM, intramuscular; IV, intravenous; PO, oral; p.r.n., as needed; SC, subcutaneous.

4 hours) is preferred for a quick result. Frequently, in this setting, consultation with a neurologist or gerontologist will aid in the management of the patient. Care should be taken in the administration of haloperidol; extrapyramidal reactions, QT interval prolongation, and torsades de pointes (a form of ventricular tachycardia) may occur during treatment.

In the evaluation of the agitated patient it must be remembered that the *patient who becomes restless or apprehensive may actually be hypoxic, acidotic, or in a low cardiac output state.* If this is the case, the administration of analgesics or sedatives will be hazardous. Evaluation of a possible metabolic abnormality by blood gas and electrolyte determination should be performed.

DIURETIC THERAPY

Patients who require cardiac surgery often suffer preoperative congestive heart failure and/or hypertension and are being treated with diuretic drugs prior to surgery. After surgery, most patients have acquired total body excesses of sodium and water and therefore diuretics are frequently prescribed on a temporary basis. The mechanism of action of the commonly used diuretic agents is to inhibit sodium reabsorption in the kidney tubules, resulting in increased sodium excretion. The major groups of diuretic drugs used clinically are (i) loop diuretics (furosemide, ethacrynic acid, or bumetanide), (ii) thiazide diuretics (hydrochlorothiazide, chlorthalidone, or metolazone), (iii) potassium-sparing diuretics (spironolactone, triamterene, or amiloride), and (iv) combination products (hydrochlorothiazide plus spironolactone, triamterene, or amiloride).

On the first morning after uncomplicated heart surgery, when cardiac function has returned toward the preoperative level and the patient is fully rewarmed, a dose of furosemide, 10 to 40 mg IV for adults, 0.5 to 1.0 mg/kg IV for infants) is often given to promote diuresis. Patients with cardiac failure, high filling pressures, and pulmonary edema are treated with higher doses of IV furosemide with careful monitoring of the ventricular filling pressures and serum potassium levels. Patients on preoperative diuretic therapy may require higher doses after surgery, particularly if they were receiving high doses for a long period of time. After extubation, when the patient is able to take medications orally, it is common practice to administer either furosemide or a combination diuretic (such as triamterene 50 mg plus hydrochlorothiazide 25 mg) for several days. The combination diuretic helps prevent hypokalemia, although the patient's potassium level should still be checked regularly. Concurrent administration of a daily dose of potassium with a combination diuretic containing a potassium-sparing agent is contraindicated because of the possibility of dangerous hyperkalemia. The patient is weighed daily; when the preoperative weight is approached, the diuretic is discontinued. Important diuretic drug interactions include potassium sparing diuretics plus ACE inhibitors such as captopril (may cause dangerous hyperkalemia), spironolactone plus digoxin (raises digoxin levels), and furosemide plus ketorolac (may cause hyperkalemia or renal insufficiency) (65).

DIABETES MANAGEMENT

Patients with diabetes mellitus have an increased incidence of cardiovascular disease; approximately 30% to 40% of adult patients undergoing heart surgery are diabetic. Patients with diabetes (insulin-dependent, on oral agents, or diet-controlled), as well as patients not previously recognized as being glucose intolerant, may become very hyperglycemic during the early postoperative period, in part due to the stress of surgical trauma and the use of catecholamine support medications. Cardiac surgery patients who experience elevated perioperative serum glucose levels have increased incidences of perioperative wound infections, stroke and death, and reduced 10-year survival (155–157). It appears that it is the perioperative hyperglycemia, with resultant adverse effects on myocardial metabolism and the proinflammatory effects of glucose and free fatty acids, that contributes to the observed morbidity and mortality in these patients, not the diagnosis of diabetes mellitus as such (158). Thus, close monitoring of glucose levels and the use of insulin to prevent hyperglycemia is associated with significantly improved outcomes, including survival, in patients undergoing cardiac surgery (159,160). Identification of patients who are glucose-intolerant ("prediabetic") or clearly diabetic and determining their level of glucose control prior to surgery is of value and is accomplished by measuring the patient's glycosylated hemoglobin ($HgbA_{1c}$) level. This topic is also discussed in Chapter 1. It should be noted that the $HbgA_{1c}$ level is inaccurate in patients who have recently received RBC transfusion.

The degree to which glycemic control should be achieved in the critically ill and perioperative patient has become a matter of some debate with contradictory reports appearing in the literature. While the adverse effects of poorly controlled perioperative serum glucose levels (above 180 mg/dL) appear to be clear, the advantages and safety of very tight control (80 to 110 mg/dL) are not as evident (161). Concern has been raised regarding adverse effects of the hypoglycemic events, including increased mortality that may accompany efforts to tightly control patients' serum glucose levels in critically ill patients (162). The Society of Thoracic Surgeons has recently published guidelines regarding blood glucose management in patients undergoing cardiac surgery (163).

Patients with diabetes are advised to discontinue oral antiglycemic drugs 24 hours before surgery. Insulin-dependent patients are instructed to not take their nutritional (regular, lispro, aspart, or glulisine) insulin following dinner the night before surgery. The basal (glargine, detemir, or NPH) insulin is continued, but at a reduced (usually one-half to two-thirds) dose. If the patient is hyperglycemic during the hours preoperatively, IV insulin therapy is begun to maintain the glucose level below 180 mg/dL.

Many different strategies for controlling the serum glucose level, both during surgery and after, have been developed. Frequent (every 30 minutes) monitoring of the patient's glucose level is begun in the operating room. In our practices, IV insulin administration is begun during surgery if the patient's glucose level exceeds 150 mg/dL. For these patients, this may be accomplished with small bolus doses of insulin, although persistent elevations may require beginning a continuous infusion. Patients with known diabetes are treated more aggressively and most often do require the continuous insulin infusion with the goal being to keep the glucose level below 150 mg/dL. When administering insulin during surgery, frequent determinations of the patient's glucose level should be made as the insulin requirement may change quickly. For example, while hypothermic on CPB, the patient may require a higher rate of insulin administration to achieve the desired goal. If this higher rate is continued as the patient is rewarmed, hypoglycemia can result.

Most hospitals have developed hyperglycemia protocols with standardized preprinted orders to facilitate insulin administration to critically ill and postoperative patients, which are useful for the patient following cardiac surgery. Generally, a concomitant infusion of a glucose-containing fluid is administered, although some protocols do not include this. The Portland Protocol is a popular, validated and updated protocol that is available on the Internet at www.portlandprotocol.org (164). A glucose target level range is selected and continuous IV insulin is infused per the protocol with serum glucose level determinations being made at 30- to 60-minute intervals. Some institutions will treat to keep the glucose level below 180 mg/dL although many aim for lower levels. At our hospitals the goal is to generally maintain the patient's glucose level below 150 mg/dL. Adjustments are made to the insulin infusion rate by the nurses as per the protocol.

When the patient begins to receive enteral caloric support (either in the form of oral intake or tube feedings), conversion to longer-acting insulin preparations may be accomplished (165). During this transition phase, subcutaneous insulin is administered on a sliding scale basis with frequent blood glucose measurements (every 4 to 6 hours) and charting of the results and doses of insulin. The goal for the postoperative patient on a regular hospital ward is for a serum glucose level

< 110 mg/dL before meals and < 180 mg/dL postprandial or randomly (163). Most patients are discharged to home on the same diabetic drug regimen they were taking when they were admitted, although some oral agent–dependent diabetics may require conversion to insulin during the hospitalization to improve their glucose control. Consultation with an endocrinologist for tailoring of the patient's discharge antiglycemic drug regimen and arranging for further follow-up is frequently useful, particularly for the patient who was not requiring diabetic therapy prior to admission to the hospital.

Hypoglycemia in adult patients is unusual, except for that resulting from excessive exogenous insulin administration. If it does occur, it is treated by the IV administration of 50% dextrose. Infants, due to decreased hepatic glycogen stores, are at increased risk for hypoglycemia, particularly with stress. Severe perioperative hypoglycemia may occur in newborns (below 30 mg/dL in full-term infants, below 20 mg/dL in the premature), leading to seizures and the potential for neurologic injury. This is prevented by administering an IV maintenance solution with adequate glucose (10% dextrose) and frequent determinations of the baby's blood glucose level.

NUTRITIONAL SUPPORT

Severe nutritional deficiencies can lead to heart failure, and heart failure can result in nutritional deficiencies. The protein-calorie malnutrition syndrome associated with severe chronic congestive heart failure is known as cardiac cachexia. Preoperative malnutrition is a risk factor for postoperative complications and prolonged hospital stay in patients undergoing cardiac surgery. A preoperative albumin level < 3.5 g/dL in elderly patients or <2.5 g/dL in all patients is associated with an increased frequency of postoperative complications (166,167). Preoperative nutritional supplementation, however, is rarely feasible due to the urgency of operation. The realization that preoperative deficiency may exist, however, should lead to early postoperative nutritional assessment and supplementation.

Many infants with congenital heart disease and heart failure are unable to feed normally, and "failure to thrive" frequently enters into the decision to recommend surgical repair for the underlying cardiac lesion. After operation, feeding problems are not uncommon and these patients need early protein and caloric supplementation (168). Routinely, a nasogastric tube is inserted after operation. Initially this is used for gastric drainage, but, as soon as bowel activity returns, tube feedings may be started if extubation is delayed. The tube should be fine-bore to prevent obstruction of the nares (infants are nose-breathers) and soft to prevent gastric perforation or nasal erosion. Initial feedings in infants consist of a clear fluid such as 5% dextrose at 5 to 10 mL per hour. The residual amount left in the stomach after each hour is determined by aspiration. If low residual amounts are present, tube feedings are advanced both in amount and substance. For newborns, expressed breast milk may be available; this is preferable to commercially available formulas. The infant may need a pacifier to satisfy the urge to suck. Once on full tube feedings and sucking well (usually after just a few days), the infant is allowed oral intake with the tube in place. Supplements are given by tube until full calories are ingested by mouth.

Likewise, adults who are experiencing postoperative complications (such as difficulty weaning from the ventilator) should receive early postoperative alimentation. In general, adults require about 25 kcal and 1 g protein per kilogram of usual body weight per day (169,170). The enteral route is preferred to the IV to avoid the problems of maintaining venous access, fluid overload, and infection associated with central venous hyperalimentation. The ileus associated with cardiac surgery usually clears within a few days and once intestinal activity is present, a small bore feeding tube is placed through the nose into the stomach or, preferably, advanced into the duodenum. For patients with delayed slow gastric emptying, treatment with metoclopramide (10 mg per the tube once a day) is of value (171). A multitude of commercially available enteral formulas are available and the type of formula can be tailored to the needs of the patient. Tube feedings are initiated with small volumes of full strength formula and the volume is gradually increased until the target volume is reached. Diarrhea is the main side effect and this may be reduced by the addition of pectin to the formula. Patients should be fed with the head of the bed raised 15 to 30 degrees and periodic measurement of the gastric residual volume should be made. If the residual exceeds 100 to 150 mL, the feeding rate should be decreased. As the patient's general condition improves, he or she can be converted gradually to a full oral diet with continued tube feeding at a lower rate. Monitoring of the patient's caloric intake ("calorie count") guides the timing of tube feeding discontinuation.

Parenteral ("hyperalimentation") nutrition is required for patients who require nutritional support and are unable to be fed by a feeding tube. This is usually delivered via a central vein, although peripheral vein hyperalimentation is possible. Parenteral feeding solutions typically contain glucose, fat, amino acids, electrolytes, vitamins, and trace minerals. At our hospitals, we use standardized protocols regarding the composition, preparation, and administration of parenteral nutrition. The hospital pharmacists have an active and important role in the formulation of the parenteral nutrition solutions. The patient is monitored closely regarding urine output, serum electrolytes, glucose and blood urea nitrogen levels, liver enzymes, and blood cell count. Common complications include hyperglycemia and catheter infection.

Patients with normal preoperative nutritional status and uncomplicated postoperative courses typically have depressed appetites and occasional nausea early after surgery, and this is of little consequence. Generally, they are prescribed a low-sodium (2 g sodium) diet as their total body sodium is usually elevated, and they are discharged home on a "no-added" salt diet. After about a week, the appetite usually returns with discharge from the hospital and the return to "home cooking." Patients with coronary artery disease or heart failure undergo dietary counseling by a registered dietician prior to discharge from the hospital.

CARE OF THE RADIAL ARTERY HARVEST SITE

Complications related to the removal of the radial artery for use as a bypass graft conduit are rare but special measures to closely monitor and document the status of the patient's incision, arm and hand during the early postoperative period are in order. An unrecognized forearm hematoma could lead to finger ischemia and permanent damage. As a part of the initial assessment of the patient performed upon arrival in the ICU, the hand should be examined for color, capillary refill, temperature, and ulnar artery pulse. The patient's nurse performs this evaluation every hour for the first 4 hours after surgery and the results are charted on the ICU flow sheet. Assessment for fingertip viability and sensation abnormalities is then performed every 4 hours for 24 hours. The arm and hand should be elevated on a pillow to help reduce edema surgery. After 24 hours, the radial artery harvest site incision dressing is removed.

References

1. O'Brien WO, Karski JM, Cheng D, et al. Routine chest roentgenography on admission to intensive care unit after heart operations: is it of any value? *J Thorac Cardiovasc Surg* 1197;113:130–133.
2. Augoustides J, Weiss SJ, Pochettino A. Hemodynamic monitoring of the postoperative adult cardiac surgical patient. *Sem Thorac Cardiovasc Surg* 2000;12:309–315.
3. Flores ED, Lange RA, Hillis RD. Relation of mean pulmonary artery wedge pressure and left ventricular end-diastolic pressure. *Am J Cardiol* 1990;66: 1532–1533.
4. Stewart RD, Psyhojos T, Levitsky S, et al. Central venous catheter use in low-risk coronary artery bypass grafting. *Ann of Thorac Surg* 1998;66:1306–1311.
5. Pulmonary Artery Catheter Consensus Conference Participants. Pulmonary Artery Catheter Consensus Conference: consensus statement. *Crit Care Med* 19907;25:910–925.
6. American Society of Anesthesiologists Task Force. Practice guidelines for pulmonary artery catheterization. *Anesthesiology* 2003;99:988–1014.

7. Bossert T, Gummert JF, Bittner HB, et al. Swan-Ganz catheter-induced severe complications in cardiac surgery: right ventricular perforation, knotting, and rupture of a pulmonary artery. *J Cardiac Surg* 2006;21:292–295.

8. Mullerworth MH, Angelopoulos P, Couyant MA, et al. Recognition and management of catheter-induced pulmonary artery rupture. *Ann Thorac Surg* 1998;66:1242–1245.

9. Sirivella S, Gielchinsky I, Parsonnet V. Management of catheter-induced pulmonary artery perforation: a rare complication in cardiovascular operations. *Ann Thorac Surg* 2001;72:2056–2059.

10. Abrue AR, Campos MA, Krieger BP. Pulmonary artery rupture induced by a pulmonary artery catheter: a case report and review of the literature. *J Intensive Care Med* 2004;19:291–296.

11. Reinhart K, Bloos F. The value of venous oximetry. *Curr Opin Crit Care* 2005;11:259–263.

12. Egi M, Bellomo R, Langenberg C, et al. Selecting a vasopressor drug for vasoplegic shock after adult cardiac surgery: a systematic literature review. *Ann Thorac Surg* 2007;83:715–723.

13. Mekontso-Dessap A, Houel R, Soustell EC, et al. Risk factors for post-cardiopulmonary bypass vasoplegia in patients with preserved left ventricular function. *Ann Thorac Surg* 2001;71:1428–1432.

14. Landry DW, Oliver JA. The pathogenesis of vasodilatory shock. *N Engl J Med* 2001;345:588–595.

15. Treschan TA, Peters J. The vasopressin system. *Anesthesiology* 2006;105: 599–612.

16. Morales DLS, Gregg D, Helman DN, et al. Arginine vasopressin in the treatment of 50 patients with postcardiotomy vasodilatory shock. *Ann Thorac Surg* 2000;69:102–106.

17. Rosenzweig EB, Starc TJ, Chen JM, et al. Intravenous arginine-vasopressin in children with vasodilatory shock after cardiac surgery. *Circulation* 1999;100 (suppl):II182–II186.

18. Albright TN, Zimmerman MA, Selzman CH. Vasopressin in the cardiac surgery intensive care unit. *Am J Crit Care* 2002;11:326–332.

19. Luckner G, Mayr VD, Jochberger S, et al. Comparison of two dose regimens of arginine vasopressin in advanced vasodilatory shock. *Crit Care Med* 2007; 35:2280–2285.

20. Shanmugam G. Vasoplegic syndrome-the role of methylene blue. *Eur J Cardiothorac Surg* 2005;28:705–710.

21. Varon J. Treatment of acute severe hypertension: current and newer agents. *Drugs* 2008;68:283–297.

22. Cheung AT. Exploring an optimum intra/postoperative management strategy for acute hypertension in the cardiac surgery patient. *J Card Surg* 2006;(suppl 1):S8–S14.

23. Zabeeda D, Medalion B, Jackobshvilli S, et al. Comparison of systemic vasodilators: effects on flow in internal mammary and radial arteries. *Ann Thorac Surg* 2001;71(1):138–141.

24. Kaplan JA, Jones EL. Vasodilator therapy during coronary artery surgery. A comparison of nitroglycerin and nitroprusside. *J Thorac Cardiovasc Surg* 1979;77:301–309.

25. Reves JG, Croughwell ND, Hawkins E, et al. Esmolol for treatment of intraoperative tachycardia and/or hypertension in patients having cardiac operations. *J Thorac Cardiovasc Surg* 1990;100:221–227.

26. Wiest DB. Esmolol: a review of its therapeutic efficacy and pharmacokinetic characteristics. *Clin Pharmacokinet* 1995;28:190–202.
27. Wiest DB, Garner SS, Uber WE, et al. Esmolol for the management of pediatric hypertension after cardiac operations. *J Thorac Cardiovasc Surg* 1998;115: 890–897.
28. Sladen RN, Klamerus KJ, Swafford MW, et al. Labetalol for the control of elevated blood pressure following coronary artery bypass grafting. *J Cardiothorac Anesth* 1990;4:210–221.
29. Wagner F, Yeter R, Bisson S, et al. Beneficial hemodynamic and renal effects of intravenous enalaprilat following coronary artery bypass surgery complicated by left ventricular dysfunction. *Crit Care Med* 2003;31:1421–1428.
30. Abernethy DR, Schwartz JB. Calcium-antagonist drugs. *N Engl J Med* 1999; 341:1447–1457.
31. Vincent J-L, Berlot G, Preiser J-C, et al. Intravenous nicardipine in the treatment of postoperative hypertension. *J Cardiothorac Vasc Anesth* 1997;11: 160–164.
32. Leslie J, Brister N, Levy JH, et al. Treatment of postoperative hypertension after coronary artery bypass surgery. *Circulation* 1994;90(part 2):II-256–II-261.
33. Curran MP, Robinson DM, Keating GM. Intravenous nicardipine: its use in the short-term treatment of hypertension and various other indications. *Drugs* 2006;66:1755–1782.
34. Singla N, Warltier DC, Gandhi SD, et al. Treatment of acute postoperative hypertension in cardiac surgery patients: an efficacy study of clevidipine assessing its postoperative antihypertensive effect in cardiac surgery (ESCAPE-2), a randomized, double-blind, placebo-controlled study. *Anesth Analg* 2008;107: 59–67.
35. Aronson S, Dyke CM, Stierer, KA, et al. The ECLIPSE trials: comparative studies of clevidipine to nitroglycerin, sodium nitroprusside, and Nicardipine for acute hypertension in treatment in cardiac surgery patients. *Anesth Analg* 2008;107:1110–1121.
36. Brogden RN, Markham A. Fenoldopam. A review of its pharmacodynamic and pharmacokinetic properties and intravenous clinical potential in the management of hypertensive urgencies and emergencies. *Drugs* 1997;54: 634–650.
37. Gombotz H, Plkaza J, Mahla E, et al. DA1-receptor stimulation by fenoldopam in the treatment of postcardiac surgical hypertension. *Acta Anaesthesiol Scand* 1998;42:834–840.
38. Hill AJ, Feneck RO, Walesby RK. A comparison of fenoldopam and nitroprusside in the control of hypertension following coronary artery surgery. *J Cardiothorac Vasc Anesth* 1993;7:279–284.
39. Halpenny M, Lakshmi S, O'Donnel A, et al. Fenoldopam: renal and splanchnic effects in patients undergoing coronary artery bypass grafting. *Anaesthesia* 2001;56:953–960.
40. McNaughton PD, Braude S, Hunter D, et al. Changes in lung function and pulmonary capillary permeability after cardiopulmonary bypass. *Crit Care Med* 1992;20:1289–1294.
41. Ranieri VM, Vitale N, Grasso S, et al. Time-course of impairment of respiratory mechanics after cardiac surgery and cardiopulmonary bypass. *Crit Care Med* 1999;27:1454–1460.
42. Filsoufi F, Rahmanian PB, Castillo JG, et al. Predictors and late outcomes of respiratory failure in contemporary cardiac surgery. *Chest* 2008;133:713–721.

43. Mickleborough LL, Maruyama H, Mohamed S, et al. Are patients receiving amiodarone at increased risk for cardiac operations? *Ann Thorac Surg* 1994;58:622–629.
44. Rady MY, Ryan T, Starr NJ. Preoperative therapy with amiodarone and the incidence of acute organ dysfunction after cardiac surgery. *Anesth Analg* 1997;85:489–497.
45. Reddy SLC, Grayson AD, Griffiths EM, et al. Logistic risk model for prolonged ventilation after cardiac surgery. *Ann Thorac Surg* 2007;84:528–536.
46. MacNee W. Update in chronic obstructive pulmonary disease 2007. *Am J Respir Crit Care Med* 2008;177(8):820–829.
47. Reis J, Mota JC, Ponce P, et al. Early extubation does not increase complication rates after coronary artery bypass graft surgery with cardiopulmonary bypass. *Eur J Cardiothorac Surg* 2002;21:1026–1030.
48. Guller U, Anstrom KJ, Holman WL, et al. Outcomes of early extubation after bypass surgery in the elderly. *Ann Thorac Surg* 2004;77:781–788.
49. Cheng DCH, Karski J, Peniston C, et al. Morbidity outcome in early versus conventional tracheal extubation after coronary artery bypass grafting: a prospective randomized controlled trial. *J Thorac Cardiovasc Surg* 1996;112: 755–764.
50. Ovrum E, Tangen G, Schiott C, et al. Rapid recovery protocol applied to 5658 consecutive "on pump" coronary bypass patients. *Ann Thorac Surg* 2000;70: 2008–2012.
51. Kloth RL, Baum VC. Very early extubation in children after cardiac surgery. *Crit Care Med* 2002;30:787–791.
52. Heinle S, Diaz K, Fox LS. Early extubation after cardiac operations in neonates and young infants. *J Thorac Cardiovasc Surg* 1997;114:413–418.
53. Ward NS, Dushay KM. Clinical concise review: mechanical ventilation of patients with chronic obstructive pulmonary disease. *Crit Care Med* 2008;36: 1614–1619.
54. Tobin MJ. Advances in mechanical ventilation. *N Engl J Med* 2001;344: 1986–1994.
55. Mallhotra A. Low-tidal-volume ventilation in the acute respiratory distress syndrome. *N Engl J Med* 2007;357:1113–1120.
56. Meade MO, Guyatt G, Butler R, et al. Trials comparing early vs. late extubation following cardiovascular surgery. *Chest* 2001;120:445S–453S.
57. Krieger BP, Isber J, Breitenbucher A, et al. Serial measurements of the rapid-shallow-breathing index as a predictor of weaning outcome in elderly medical patients. *Chest* 1997;112:1029–1034.
58. Oikkonen M, Karjalainen K, Kahara V, et al. Comparison of incentive spirometry and intermittent positive pressure breathing after coronary artery bypass graft. *Chest* 1991;99:60–65.
59. Davies LK. Cardiopulmonary bypass in infants and children: how is it different? *J Cardiothorac Vasc Anesth* 1999;13:330–345
60. American Thoracic Society. Evidence-based colloid use in the critically ill: American Thoracic Society consensus statement. *Am J Respir Crit Care Med* 2004;170:1247–1259.
61. The SAFE Study Investigators. A comparison of albumin and saline for fluid resuscitation in the intensive care unit. *N Engl J Med* 2004;350: 2247–2256.
62. Schramko AA, Suojaranta-Ylinen RT, Kuitunen AH, et al. Rapidly degradable hydroxyethyl starch solutions impair blood coagulation after cardiac surgery: a prospective randomized trial. *Anesth Analg* 2009;108:30–36.

63. Wilkes MM, Navickis RJ, Sibbald WJ. Albumin versus hydroxyethyl starch in cardiopulmonary bypass surgery: a meta-analysis of postoperative bleeding. *Ann Thorac Surg* 2001;72:527–533.
64. Kozek-Langenecker SA. Effects of hydroxyethyl starch solutions on hemostasis. *Anesthesiology* 2005;103:654–660.
65. Brater DC. Diuretic therapy. *N Engl J Med* 1998;339:387–395.
66. Gulbis BE, Spencer AP. Efficacy and safety of a furosemide continuous infusion following cardiac surgery. *Ann Pharmacother* 2006;40:1797–1803.
67. Gennari FJ. Hypokalemia. *N Engl J Med* 1998;339:451–458.
68. Johnson RG, Shafique T, Sirois C, et al. Potassium concentrations and ventricular ectopy: a prospective observational study in post-cardiac surgery patients. *Crit Care Med* 1999;27:2430–2434.
69. Weber T, Berent R, Lamm G, et al. Serum potassium level and risk of postoperative atrial fibrillation in patients undergoing cardiac surgery. *J Am Coll Cardiol* 2004;44:938–939.
70. Parham WA, Mehdirad AA, Biermann KM, et al. Hyperkalemia revisited. *Tex Heart Inst J* 2006;33:40–47.
71. American Heart Association. 2005 Guidelines for cardiopulmonary resuscitation and emergency cardiovascular care: life-threatening electrolyte abnormalities. *Circulation* 2005;112:IV-121–IV-125.
72. Wait RB, Kahng KU, Dresner LS. Fluids and electrolytes and acid-base balance. In: Greenfield LJ, Mulholland M, Oldham KT, et al., eds. *Surgery: scientific principles and practice.* New York: Lippincott-Raven, 1997:254
73. Gray R, Braunstein G, Krutzik S, et al. Calcium homeostasis during coronary bypass surgery. *Circulation* 1980;62(suppl I):I-57–I-61.
74. Reiner AP. Massive transfusion. In: Spiess BD, Counts RB, Gould SA, eds. *Perioperative transfusion medicine.* Baltimore: Lippincott Williams & Wilkins, 1998:360.
75. Meldrum DR, Cleveland JC, Sheridan BC, et al. Cardiac surgical implications of calcium dyshomeostasis in the heart. *Ann Thorac Surg* 1996;61:1273–1280.
76. Chen RH. The scientific basis for hypocalcemic cardioplegia and reperfusion in cardiac surgery. *Ann Thorac Surg* 1996;62:910–914.
77. Dyike PC, Yates AR, Cua CL, et al. Increased calcium supplementation is associated with morbidity and mortality in the infant postoperative cardiac patient. *Pediatr Crit Care Med* 2007;8:254–257.
78. Prielipp R, Butterworth J. Con: Calcium is not routinely indicated during separation from cardiopulmonary bypass. *J Cardiothorac Vasc Anesth* 1997;11:908–912.
79. Munoz R, Laussen PC, Palacio G, et al. Whole blood ionized magnesium: age-related differences in normal values and clinical implications of ionized hypomagnesemia in patients undergoing surgery for congenital cardiac disease. *J Thorac Cardiovasc Surg* 2000;119:891–898.
80. Pasternak K, Dabrowski W, Wronska J, et al. Changes in blood magnesium concentration in patients undergoing surgical myocardial revascularization. *Magnes Res* 2006;19:107–112.
81. Storm W, Zimmerman JJ. Magnesium deficiency and cardiogenic shock after cardiopulmonary bypass. *Ann Thorac Surg* 1997;64:572–577.
82. Caspi J, Rudis E, Bar I, et al. Effects of magnesium on myocardial function after coronary artery bypass grafting. *Ann Thorac Surg* 1995;59:942–947.
83. Miller S, Crystal E, Garfinkle M, et al. Effects of magnesium on atrial fibrillation after cardiac surgery: a meta-analysis. *Heart* 2005;91:618–623.

84. Ritter JM, Doktor HS, Benjamin N. Paradoxical effect of bicarbonate on cytoplasmic pH. *Lancet* 1990;336:372–373.
85. Androgue HJ, Madias NE. Management of life-threatening acid-base disorders: first of two parts. *N Engl J Med* 1998;338:26–34.
86. Viitanen A, Salmenpera M, Heinonen J, et al. Pulmonary vascular resistance before and after cardiopulmonary bypass: the effect of PaCO2. *Chest* 1989;95:773–778.
87. Fullerton DA, McIntyre RC, Kirson LE, et al. Impact of respiratory acid-base status in patients with pulmonary hypertension. *Ann Thorac Surg* 1996;61:696–701.
88. Androgue HJ, Madias NE. Management of life-threatening acid-base disorders: second of two parts. *N Engl J Med* 1998;338:107–111.
89. The Society of Thoracic Surgeons Blood Conservation Guideline Task Force, Ferraris VA, Ferraris SP, et al. Perioperative Blood Transfusion and Blood Conservation in Cardiac Surgery: the Society of Thoracic Surgeons and The Society of Cardiovascular Anesthesiologists clinical practice guideline. *Ann Thorac Surg* 2007;83:S27–S86.
90. Jawa RS, Anillo S, Kulaylat MN. Transfusion-related acute lung injury. *J Intensive Care Med*. 2008;23:109–121.
91. Rebollo MH, Bernal JM, Llorca J, et al. Nosocomial infections in patients having cardiovascular operations: a multivariate analysis of risk factors. *J Thoracic Cardiovasc Surg* 1996;112:908–913.
92. Leal-Noval SR, Rincon-Ferrari MD, Garcia-Curiel A, et al. Transfusion of blood components and postoperative infection in patients undergoing cardiac surgery. *Chest* 2001;119:1461–1468.
93. Chelemer SB, Prato BS, Cox PM Jr, et al. Association of bacterial infection and red blood cell transfusion after coronary artery bypass surgery. *Ann Thorac Surg* 2002;73:138–142.
94. van de Watering LM, Hermans J, Houbiers JG, et al. Beneficial effects of leukocyte depletion of transfused blood on postoperative complications in patients undergoing cardiac surgery. *Circulation* 1998;97:562–568.
95. Scott BH, Seifert FC, Grimson R. Blood transfusion is associated with increased resource utilization, morbidity and mortality in cardiac surgery. *Ann Card Anaesth* 2008;11:15–19.
96. Murphy GJ, Reeves BC, Rogers CA, et al. Increased mortality, postoperative morbidity, and cost after red cell blood transfusion in patients having cardiac surgery. *Circulation* 2007;116:2544–2552.
97. Koch CG, Li L, Van Wagoner DR, et al. Red cell transfusion is associated with an increased risk for postoperative atrial fibrillation. *Ann Thorac Surg* 2006;82:1747–1757.
98. Koch CG, Li L, Duncan AI, et al. Transfusion in coronary artery bypass grafting is associated with reduced long-term survival. *Ann Thorac Surg* 2006;81:1650–1657.
99. American Society of Anesthesiologists Task Force on Perioperative Blood Transfusion and Adjuvant therapies. Practice guidelines for perioperative blood transfusion and adjuvant therapies. *Anesthesiology* 2006;105:198–208.
100. Kerendi F, Thourani VH, Puskas JD, et al. Impact of heparin-induced thrombocytopenia on postoperative outcomes after cardiac surgery. *Ann Thorac Surg* 2007;84:1548–1555.
101. Baldwin ZK, Spitzer AL, Ng VL, et al. Contemporary standards for the diagnosis and treatment of heparin-induced thrombocytopenia. *Surgery* 2008;143: 305–312.

102. Warkenttin TE, Greinacher A. Heparin-induced thrombocytopenia and cardiac surgery. *Ann Thorac Surg* 2003;76:2121–2131.
103. Levy JH, Tanaka KA, Hursting MJ. Reducing thrombotic complications in the perioperative setting: an update on heparin-induced thrombocytopenia. *Anesth Analg* 2007;105:570–582.
104. Alghamdi AA, Davis A, Brister S, et al. Development and validation of Transfusion Risk Understanding Scoring Tool (TRUST) to stratify cardiac surgery patients according to their blood transfusion needs. *Transfusion* 2006;46: 1120–1129.
105. Arora RC, Légaré JF, Buth KJ, et al. Identifying patients at risk of intraoperative and postoperative transfusion in isolated CABG: toward selective conservation strategies. *Ann Thorac Surg* 2004;78:1547–1554.
106. Moskowitz DM, Klein JJ, Shander A, et al. Predictors of transfusion requirements for cardiac surgical procedures at a blood conservation center. *Ann Thorac Surg* 2004;77:626–634.
107. Bybee KA, Powell BD, Valeeti U, et al. Preoperative aspirin therapy is associated with improved postoperative outcomes in patients undergoing coronary artery bypass grafting. *Circulation* 2005;112(suppl I):I-286–I-292.
108. Purkayastha S, Athanasiou T, Malinovski V, et al. Does clopidogrel affect outcome after coronary artery bypass grafting? A meta-analysis. *Heart* 2006;92: 531–532.
109. Dunning J, Versteegh M, Fabbri A, et al. Guideline on antiplatelet and anticoagulation management in cardiac surgery. *Eur J Cardiothorac Surg* 2008;34: 74–92.
110. Berger JS, Frye CB, Harshaw Q, et al. Impact of clopidogrel in patients with acute coronary syndrome requiring coronary artery bypass surgery. *J Am Coll Cardiol* 2008;52:1693–1701.
111. Vaccarino GN, Thierer J, Albertal M, et al. Impact of preoperative clopidogrel in off pump coronary artery bypass surgery: a propensity score analysis. *J Thorac Cardiovasc Surg* 2009;137:309–313.
112. Parolari A, Antona C, Rona P, et al. The effect of multiple blood conservation techniques on donor blood exposures in adult coronary and valve surgery performed with a membrane oxygenator: a multivariate analysis on 1310 patients. *J Card Surg* 1995;10:227–235.
113. Lewis CE, Hiratzka LF, Woods SE, et al. Autologous blood transfusion in elective cardiac valve operations. *J Card Surg* 2005;20:513–518.
114. Dietrich W, Thuermel K, Heyde S, et al. Autologous blood donation in cardiac surgery: reduction of allogenic blood transfusion and cost-effectiveness. *J Cardiothorac Vasc Anesth* 2005;19:589–596.
115. Goodnough LT, Brecher ME, Kanter MH, et al. Transfusion medicine: blood conservation. *N Engl J Med* 1999;340:525–533.
116. Hardy J-F, Belisle S, Janview G, et al. Reduction in requirements for allogenic blood products: nonpharmacologic methods. *Ann Thorac Surg* 1996;62: 1935–1943.
117. Shimpo H, Mizumoto T, Onoda K, et al. Erythropoietin in pediatric cardiac surgery: clinical efficacy and effective dose. *Chest* 1997;111:1565–1570.
118. Alghamdi AA, Albanna MJ, Guru V, et al. Does the use of erythropoietin reduce the risk of exposure to allogeneic blood transfusion in cardiac surgery? A systematic review and meta-analysis. *J Card Surg* 2006;21:320–326.
119. Corwin HL, Gettinger A, Fabian TC, et al. Efficacy and safety of epoetin alfa in critically ill patients. *N Engl J Med* 2007;357:965–976.

120. Schved JF. Preoperative autologous blood donation: a therapy that needs to be scientifically evaluated. *Transfus Clin Biol* 2005;12:365–369.

121. Ascione R, Williams S, Lloyd CT, et al. Reduced postoperative blood loss and transfusion requirement after beating-heart coronary operations: a prospective randomized study. *J Thorac Cardiovasc Surg* 2001;121:689–696.

122. Sellke FW, DiMaio M, Caplan LR, et al. Comparing on-pump and off-pump coronary artery bypass grafting. Numerous studies but few conclusions. A scientific statement from the American Heart Association Council on Cardiovascular Surgery and Anesthesia in collaboration with the Interdisciplinary Working Group on Quality of Care and Outcomes Research. *Circulation* 2005;111:2858–2864.

123. Laffey JG, Boylan JF, Cheng DCH. The systemic inflammatory response to cardiac surgery. *Anesthesiology* 2002;97:215–252.

124. Hsu L-C. Biocompatibility in cardiopulmonary bypass. *J Cardiothorac Vasc Anesth* 1997;11:376–382.

125. Shann KG, Likosky DS, Murkin JM, et al. An evidence-based review of the practice of cardiopulmonary bypass in adults: a focus on neurologic injury, glycemic control, hemodilution, and the inflammatory response. *J Thorac Cardiovasc Surg* 2006;132:283–290.

126. Aldea GS, Doursounian M, O'Gara P, et al. Heparin-bonded circuits with a reduced anticoagulation protocol in primary CABG: a prospective randomized study. *Ann Thorac Surg* 1996;62:410–418.

127. Bannan S, Danby A, Cowan D, et al. Low heparinization with heparin-bonded bypass circuits: is it a safe strategy? *Ann Thorac Surg* 1997;63:663–668.

128. Balachandran S, Cross MH, Karthikeyan S, et al. Retrograde autologous priming of the cardiopulmonary bypass circuit reduces blood transfusion after coronary artery surgery. *Ann Thorac Surg* 2002;73:1912–1918.

129. Rosengart TK, Debois W, O'Hara, et al. Retrograde autologous priming for cardiopulmonary bypass: a safe and effective means of decreasing hemodilution and transfusion requirements. *J Thorac Cardiovasc Surg* 1998;115: 426–439.

130. DeFoe GR, Ross CS, Olmstead EM, et al. Lowest hematocrit on bypass and adverse outcomes associated with coronary artery bypass grafting. Northern New England Cardiovascular Disease Study Group. *Ann Thorac Surg* 2001;71: 769–776.

131. Habib RH, Zacharaias A, Schwann TA, et al. Adverse effects of low hematocrit during cardiopulmonary bypass in the adult: should current practices be changed? *J Thorac Cardiovasc Surg* 2003;125:1438–1450.

132. Jamnicki M, Kocian R, van der Linden P, et al. Acute normovolemic hemodilution: physiology, limitations, and clinical use. *J Cardiothorac Vasc Anesth* 2003;17:276–282.

133. Fergusson DA, Hébert PC, Mazer CD, et al. A comparison of aprotinin and lysine analogues in high-risk cardiac surgery. *N Engl J Med* 2008;358:2319–2331.

134. Umscheid CA, Kohl BA, Williams K. Antifibrinolytic use in adult cardiac surgery. *Curr Opin Hematol* 2007;14:455–467.

135. Vander Salm TJ, Kaur S, Lancey RA, et al. Reduction of bleeding after heart operations through the prophylactic use of epsilon-aminocaproic acid. *J Thorac Cardiovasc Surg* 1996;112:1098–1107.

136. Casati V, Guzzon D, Oppizi M, et al. Tranexamic acid compared with high-dose aprotinin in primary elective heart operations: effects on perioperative bleeding and allogeneic transfusion. *J Thorac Cardiovasc Surg* 2000;120:520–527.

137. Henry DA, Carless PA, Moxey AJ, et al. Anti-fibrinolytic use for minimizing perioperative allogeneic blood transfusion. *Cochrane Database Syst Rev* 2007;(4): CD001886.
138. Brown RS, Thwaites BK, Mongan PD. Tranexamic acid is effective in reducing postoperative bleeding and transfusions in primary coronary artery bypass operations: a double-blind, randomized, placebo-controlled trial. *Anesth Analg* 1997;85:963–970.
139. Andreasen JJ, Nielsen C. Prophylactic tranexamic acid in elective, primary coronary artery bypass surgery using cardiopulmonary bypass. *Eur J Cardiothoracic Surg* 2004;26:311–317.
140. Dunn CJ, Goa KL. Tranexamic acid: a review of its use in surgery and other indications. *Drugs* 1999;57:1005–1032.
141. Eaton MP. Antifibrinolytic therapy in surgery for congenital heart disease. *Anesth Analg* 2008;106:1087–1100.
142. Despotis GJ, Levine V, Saleem R, et al. DDAVP reduces blood loss and transfusion in cardiac surgical patients with impaired platelet function identified using a point-of-care test: a double-blind, placebo controlled trial. *Lancet* 1999;254:106–110.
143. Koscielny J, von Tempelhoff GF, Ziemer S, et al. A practical concept for preoperative management of patients with impaired primary hemostasis. *Clin Appl Thromb Hemost* 2004;10:155–166.
144. Ong CKS, Lirk P, Tan CH, et al. An evidence-based update on nonsteroidal anti-inflammatory drugs. *Clin Med Res* 2007;5:19–34.
145. Jones SF, Power I. Postoperative NSAIDs and COX-2 inhibitors: cardiovascular risks and benefits. *Br J Anaesth* 2005;95:281–284.
146. Ott E, Nussmeier NA, Duke PC, et al. Efficacy and safety of the cyclooxygenase 2 inhibitors parecoxib and valdecoxib in patients undergoing coronary artery bypass surgery. *J Thorac Cardiovasc Surg* 2003;125:1481–1492.
147. Roche Laboratories, Inc [package insert]. Ketorolac Tromethamine Tablets Product Information.
148. Hospira, Inc [package insert]. Ketorolac Tromethamine Injection USP IV/IM Product Information. January 2007.
149. Fudickar A, Bein B, Tonner PH. Propofol infusion syndrome in anaesthesia and intensive care medicine. *Curr Opin Anaesthesiol* 2006;19:404–410.
150. Papaioannou V, Dragoumanis C, Theodorou V, et al. The propofol infusion "syndrome" in intensive care unit: from pathophysiology to prophylaxis and treatment. *Acta Anaesthesiol Belg* 2008;59:79–86.
151. Herr DL, Sum-Ping J, England M. ICU sedation after coronary artery bypass graft surgery: dexmedetomidine-based versus propofol-based sedation regimens. *J Cardiothorac Vasc Anesth* 2003;17:576–584.
152. Aantaa R, Jalonen J. Perioperative use of alpha2-adrenoceptor agonists and the cardiac patient. *Eur J Anaesthesiol* 2006;23:361–372.
153. Young C, Knudsen N, Hilton A, et al. Sedation in the intensive care unit. *Crit Care Med* 2000;28:854–866.
154. Dowling R, Thielmeier K, Ghaly A, et al. Improved pain control after cardiac surgery: results of a randomized, double-blind, clinical trial. *J Thorac Cardiovasc Surg* 2003;126:1271–1278.
155. Thourani VH, Weintraub WS, Stein B, et al. Influence of diabetes mellitus on early and late outcome after coronary artery bypass grafting. *Ann Thorac Surg* 1999;67:1045–1052.

156. Brown JR, Edwards FH, O'Connor GT, et al. The diabetic disadvantage: historical outcomes measures in diabetic patients undergoing cardiac surgery–the pre-intravenous insulin era. *Semin Thorac Cardiovasc Surg* 2006;18:281–288.

157. Doenst T, Wijeysundera D, Karkouti K, et al. Hyperglycemia during cardiopulmonary bypass is an independent risk factor for mortality in patients undergoing cardiac surgery. *J Thorac Cardiovasc Surg* 2005;130:1144.

158. Ascione R, Rogers CA, Rajakaruna C, et al. Inadequate blood glucose control is associated with in-hospital mortality in diabetic and nondiabetic patients undergoing cardiac surgery. *Circulation* 2008;118:113–123.

159. Furnary AP, Xu YX. Eliminating the diabetic disadvantage: the Portland diabetic project. *Semin Thorac Cardiovasc Surg* 2006;18:302–306.

160. Lazar HL, Chipkin SR, Fitzgerald CA, et al. Tight glycemic control in diabetic coronary artery bypass graft patients improves perioperative outcomes and decreases recurrent ischemic events. *Circulation* 2004;109:1497–1502.

161. Lipschutz AKM, Gropper MA. Perioperative glycemic control: an evidence-based review. *Anesthesiology* 2009;110:408–421.

162. The NICE-SUGAR Study Investigators. Intensive versus conventional glucose control in critically ill patients. *N Engl J Med* 2009;260:1283–1297.

163. Lazar HL, Mcdonnell M, Chipkin SR, et al. The Society of Thoracic Surgeons practice guideline series: blood glucose management during adult cardiac surgery. *Ann Thorac Surg* 2009;87:663–669.

164. Kelly JL, Hirsch IB, Furnary AP. Implementing an intravenous insulin protocol in your practice: practical advice to overcome clinical, administrative and financial barriers. *Semin Thorac Cardiovasc Surg* 2006;18:346–358.

165. Schmeltz LR, DeSantis AJ, Thiyagarajan V, et al. Reduction of surgical mortality and morbidity in diabetic patients undergoing cardiac surgery with a combined intravenous and subcutaneous insulin glucose management strategy. *Diabetes Care* 2007;30:823–828.

166. Rich MW. Keller AJ, Schechtman, et al. Increased complications and prolonged hospital stay in elderly cardiac surgical patients with low serum albumin. *Am J Cardiol* 1989;63:714–718.

167. Engelman DT, Adams DH, Byrne JG, et al. Impact of body mass index and albumin on morbidity and mortality after cardiac surgery. *J Thorac Cardiovasc Surg* 1999;118:866–873.

168. Kogon BE, Ramaswamy V, Todd K, et al. Feeding difficulty in newborns following congenital heart surgery. *Congenit Heart Dis* 2007;2:332–337.

169. Cerra FB, Benitez MR, Blackburn GL, et al. Applied nutrition in ICU patients: a consensus statement of the American College of Chest Physicians. *Chest* 1997;111:769–778.

170. Souba WW. Nutritional support. *N Engl J Med* 1997;336:41–48.

171. Genton L, Jolliet P, Pichard C. Feeding the intensive care patient. *Curr Opinion Anaesthesiol* 2001;14:131–136.

4 Postoperative Complications Involving the Heart and Lungs

Despite advances in cardiac surgery and perioperative care, the prevention and treatment of postoperative complications continue to be an integral part of the care of the cardiac surgery patient. As older, sicker, and more complicated adult patients undergo surgery with greater frequency, the opportunity for postoperative morbidity and mortality has increased. Likewise, infants with congenital heart conditions are undergoing total repair operations at an earlier age than in previous years, with a concomitant increase in the potential difficulties encountered in their early postoperative care. Recognition and treatment of perioperative complications are as important as the performance of the surgery itself. A technically perfect operation can be ruined by poor postoperative care, and a less-than-perfect technical operative result can often be "saved" by appropriate management of postoperative problems.

LOW CARDIAC OUTPUT (CARDIOGENIC SHOCK)

Although various definitions exist, low cardiac output or cardiogenic shock may be considered to be present when the patient has hypotension (systolic blood pressure <80 mm Hg), reduced cardiac index (<1.8 L/min/M^2 without pharmacologic support or 2.0 L/min/M^2 with support), with adequate filling pressures [the left ventricular (LV) end-diastolic pressure being >18 mm Hg and/or right atrial pressure >15 mm Hg] (1). Likewise, low cardiac output following heart surgery is considered to be present if the patient requires intra-aortic balloon counterpulsation or significant doses of inotropic drug support for longer than 30 minutes to maintain the systolic blood pressure higher than 90 mm Hg and the cardiac index >2.2 L/min/M^2 (2). Low cardiac output occurs during the early postoperative period in approximately 10% to 20% of patients who undergo cardiac surgery. The incidence is dependent on the type and severity of the cardiac lesion undergoing repair, preoperative ventricular function, adequacy of myocardial preservation during the procedure, and the adequacy of the surgical repair. For example, coronary artery bypass graft (CABG) procedures on patients with normal LV function have a low incidence of postoperative low cardiac output, whereas patients with ischemic mitral valve regurgitation and poor LV function have a notoriously high incidence of low cardiac output after mitral valve replacement and CABG. Preoperative risk factors for postoperative low cardiac output include poor LV function [ejection fraction (EF) <30%], repeat operation, emergency operation, diabetes mellitus, age above 70 years, and recent myocardial infarction (MI) (2).

Although intraoperative technical mishaps or inadequate myocardial protection during surgery can cause damage to a previously normal ventricle, the most important factor determining the incidence of postoperative low cardiac output is preoperative ventricular function. Thus, preoperative evaluation of ventricular function is important. Careful review of the patient's cardiac catheterization study—both the hemodynamic measurements (cardiac output, LV end-diastolic pressure, and pulmonary artery pressures) and the left ventriculogram—provides a good indication of the presence or absence of preoperative ventricular dysfunction. Very useful is the preoperative echocardiogram, which provides information of global and segmental myocardial contractility, chamber sizes, and valvular function.

Normal systolic function is associated with an EF of 60% to 75%. Moderate LV dysfunction is present when the EF is 35% to 50%, and severe impairment of contractility is associated with an EF below 35%. The EF is dependent on preload and afterload; therefore, the value should be assessed in the context of the patient's history and other data. The EF, however, reflects only the systolic (ejection) function of the heart. Diastolic dysfunction, reflected as abnormalities in ventricular relaxation and filling, also can result in heart failure and even pulmonary edema despite the presence of a normal systolic EF (3). Patients with LV hypertrophy are particularly susceptible to diastolic dysfunction.

Preoperative recognition of poor ventricular function leads to modifications in the management of technical aspects of the operative procedure. For example, for patients with poor preoperative LV function we frequently use the technique of combined antegrade and retrograde cardioplegia to optimize cardioplegia delivery (see Chapter 2). Likewise, a lower perfusion temperature on bypass (such as 28°C to 30°C) may be employed. For the patient with poor preoperative ventricular function, we routinely introduce a femoral artery catheter in the operating room just before beginning surgery to provide access for the expeditious introduction of an intra-aortic balloon pump should one is required in the operating room or during the early postoperative period. Patients with preoperative left ventricular ejection fraction of <20% to 25% often have an intra-aortic balloon pump placed prior to surgery, either in the catheterization laboratory (under fluoroscopic guidance) or in the operating room prior to making the chest incision (4,5).

Management of Low Cardiac Output

When low cardiac output is present early after cardiac surgery, management should follow a logical order of analysis and treatment (Fig. 4.1). First, consideration should be given to the possibility of reversible mechanical factors causing the poor cardiac performance. This is especially true for the patient who had good preoperative ventricular function and who was weaned from cardiopulmonary bypass (CPB) without difficulty. Inadequate preload is a common, and easily reversible, cause of low cardiac output. The left and right heart filling pressures should be measured and compared with those found to be optimal in the operating room and before surgery. Cardiac tamponade must be ruled out (see Chapter 5). Consideration should be given to the possibility of technical problems related to the operation: incomplete revascularization, occlusion of bypass grafts, embolic obstruction of a coronary artery, prosthetic valve dehiscence or obstruction, residual shunts, or obstruction of a conduit or baffle (6).

The physical examination should be repeated. Patients with severe low cardiac output have cold, poorly perfused extremities and absent peripheral pulses. In infants, an elevated core temperature is often present with a cool periphery. Auscultation should be performed to listen especially for valvular regurgitation murmurs, abnormal prosthetic valve sounds (if one is present), and muffled heart tones. The arterial blood pressure tracing should be inspected for the presence of an abnormally wide pulse pressure indicative of possible aortic valve regurgitation; paradoxical variation with ventilation suggests hypovolemia. The pulmonary artery wedge pressure tracing should be examined for the presence of "V" waves suggesting mitral valve regurgitation. The 12-lead electrocardiogram (ECG) should be studied for evidence of ischemia.

Echocardiography provides essential information about both valvular and ventricular function. In infants, transthoracic echocardiography can be used to visualize the ventricles, assess their contractility, and determine the presence or absence of significant mediastinal blood clots; color flow Doppler can be used to identify residual intracardiac shunts. A bolus of saline injected through a right atrial or central venous catheter will produce a cloud of visible microbubbles ("echo contrast") in the right atrium and ventricle that will appear immediately in the left atrium or ventricle if there is a right-to-left shunt. Likewise, agitated saline injected into the left atrial line (if present) will produce echo contrast in the right side if there is a left-to-right shunt.

Early after surgery, transthoracic echocardiography is not as useful in adults as it is in infants. Inability to turn the patient, bandages, mediastinal air, chest tubes, and the adult chest configuration combine to make assessment of the heart by this technique difficult. Transesophageal

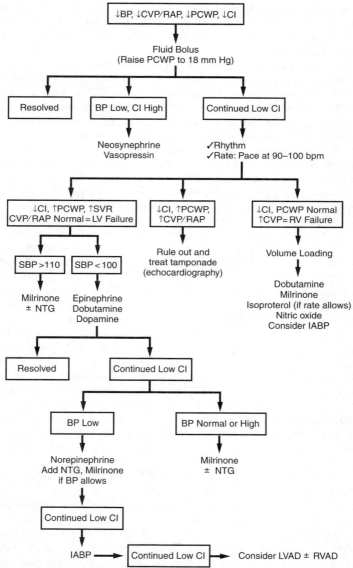

FIGURE 4.1 Management algorithm for low cardiac output. BP, blood pressure; CI, cardiac index; CVP, central venous pressure; IABP, intra-aortic balloon pump; LV, left ventricle; LVAD, left ventricular assist device; NTG, nitroglycerin; PCWP, pulmonary capillary wedge pressure; PGE$_1$, prostaglandin E$_1$; RAP, right atrial pressure; RV, right ventricle; RVAD, right ventricular assist device; SBP, systolic blood pressure; SVR, systemic vascular resistance.

echocardiography, however, is easily performed by the experienced operator and provides reliable information regarding ventricular filling and function, valvular function, and the presence or absence of tamponade (7–9).

Occasionally, emergency cardiac catheterization may be indicated to rule out reparable abnormalities. Coronary arteriography may reveal native artery or bypass graft spasm or occlusion. If a mechanical cause for the low cardiac output state is identified, immediate surgical repair is usually indicated despite the emotional trauma experienced by both the patient's family and by the surgeon in these situations.

While this evaluation is proceeding, efforts to improve the cardiac output and systemic perfusion are begun. The treatment of low cardiac output involves consideration of the heart rhythm, heart rate, status of the ventricular filling pressure (preload), myocardial contractility, and systemic (and pulmonary) vascular resistance (afterload).

Attention should be given to the patient's cardiac rhythm and rate. Cardiac output is reduced in the presence of arrhythmias such as heart block, junctional rhythm, atrial fibrillation, and sinus bradycardia. For the severely compromised patient with new-onset atrial fibrillation, synchronized electrical cardioversion is indicated; restoration of normal sinus rhythm or pharmacologic control of a rapid ventricular response to atrial fibrillation will improve the cardiac output. For patients with heart block or junctional rhythm, sequential atrioventricular pacing will restore the atrial contribution to the stroke volume, increasing the patient's cardiac output by 15% to 35% (10). Proper capture of the atrium must be ensured, and, for adults, the atrioventricular interval (the time between the pacing impulse to the atrium and the impulse to the ventricle) should be set at 150 to 180 milliseconds; shorter intervals are used for pediatric patients. Even for patients in sinus rhythm, if the heart rate is substantially <100 beats per minute, pacing at the rate of 100 will usually result in an improvement in the cardiac output (11). For patients with intact atrioventricular conduction, this is accomplished best by pacing only the atrium.

During the first few hours after surgery, patients frequently have a below-normal core temperature although the importance of this abnormality is not entirely clear. During surgery, the patients are rewarmed to around 36°C (nasopharyngeal) prior to weaning from CPB; excessive or too rapid rewarming is avoided. Patients who undergo surgery without CPB may experience significant cooling, despite measures such as the use of a heated air-warming blanket during surgery. Postoperative hypothermia reduces cardiac output and increases systemic vascular resistance (SVR) and may be associated with increased complications although the reduction in oxygen consumption associated with hypothermia may balance the negative hemodynamic effects (12,13).

Shivering occurs in some postoperative patients as a response to hypothermia although the mechanism is not entirely clear. It does, however, result in increased metabolic rate and oxygen expenditure. For the shivering patient with low cardiac output, treatment with neuromuscular blocking agents or other drugs will decrease oxygen consumption and may improve the patient's hemodynamic status (14).

Optimal cardiac output requires adequate preload for LV filling. LV preload may be monitored by measurement of the pulmonary capillary wedge pressure (PCWP), pulmonary artery diastolic pressure, and, if a catheter was placed intraoperatively, left atrial pressure. Although the normal heart functions well with a PCWP of 6 to 12 mm Hg, failing hearts require higher filling pressures because of poor compliance of the left ventricle. Even a relatively normal left ventricle may exhibit reduced compliance postoperatively and may have improved output with a PCWP of 15 to 16 mm Hg. A trial infusion of 250 to 500 mL of crystalloid or colloid fluid to the adult patient, given over a short period, is an important early maneuver in the management of low cardiac output. Raising the LV filling pressure to 15 to 18 mm Hg frequently improves the cardiac output. Patients with LV hypertrophy and diastolic (relaxation) dysfunction require higher-than-normal filling pressures even though the systolic function is normal. In some patients, very high filling pressures, even up to 25 to 30 mm Hg, are required to optimize LV performance. Knowledge of the patient's preoperative filling pressures is useful as well as the patient's hemodynamic status after weaning from CPB. Volume infusion should be administered with care; overfilling of the heart leads to ventricular distention, worsening of the myocardial performance, and pulmonary edema. Either crystalloid (often as 5% dextrose/one half normal saline) or colloid may be used for volume expansion. Although avoidance of unnecessary blood product transfusion is important, severe anemia in the presence of impaired ventricular function (and loss of ability to compensate for the anemia) results in diminished systemic oxygen delivery. Thus, for patients with low cardiac output after surgery, we often transfuse red blood cells to raise the hematocrit level to at least 24%. Transfusion to a higher hematocrit level is likely not of further benefit.

Inotropic Drug Treatment of Low Cardiac Output

Various drugs optimize cardiac output through their effects on myocardial contractility (inotropic effect), their effects on the SVR or both. Table 4.1 summarizes the commonly used drugs. No one drug is best for all patients with low cardiac output. Several drugs may be equally effective in the same hemodynamic setting, and the combined use of several drugs may prove to be most efficacious. Local institutional custom,

TABLE 4.1 Effects of Pharmacologic Agents Used to Treat Hypotension and Low Cardiac Output

Drug	Inotropic Effect	Chronotropic Effect	Peripheral Resistance	Cardiac Output	Intravenous Dose Range	Comment
Dobutamine (Dobutrex)	++	+	−	++	2–20 µg/kg/min	May produce more tachycardia than dopamine
Dopamine	++	+	0 or + (dose dependent)	+	2–15 µg/kg/min	Usefulness in renal insufficiency not confirmed
Ephedrine	++	++	0 or +	++	5–25 mg q 10 min (adult dose)	Short-term use only
Epinephrine (Adrenalin)	+++	++	− or 0 or + (dose dependent)	++	0.01–2.0 µg/kg/min (adult: 1–10 µg/min)	β-Receptor agonist at low dose, more α at higher doses; less tachycardia than dobutamine
Isoproterenol (Isuprel)	++	+++	−	++	0.01–2.0 µg/kg/min (adult: 2–10 µg/min)	Usefulness limited by tachycardia
Milrinone (Primacor)	++	0	− −	+	Load 50 µg/kg over 10 min, then 0.375–0.75 µg/kg/min	Reduces PA resistance and pressure; increases flow in arterial grafts; useful for RV failure
Norepinephrine (Levophed)	++	0 or −	+++	++	0.01–0.2 µg/kg/min (adult: 0.5–30 µg/min)	Particularly useful with milrinone or nitroglycerin
Phenylephrine (Neosynephrine)	0	0 or −	+++	0 or −	0.15–0.5 µg/kg/min (adult: 20–180 µg/min)	Used for high–cardiac output/ low–blood pressure situation
Vasopressin	0	0 or −	+++	0 or −	1–4 IU/h (adult dose)	Used for high–cardiac output/ low–blood pressure situation; may cause graft vasospasm

personal opinion, and, at times, a bit of superstition are often involved in the decision as to which agents are used for which circumstances. Despite widespread use of the positive inotropic drugs, guidelines for their use are lacking (15,16). Rational selection of drugs to treat low cardiac output requires a basic understanding of the agents available, careful analysis of the hemodynamic abnormalities present, tailoring of the therapy to fit the individual hemodynamic setting, and realization that the patient's state is dynamic and thus alterations in the type of drug support administered may be required with the passage of time (17). In general, the drugs used to treat low cardiac output are administered at doses sufficient to achieve a certain end-point (e.g., normalization of blood pressure, cardiac output, and heart rate) rather than at certain specific doses.

All of the available inotropic drugs should be administered via a central vein to ensure delivery into the circulation, to avoid vein irritation, and to prevent extravasation. These agents are usually administered via a catheter in the internal jugular vein or right atrium. Continuous blood pressure monitoring via a radial or femoral artery catheter is advised for patients receiving significant doses of vasoactive drugs.

The catecholamine type positive inotropic drugs used during the early postoperative period act by increasing the level of intracellular cyclic adenosine monophosphate (cAMP), which has a direct role in the contractile state of the myocardial cells (18). Increased intracellular cAMP results in increased contractility and relaxation, resulting in improved ventricular function. β-Adrenergic agonists (dopamine, dobutamine, epinephrine, norepinephrine, and isoproterenol) stimulate cell surface β1- and β2-receptors resulting in increased adenylate cyclase activity with increased production of cAMP. β1-Receptors exist predominantly in the myocardium; their activation results in increased speed and force of myocardial contraction, increased rate of automaticity of the sinoatrial node, and faster atrioventricular conduction. The β2-receptors are present predominantly in the smooth muscles of blood vessels and bronchi; their activation results in vasodilation and bronchodilation. α-Adrenergic receptors exist primarily in the peripheral and pulmonary vasculature; α-receptor stimulation causes vasoconstriction.

Dopamine is frequently used for the treatment of reduced cardiac output. A unique feature of this agent is that it has distinctly different hemodynamic effects at different doses. When administered at low doses, 1 to 3 μg/kg per minute, dopamine stimulates the dopamine (DA1) receptors in the renal, mesenteric, coronary, and cerebral circulations resulting in vasodilation of these vascular beds. Improved renal and mesenteric blood flow results although the effectiveness of "renal dose" dopamine for the treatment of renal insufficiency is unsupported

(19,20). At moderate dopamine doses, 3 to 5 µg/kg per minute, dopamine activates β1-receptors causing increases in myocardial contractility and cardiac output, often without a significant change in the blood pressure. Myocardial oxygen consumption is increased. At high dopamine doses, above 10 to 15 µg/kg per minute, α-adrenergic activation predominates, resulting in vasoconstriction of most vascular beds, tachycardia, increased blood pressure, and increased SVR. In some patients, tachycardia may develop even at moderate doses, thus limiting the effectiveness of dopamine as a positive inotropic agent. Although useful, dopamine is not a strong inotropic agent and it may be associated with tachycardia and tachyarrhythmias. We use it infrequently.

Dobutamine is a popular, effective short-acting agent for treatment of postoperative low cardiac output syndrome. A synthetic sympathomimetic amine, dobutamine acts through stimulation of β1-receptors with no α-receptor effects at any dose (unlike dopamine). It has moderate positive inotropic effects, causes a decrease in peripheral vascular and pulmonary vascular resistances (PVRs), and increases the heart rate. This combination of increased contractility and decreased afterload can be useful in many patients; thus, dobutamine is often a good first-choice drug for the treatment of mild-to-moderate low cardiac output (21). Dobutamine is preferable to moderate- or high-dose dopamine because it increases the cardiac output with a smaller increase in myocardial oxygen consumption (22,23). Frequently, however, dobutamine usefulness may be limited by the concomitant tachycardia and/or tachyarrhythmias produced. It is administered in a starting dose of 2 to 5 µg/kg per minute, which may be increased to achieve the desired hemodynamic effect (usually up to no more than 12 to 15 µg/kg per minute) or until the heart rate exceeds 100 beats per minute.

Epinephrine is the naturally occurring catecholamine released from the adrenal medulla. Epinephrine acts directly on both α- and β-receptors. At low doses (<0.02 µg/kg per minute), epinephrine predominantly activates β1-receptors in the heart and β2-receptors in skeletal muscle blood vessels causing vasodilation. Myocardial contractility and oxygen consumption, cardiac index, and heart rate all increase while SVR is often decreased. At low doses, blood may be shunted away from the kidneys and mesentery. At higher doses, the β2-effect is lost, and β1- and α-receptor stimulation predominates. This results in further positive inotropic and chronotropic effects and elevation of the blood pressure but at the cost of increased myocardial oxygen consumption, increased pulmonary artery pressure, and significant increases in vascular resistance that may compromise kidney and other vital organ perfusion. Vasoconstriction, tachycardia, and arrhythmias limit the usefulness of epinephrine at high doses. Epinephrine also reduces tissue glucose uptake and inhibits insulin release in the pancreas, often resulting in hyperglycemia that may require insulin administration. Furthermore, lactic acidosis may result from epinephrine administration (24,25). Despite these limitations, epinephrine is a popular agent and is often our first choice for the treatment of moderate low cardiac output syndrome as it compares quite favorably with dobutamine (26,27). Combined with a vasodilator (such as nitroglycerin), the vasoconstriction caused by higher dose epinephrine may be lessened with improvement in the overall hemodynamic state.

Norepinephrine, an endogenous neurotransmitter, acts primarily to stimulate β1- and α-receptors with little or no effect on β2-receptors. This results in cardiac stimulation and vasoconstriction. The cardiac effects result in increased cardiac output and increased myocardial oxygen consumption with increased myocardial perfusion as the coronary vessels have a low density of α-receptors. The vasoconstriction effect causes the blood pressure to be increased (often dramatically) and, through increased reflex vagal activity, the heart rate usually falls or remains the same. This combination of improved inotropic state, increased blood pressure, improved myocardial blood flow, and reduced heart rate is often quite favorable for the patient suffering severe low cardiac output. The perfusion of different organ systems is variable and depends largely on the relative concentration of α-receptors. Blood flow is redistributed so as to increase heart and brain perfusion, while blood flow to skeletal muscle, skin, and splanchnic beds decreases. Norepinephrine is less arrhythmogenic than epinephrine.

These properties make norepinephrine particularly useful for treating severe low cardiac output states, especially when associated with hypotension. A starting dose of 0.05 μg/kg per minute is increased as needed to raise the blood pressure and cardiac index. The goal is to return the patient's blood pressure to a level slightly less than his or her usual pressure. For adult patients who were normotensive prior to surgery, this would be a systolic pressure of 80 to 100 mm Hg. Norepinephrine should not be used to raise the blood pressure to supranormal levels. At high doses, the usefulness of norepinephrine is limited by severe peripheral and visceral vasoconstriction that may cause renal insufficiency, intestinal hypoperfusion, and limb ischemia. This is more likely to occur if the patient is hypovolemic; sufficient volume loading should always be accomplished prior to the administration of significant doses of any catecholamine agent.

The concomitant administration of norepinephrine plus a vasodilator such as a phosphodiesterase inhibitor (namely milrinone) or nitroglycerin is logical, results in further improvement in the cardiac index, and has proven useful for assistance in weaning patients from CPB (28). The combination of norepinephrine and milrinone is used frequently in our practices for the treatment of severe postoperative low cardiac output syndrome.

As a rule, norepinephrine should be administered at the lowest effective dose for the shortest necessary period of time. As the patient's cardiac function improves, it is our practice to switch the patient over to a less potent inotropic drug, most commonly dobutamine.

Dopexamine has both β2- and dopamine receptor agonist activity thus increasing the inotropic state of the heart while also producing a reduction in SVR. It is, however, less effective than dopamine and is more likely to cause tachycardia (21). We do not have experience in using this drug.

Isoproterenol stimulates β1-receptors in the heart and β2-receptors in the peripheral vessels, resulting in increases in heart rate, contractility, cardiac output, and myocardial oxygen consumption with a decrease in peripheral vascular resistance. The result is an increase in the cardiac index, largely due to the increased heart rate, with little change in blood pressure. In general, isoproterenol is not recommended for the treatment of postoperative myocardial dysfunction, especially in patients with ischemic heart disease, because it causes a significant increase in myocardial oxygen consumption and is very arrhythmogenic (17). One benefit of isoproterenol is that it lowers PVR, an especially helpful action when reactive pulmonary hypertension and right heart dysfunction are present. This may be particularly useful for cardiac transplant patients who may have a slow heart rate and diminished contractility for several days after implantation.

Milrinone increases intracellular cAMP levels by inhibiting the enzyme responsible for cAMP degradation (phosphodiesterase). This results in increased myocardial cell contractility and improved relaxation plus significant vascular smooth muscle cell relaxation resulting in vasodilation. This combination is favorable for the treatment of low cardiac output. Milrinone infusion causes increased cardiac output with decreased SVR and PVR and minimal or no effect on myocardial oxygen consumption (29). Milrinone also improves internal mammary artery flow and may help prevent spasm (30). Because of vasodilation, however, arterial blood pressure may fall and heart rate may increase during treatment. Concomitant treatment with a vasoconstrictor agent, such as norepinephrine or phenylephrine, is often required. With efficacy comparable to dobutamine, milrinone can be used alone or in conjunction with a catecholamine (31–33). Having a different mechanism of action than the β-adrenergic agonists, the combined administration results in synergistic effects that are often very effective in the treatment of low cardiac output. In particular, we have found the simultaneous administration of milrinone and norepinephrine to be very effective. By titrating the relative doses of the two agents the degree of afterload reduction can be controlled while both agents provide inotropic support via differing mechanisms. For patients with poor preoperative LV function and a significant likelihood of difficulty weaning from CPB and postoperative low cardiac output, we frequently will administer a single dose of milrinone (50 μg/kg) prior to CPB weaning. As CPB support is withdrawn, norepinephrine is infused at a low dose and titrated to offset the milrinone-induced hypotension (if needed) and to provide further inotropic support. If needed, a continuous milrinone infusion of 0.5 μg/kg per minute is instituted (34). Milrinone has also been demonstrated to be effective in pediatric cardiac surgery patients and for use in heart transplantation (29).

Calcium chloride administered by slow intravenous (IV) bolus (10 mg/kg) will raise the patient's blood pressure associated with increases in myocardial contractility and peripheral vascular resistance. This effect, however, is transient, and sustained improvement in the hemodynamic state is not achieved. Continuous infusion does not result in sustained improvement in the cardiac index and risks dangerous hypercalcemia. There are multiple potential adverse effects of bolus calcium administration: ventricular irritability, coronary vasospasm, bradycardia, sinus arrest, exacerbation of myocardial reperfusion injury, and possibly pancreatitis. We recommend calcium administration only for documented hypocalcemia (see Chapter 3).

Digoxin has long been an important part of the treatment of *chronic* congestive heart failure, although its use is largely being replaced by newer drugs (35). For *acute* low cardiac output in adults, however, there is no role for digoxin due to its slow onset of action, long half-life, and narrow margin between therapeutic and toxic levels. Digoxin toxicity occurs at lower serum levels in the presence of hypokalemia, hypomagnesemia, or hypoxia—all conditions that may arise during the early postoperative period. Digoxin has multiple potential interactions with other drugs that are often unpredictable in an individual patient. For these reasons, digoxin is not recommended to treat acute postoperative low cardiac output.

Other inotropic agents have been described for use in cardiac surgical patients with postoperative low cardiac output, although their use is not widespread. Triiodothyronine, administered intra- and postoperatively in CABG surgery patients may have beneficial hemodynamic effects, be associated with fewer complications such as atrial fibrillation and myocardial ischemia, and may reduce the need for postoperative mechanical support. These results have not, however, been consistently demonstrated and widespread use of triiodothyronine administration has not been adopted (36,37). The combination of glucose (30% dextrose), insulin (50 U/L), and potassium (80 mEq/L), known as "GIK," infused intravenously at 1.0 mL/kg per hour improves cardiac output and decreases the need for other inotropic drugs in adult patients undergoing cardiac surgery (38,39). Despite these potential benefits, thyroid hormone and GIK are not used in our practices. By far, most clinical experience has involved the adrenergic agents and the phosphodiesterase inhibitors as drug treatment for postoperative low cardiac output.

Vasoactive Drugs in the Management of Low Cardiac Output

Management of low cardiac output involves optimization of preload (ventricular filling), contractility (inotropic state), and afterload (SVR and PVR). Drugs that alter the SVR and, thus, the patient's blood pressure are used frequently in the treatment of low cardiac output. Vasodilating drugs decrease the resistance against which the left ventricle ejects (the afterload), thus increasing the cardiac output. If the ventricular preload is adequate, little or no reduction in systemic arterial pressure should result. However, if the blood volume is low, hypotension may occur. This potential complication of vasodilator therapy is, of course, reversible by volume expansion. It is important to remember that blood volume may be low even when central venous or left atrial pressure is normal in the vasoconstricted patient. Afterload reduction results in a decrease in the PCWP, reflecting decreases in ventricular filling pressure and myocardial wall tension. Afterload-reducing drugs should be used only when ventricular preload is adequate, generally with the PCWP (or left atrial pressure) being 10 to 15 mm Hg. Continuous blood pressure monitoring is employed when using significant doses of vasodilators.

The agents most commonly used for afterload reduction in the setting of acute low cardiac output are nitroglycerin and milrinone. Nitroglycerin is administered by continuous IV infusion, has a short half-life, and effectively reduces SVR. It is particularly useful for CABG surgery patients. As discussed previously, milrinone has both vasodilatory and inotropic properties making it particularly use for the treatment of high vascular resistance in the presence of low cardiac output.

Nesiritide is recombinant human B-type natriuretic peptide (BNP). Endogenous BNP is secreted by the ventricles in response to myocardial stretch, as a response to heart failure. BNP effects include arterial vasodilation and sodium and water excretion. When administered to patients with impaired ventricular function undergoing cardiac surgery, improved postoperative renal function, improved cardiac output, and possible reduced mortality have been reported (40–43). Other reports regarding the use of nesiritide for the treatment of heart failure and for cardiac surgery patients are, however, less favorable. The role of nesiritide in the management of cardiac surgery patients remains undetermined at this time (44,45). The use of nesiritide in children is limited (46).

The use of vasodilators alone in the treatment of low cardiac output is often limited by hypotension; frequently these drugs are used with an inotropic agent to augment cardiac output and maintain the systemic arterial pressure. Various combinations of an inotropic drug (dopamine, dobutamine, epinephrine, or norepinephrine) plus a vasodilator drug (nitroglycerin or milrinone) are used with clinical success.

Drugs that cause peripheral vasoconstriction are sometimes required in the management of patients early after cardiac surgery, usually when the arterial pressure is low, the SVR is low, and the cardiac output is relatively normal or high. Chapter 3 discusses the use of phenylephrine and vasopressin for the treatment of postoperative hypotension. In general, however, pure vasoconstricting drugs are not used for patients with hypotension that occurs in association with low cardiac output. Although the arterial pressure may rise, the cardiac output may fall further due to the increased SVR, which results in decreased organ perfusion. More often, these drugs are indicated to treat "high output" hypotensive states where the arterial pressure is low but cardiac output is above normal.

Overall, drug therapy for low cardiac output requires assessment of the hemodynamic situation based on physical examination and invasive measurements. Some patients with postoperative mild-to-moderate low cardiac output have a depressed cardiac index and normal peripheral vascular resistance. Many of these are successfully treated with moderate-dose dobutamine or a low-dose epinephrine infusion. More severe states of low cardiac output may require higher-dose epinephrine or norepinephrine with the addition of milrinone and/or a pure vasodilator. For patients with coronary artery disease, nitroglycerin is useful as the initial agent for afterload reduction. The simultaneous, but separately controlled, administration of an inotropic/vasopressor drug (such as norepinephrine) and a vasodilator (such as nitroglycerin or milrinone) agent allows for separate control of myocardial stimulation and vascular resistance with the goal being a balance that provides optimal systemic oxygen delivery.

It should be recognized that all patients do not react uniformly to the same inotropic agents and that the patient's hemodynamic status may change over the course of hours. Thus, flexibility, often with some experimentation, is necessary to determine the most suitable agent or combination of agents for a given patient. The recovering patient is weaned from the drugs one by one with careful monitoring of hemodynamic parameters.

Patients suffering significant low cardiac output despite moderate doses of drug support may require mechanical support of the failing heart. By far the most common initial form of mechanical support after cardiac surgery is intra-aortic balloon counterpulsation, the so-called

"balloon pump" (47). In general, an intra-aortic balloon pump is inserted when the patient's cardiac index is <1.8 to 2.0 L/min/M^2 despite
moderate doses of inotropic drugs in the absence of hypovolemia or reversible conditions such as tamponade. The topic of mechanical cardiac support is discussed in Chapter 8.

Low Cardiac Output Due to Right Ventricular Failure

Not all instances of postoperative low cardiac output are due to failure
of the left ventricle. Inadequate output from the right ventricle (RV), decompensated RV failure, results in inadequate filling of the left ventricle, decreased LV cardiac output, and poor systemic perfusion. Patients
with pre-existing pulmonary hypertension (such as those with long-
standing mitral valve disease, some transplant patients, or those with
chronic left-to-right shunts) or RV hypertrophy are at particular risk for
right ventricular failure. Other causes of RV dysfunction include RV infarction, the performance a right ventriculotomy necessary for cardiac
repair (as in the correction of tetralogy of Fallot), inadequate intraoperative RV protection during aortic crossclamping, and air embolism into
the right coronary artery or bypass graft. Elevation of pulmonary artery
pressure, either acute or chronic, produces increased afterload to ejection of the RV with reduced RV output. Mechanical ventilation may contribute to the workload of the RV.

The diagnosis of RV failure is based on the demonstration of a low
cardiac output with elevated right-sided filling pressures (central venous or right atrial) and relatively normal or decreased left-sided filling
pressures (PCWP or left atrial). Echocardiography can be confirmatory
by demonstrating poor RV contractility and dilatation in the presence
of relatively normal LV wall motion. Associated findings include tricuspid regurgitation, right atrial enlargement, and paradoxical septal motion.

Principles in the management of RV failure are (i) provide adequate
preload, (ii) reduce RV afterload (PVR), and (iii) maintain systemic blood
pressure (48). Right ventricular output is very dependent on its preload.
Volume loading, to a right atrial pressure of 8 to 15 mm Hg (or to 80% of
the PCWP), may be necessary to increase the right heart output. The
goal of inotropic drug support is to improve RV contractility and RV
myocardial perfusion without increasing PVR. Isoproterenol infusion
results in improved contractility and a decrease in PVR. Its usefulness is
frequently limited, however, by the tachycardia and systemic vasodilation it causes. In contemporary practice it is used primarily following
heart transplantation. Dobutamine is often useful, as it usually does not
cause elevation of the pulmonary artery pressure. Milrinone, by providing inotropic support to the myocardium while simultaneously decreasing PVR, is particularly useful for treating postoperative RV failure. In

addition to drug treatment, it is also useful to adjust ventilatory support to minimize mean airway pressure in the management of right ventricular failure. Finally, even though LV function may be normal, intra-aortic balloon counterpulsation may prove helpful, possibly due to improved coronary blood flow.

When aggressively treated, low cardiac output due to acute right heart failure will frequently be temporary and abate over a few days as the RV recovers. Please see Chapter 2 for further discussion.

Low Cardiac Output Due to Diastolic Dysfunction

LV diastolic dysfunction is due to the inability of the left ventricle to fill sufficiently at low atrial filling pressures, that is not due to valvular or pericardial causes (49). Common contributors include LV hypertrophy, atrial fibrillation, myocardial ischemia, tachycardia, positive pressure ventilation, and ventricular pacing. The basic problem is impaired LV relaxation with elevated end-diastolic pressure but unchanged or reduced end-diastolic volume. Therefore, the cardiac output is reduced, despite relatively normal LV systolic function. Diagnostic features include elevated PCWP, EF the same or greater than preoperative measurement, and small LV size with low end-diastolic volume.

Treatment of postoperative diastolic dysfunction is often difficult (50). Positive inotropic drugs will likely worsen the situation by causing tachycardia with resultant decrease in LV filling time and so should be used at low dose only as needed. Diuretics should be used with caution, as higher filling pressures are generally required to maintain the cardiac output. Maintenance of sinus rhythm, reducing positive end-expiratory pressure (PEEP), avoidance of hypercarbia, and the use of low-dose vasoconstrictor (e.g., neosynephrine) or vasodilator (e.g., nitroglycerine or milrinone) drug therapy to maintain the SVR in the normal range may all be of benefit for this situation. Finally, the acceptance of lower-than-usual hemodynamic goals (cardiac index 1.8 to 2.2 L/min/M^2), as long as perfusion is relatively well maintained, is recommended. The roles of β-blockers, nesiritide, and levosimendan in the treatment of postoperative diastolic dysfunction are not clear (50).

PULMONARY HYPERTENSION

In adults, pulmonary hypertension may develop as a consequence of long-standing valvular heart disease. With time, the pulmonary artery pressure approaches the systemic blood pressure and the risk of cardiac surgery is greatly increased, particularly if the hypertension is not reversible (51). Pulmonary hypertension may be considered to be present when the patient's mean pulmonary artery pressure exceeds 25 mm Hg with the pulmonary artery capillary wedge pressure being <15 mm Hg. When severe, the risk of severe postoperative right ventricular failure and death following surgery is greatly increased and therefore severe preoperative pulmonary hypertension may be a contraindication to surgery. Management of postoperative pulmonary hypertension may include the IV administration of milrinone, inhaled nitric oxide, inhaled prostacyclin, and oral sildenafil (52–58). By reducing PVR, improved right ventricular function may result with increased cardiac output and oxygenation. Managing the patient's ventilatory status to produce a relative hypocarbic alkalosis will also help to reduce the PVR (59). The management of pulmonary hypertension in children is also discussed in Chapter 7.

CARDIAC ARREST

For the hospitalized cardiac surgery patient, nearly all cardiac arrests are "witnessed" because he patient is being continuously monitored unexpectedly. These may occur unexpectedly [as in sudden development of ventricular fibrillation (VF)] or as the terminal event after a progressive downhill course (such as refractory low cardiac output syndrome). Patients who suffer unexpected cardiac arrest have the best chance of successful resuscitation, but the complication must be managed quickly and appropriately (60,61). Thus, the ECG and blood pressure are monitored constantly in all patients early after surgery (when the risk of cardiac arrest is the greatest) with alarm systems in place to alert the nursing staff if dangerous abnormalities occur. These alarms are lifesaving and must not be turned off to silence repeated irritating false sensing as this might lead to failure to recognize a potentially reversible, but otherwise fatal, arrhythmia.

Despite the many possible underlying causes of cardiac arrest in the postoperative patient (including arrhythmia, ischemia, pulmonary embolism, abrupt mechanical obstruction of a prosthetic valve, and tamponade), the initial management generally follows the Advanced Cardiovascular Life Support (ACLS) cardiopulmonary resuscitation (CPR) protocols developed by the American Heart Association (62). The technique of CPR involves chest compressions and maintenance of an open airway (with or without mouth-to-mouth breaths). Emphasis is placed on maintenance of the circulation via chest compressions with a lesser degree of initial importance being placed on ventilation. The recommended ratio of compressions to breaths for the adult is 30 to 2. The universal advanced life support algorithm specifies the following steps for management of cardiac arrest: perform chest compressions for pulseless patients, defibrillate VF or ventricular tachycardia (VT) until no longer present, gain control of the airway by (mask and bag insufflations or endotracheal intubation) and provide adequate oxygenation and ventilation, give IV boluses of epinephrine (and/or vasopressin), and correct reversible causes. CPR should be immediately resumed for 2 minutes following defibrillation shocks, even if the rhythm appears to have been changed, before stopping to study the ECG tracing. Potentially reversible causes of cardiac arrest include hypovolemia, hypoxia, myocardial ischemia, metabolic abnormalities, drug overdoses, cardiac tamponade, tension pneumothorax, and pulmonary embolism.

VF is the most common cause of sudden cardiac arrest, particularly during the early postoperative period. Pulseless VT is similarly dangerous. Prompt defibrillation is imperative; delays in defibrillation decrease the chance of successful resuscitation. Even if the patient is not being monitored, a witnessed cardiac arrest can be treated initially with an attempt at "blind" defibrillation, as it is likely that VF is the underlying rhythm. The initial defibrillation shocks should not be delayed for drug administration or CPR if the defibrillator is immediately available. The recommended initial adult defibrillation energy dose is 360 J when using a monophasic defibrillator and 150 to 200 J when using a biphasic defibrillator. It is important to place the paddles across the patient's chest in a position that will optimize the amount of energy delivered to the heart (i.e., so that the paddles face each other as well as possible with the center of the mass of the heart between them). An unsuccessful defibrillation attempt should be followed by a period of CPR (about 2 minutes) with repeat defibrillation attempt at the same or a higher energy level. For children the initial defibrillation energy dose is 2 J/kg and is increased to 4 J/kg for subsequent shocks (63). Delays in shock delivery, even for administering drugs, should not occur as the sooner defibrillation occurs, the higher the likelihood of resuscitation (64). If VF (or tachycardia) persists following one or two shocks, administration of a vasopressor (epinephrine, 1 mg IV, or vasopressin, 40 U IV) is recommended.

After endotracheal intubation, ventilation with 100% oxygen is begun. Moderate hyperventilation is best; frequent measurement of the arterial blood gases is performed if an arterial catheter is present. ECG monitoring is established if not already in progress. Secure IV access is essential, preferably through a central or femoral venous route.

CPR is maintained between shocks with hard and fast compressions of the chest at about 100 per minute with minimal interruptions. A bed board is placed beneath the patient to improve the effectiveness of closed chest cardiac massage. Closed chest cardiac massage restores cardiac output to only about 20% of normal (65). Although a normal systolic blood pressure (70 to 90 mm Hg) may be generated, the mean perfusion pressure is frequently far below normal during CPR. Adequacy of massage may be determined by observing the arterial blood pressure monitor if an arterial catheter is in place, palpating the peripheral pulses, and examining the patient's pupils, which, if previously dilated, may decrease to normal size. For neonatal patients, CPR employs the "two thumb-encircling" compression technique (with two thumbs on the sternum and fingers encircling the chest and supporting the back) with the depth of compression being approximately one third of the anterior–posterior diameter of the chest (66). The usual neonatal compression rate is approximately 90 per minute.

For some postoperative patients, adequate perfusion pressure cannot be generated by closed-chest massage because of instability of the sternum. In others, the presence of a compressing blood clot within the mediastinum may prevent effective CPR. Also, the presence of a prosthetic valve may make closed massage more hazardous because the myocardium can be perforated when compressed against the rigid prosthesis. In these instances, the chest should be reopened for open cardiac massage using the sterile thoracotomy instruments should be readily available in all properly equipped cardiac surgical intensive care units. Open-chest (or "internal") cardiac massage is often more effective than closed-chest massage, especially if tamponade is relieved on opening the chest. Care must be taken in reopening the sternotomy incision, particularly if the patient has coronary bypass grafts.

Open massage is performed by placing one hand behind the heart and one hand on the anterior surface of the right atrium and ventricle. The hands should be kept flat while pressing them together at a rate of about 80 to 90 times per minute for adults. Compression begins at the apex and is advanced toward the ventricular outflow tracts. The heart should not be kneaded or squeezed by the fingers as this may cause perforation of the myocardium. Open cardiac massage allows for direct visualization of the heart and lungs, safer compressions in the presence of a prosthetic valve, less trauma to mediastinal structures, inspection for causative factors (such as an occluded bypass graft), direct application of pacing wires or internal defibrillation paddles, and direct injection of drugs into the heart or aorta. Fear of infection should not prevent the surgeon from reopening the patient's chest for open resuscitation, as the infection rate among those who survive is low (<10%) (67).

Epinephrine is often the first drug given for the management of cardiac arrest, although vasopressin appears to be just as effective (68). The combined α- and β-adrenergic agonist properties of epinephrine result in increased SVR, which directs more of the cardiac output to the brain and heart; also, the drug increases myocardial contractility and heart rate. Epinephrine may also facilitate defibrillation. The adult dose is a 1.0-mg IV bolus, and this may be repeated every 3 to 5 minutes as needed. In the event that an IV catheter is not present, 2.0 mg of epinephrine can be mixed with 10 mL of normal saline (for adults) and in injected down the patient's endotracheal tube although bioavailability may be highly variable. The pediatric dose of IV epinephrine for cardiac arrest is 0.01 mg/kg, administered at the same frequency as for adults. If IV access is not secure, epinephrine may be administered via the child's endotracheal tube at the dose of 0.1 mg/kg (0.1 mL/kg of 1:1,000 epinephrine solution).

Vasopressin (for adults 40 U IV) may be administered instead of epinephrine, or after one or more epinephrine doses. In this setting, vasopressin may actually be more effective than epinephrine, as it has a longer half-life (10 to 20 minutes) and a lower incidence of adverse effects. Vasopressin may also be administered to children with cardiac arrest, although experience is limited (61).

Sodium bicarbonate is not recommended for the early treatment of the patient who suffers cardiac arrest and who did not have pre-existing metabolic acidosis. Adverse effects of bicarbonate administration in this setting include paradoxical intracellular acidosis and cerebrospinal fluid acidosis, plasma hyperosmolarity, impairment of oxygen delivery by increasing hemoglobin's affinity for oxygen, reduction in coronary perfusion, reduced peripheral vascular resistance, and alkalemia-induced reduction of cerebral blood flow (69,70). The acidosis that occurs early during cardiac arrest is largely respiratory in etiology, although the arterial blood gases may not accurately reflect this. Actually, it takes 20 to 30 minutes before metabolic acidosis develops during cardiac arrest unless the patient had metabolic acidosis before the arrest. The early administration of sodium bicarbonate in cardiac arrest has not been shown to improve survival, and the drug should be used only to treat a pH of <7.20 that is due to established metabolic causes. The usual dose is 1 mEq/kg; overtreatment (iatrogenic alkalosis) should be avoided.

Lidocaine is not the drug of choice for the treatment of shock-refractory VF or pulseless VT and may increase the amount of energy required for defibrillation. *Amiodarone* is, however, recommended for the treatment of patients with VF that is unresponsive to CPR, defibrillation shocks, and the administration of a vasopressor. Amiodarone is the *first arrhythmic drug of choice* for ventricular arrhythmias, rather than lidocaine (71). The initial dose for adults in this setting is 300 mg diluted in 20 to 30 cc normal saline or 5% dextrose in water given by rapid IV infusion with repeated doses of 150 mg given if required.

Magnesium is recommended for the treatment of patients who develop torsades de points, with or without cardiac arrest (72). Torsades de points is a characteristic form of VT in which the polymorphic QRS "peaks" appear to twist around the baseline. It may occur as a proarrhythmic effect of certain antiarrhythmic drugs or in association with a prolonged QT interval. Magnesium may be administered to adults with 1 to 2 g diluted in D5W, given over 5 to 30 minutes. *Procainamide* may be indicated for patients with stable VT and in the management of supraventricular arrhythmias. It should be used with caution in patients who have a prolonged QT interval. *Calcium* is of no benefit to the patient with cardiac arrest unless documented severe hypocalcemia or severe hyperkalemia is present.

Pulseless electrical activity (PEA), previously known as electromechanical dissociation, is a usually fatal cause of cardiac arrest characterized by lack of ejection of blood from the heart despite relatively normal ECG complexes. The basic problem is the inability of weak ventricular contractions to produce a detectable blood pressure or pulse. Treatment is the institution of CPR, assessment for treatable causes, and administration of epinephrine or vasopressin. If the PEA rate is quite slow, atropine (adult dose 1 mg IV) may be used following epinephrine. If PEA is due to calcium channel blocker overdose or hyperkalemia, IV calcium may be indicated. In the postoperative patient, PEA may be due to severe hypovolemia, tamponade, tension pneumothorax, prosthetic valve dysfunction obstruction, severe hypoxia, or pulmonary embolism. When one is confronted with a patient with PEA, these potentially reversible causes must be quickly considered.

Asystole is the total lack of cardiac electrical activity. In the postoperative patient this is may treated by the institution of pacing via the temporary pacing wires that were placed on the heart at the time of surgery. Failure of pacing to initiate ventricular contractions indicates nonfunctional pacing wires (due to lack of contact with the heart or breakage), inappropriate function of the temporary pacemaker, or a globally ischemic or otherwise nonfunctional heart. Transcutaneous pacing may be attempted but if the heart has irretrievably decompensated, pacing efforts by any method will fail.

After successful resuscitation from cardiac arrest, an arterial cannula should be introduced (if not already present), and the patient should be moved to the intensive care unit (if not already there). A nasogastric tube is often placed, and a pulmonary artery catheter may be useful to aid in the management of the unstable patient. If the arrest rhythm was VF, amiodarone or lidocaine is continued (or started) in an effort to prevent recurrent dysrhythmias. If the cause of the arrest is ischemia, and if the ischemia is continuing, then further stabilization can be achieved by the addition of intra-aortic balloon pump support. Serial ECGs and measurements of cardiac enzymes to rule out an MI should be ordered. If the patient remains unstable, echocardiography should be performed and, if indicated, cardiac catheterization with coronary arteriography may be ordered.

POSTOPERATIVE CARDIAC ARRHYTHMIAS

Abnormalities of the heart rhythm occur in more than one third of patients after open heart surgery and, thus, the management of these arrhythmias is an almost daily part of the care of the cardiac surgery patients. Although often a benign event, postoperative arrhythmias may be life threatening, may contribute significantly to both short- and long-term morbidity, and often lengthen the patient's duration of hospitalization. The high frequency of postoperative arrhythmias and the potential for serious adverse consequences make it important to identify them quickly and treat appropriately. Most of the common arrhythmias are successfully managed by routine measures (Table 4.2). The parenterally administered drugs useful in treating postoperative rhythm problems are summarized in Table 4.3.

Postoperative Bradyarrhythmia

A slow heart rate may be well tolerated and not require treatment or may decrease the cardiac output. The most effective combination of rate and ventricular filling time for adults is approximately 100 to 110 beats per minute although this is not the goal heart rate for most patients. A lower rate, 80 to 90 beats per minute, is likely to be more efficient with regard to myocardial oxygen consumption. The cardiac output of infants is particularly rate dependent, and bradycardia (<80 beats per minute) should be treated even if the arterial pressure is normal. Sinus bradycardia (heart rate <70 beats per minute) is frequent in adult patients who are receiving β-adrenergic antagonists in the perioperative period. Other drugs that can cause bradycardia include verapamil, diltiazem, and amiodarone. It is standard practice to attach temporary pacing wires to the RV at the time of operation; most often atrial wires are also placed. Thus, the simplest treatment of sinus bradycardia is the institution of pacing. If conduction through the atrioventricular node is preserved, pacing the atrium alone is usually preferred as this mode is more physiologic than sequential atrioventricular pacing or ventricular pacing alone.

If the patient's pacing wires fail to capture and do not provide satisfactory atrial or ventricular pacing, symptomatic bradycardia can be treated acutely with atropine (adult dose, 0.5 to 1.0 mg IV, may repeat every 3 to 5 minutes to a total dose of 3.0 mg; pediatric dose, 0.02 mg/kg, may repeat every 5 minutes to a total dose of 1.0 mg in a child, 2.0 mg in an adolescent). Longer-term treatment includes continuous IV infusion of dopamine (2 to 10 μg/kg per minute), epinephrine (2 to 10 μg per minute), or isoproterenol (adult dose, 2 to 10 μg per minute; pediatric dose, 0.01 to 0.10 μg/kg per minute); external (transcutaneous) cardiac pacing; and passage of a temporary transvenous pacing wire.

Management Strategies for Postoperative Arrhythmias

Arrhythmia	Treatment
Sinus bradycardia, some nodal bradycardias	1. Atrial pacing (DDD mode preferred) 2. Dopamine 3. Atropine
Complete heart block, slow nodal rhythm	1. Discontinue amiodarone and/or β-blocker 2. Sequential atrioventricular pacing 3. Ventricular pacing (VVI mode)
Nodal rhythm	1. Discontinue amiodarone and/or β-blocker 2. Pacing (atrial if possible) 3. Observe if rate reasonable and blood pressure satisfactory

Premature ventricular contractions	1. Observe if infrequent, chronic, asymptomatic
	2. Check blood gases, potassium, magnesium
	3. If new or frequent, consider:
	  a. Overdrive pacing
	  b. β-Blocker

Ventricular tachycardia, sustained	1. Electrical cardioversion 2. Amiodarone
Sinus tachycardia	1. Treat underlying cause 2. β-Blocker
Narrow complex paroxysmal supraventricular tachycardia	1. Adenosine to slow and observe etiology
Atrial premature beats	1. Not usually treated 2. β-Blocker

Atrial fibrillation	1. Patient stable and heart rate satisfactory:
	  a. Not always treated
	  b. Amiodarone
	  c. Anticoagulation if persists >48 h
	2. Unstable and tachycardic:
	  a. Synchronized cardioversion
	3. Hemodynamically stable but tachycardic:
	  a. Rate control: if LV good: diltiazem or esmolol infusion
	  b. Amiodarone
	4. Persistent or chronic:
	  a. Oral β-blocker
	  b. Anticoagulation if persists >48 h

Atrial flutter	1. Rapid atrial pacing 2. If ineffective: treat as for atrial fibrillation

LV, left ventricle; see text for description of DDD, DVI, and VVI modes.

TABLE
4.3

Commonly Used Parenteral Drugs for Treating Postoperative Arrhythmias

Drug	Indications	Adult Dose	Side Effects
Adenosine	Narrow complex paroxysmal supraventricular tachycardia	*IV bolus:* 6 mg; may repeat with 12 mg if indicated	Flushing, atrioventricular block; if given for wide complex tachycardia/VT, may cause deterioration
Amiodarone	VF or pulseless VT; wide QRS-complex tachycardia Atrial fibrillation	*IV bolus:* 150 mg IV, q 5–10 min (For VF: 300-mg bolus; may repeat 150 mg in 5–10 min) See Table 4.4	Hypotension, vasodilation, negative inotropic effect, bradycardia, AV block, hepato- and pulmonary toxicity, nausea, vomiting
Atropine	Symptomatic sinus bradycardia	1.0 mg IV push	May cause myocardial ischemia; pacing is preferable
Diltiazem	Atrial fibrillation/flutter	*IV load:* 0.25 mg/kg over 2 min; may repeat in 15 min *Maintenance:* 5–15 mg/h; titrate for HR 70–120 beats/min with SBP >90 mm Hg	Hypotension, AV block, bradycardia, decreased cardiac output, headache
Esmolol	Atrial fibrillation/flutter; tachycardia	*IV:* Begin at 50 μg/kg/min; increase in 50-μg/kg/min increments q 5 min to max 200 μg/kg/min; maintain HR 70–120 beats/min and SBP >90 mm Hg	Bradycardia, hypotension, atrioventricular block reduced cardiac output (transient due to short half-life)
Lidocaine	VT, VF	*IV bolus:* 1.0–1.5 mg/kg; may repeat with 0.5–1.5 mg/kg in 10 min *Maintenance:* 1–4 mg/min	Confusion, coma, seizures, hypotension, nausea, vomiting
Magnesium sulfate	Torsade de pointes; hypomagnesemia	*IV bolus:* 1–2 g	May cause hypotension; caution if renal insufficiency present
Procainamide	VT, VF, wide QRS-complex tachycardia of uncertain origin, atrial fibrillation/flutter	*IV load:* 500–1,000 mg (up to 17 mg/kg); run at 20 mg/min *Maintenance:* 1–4 mg/min; hypotension or QRS widening occurs	VT, asystole, hypotension, seizures, thrombocytopenia, lupuslike syndrome reduce if desired effect seen or
Propranolol	Atrial fibrillation/flutter	*IV:* 0.5–1.0 mg q 5 min up to 2–5 mg	Bradycardia, hypotension, reduced cardiac output

AV, atrioventricular; HR, heart rate; IV, intravenous; SBP, systolic blood pressure; VF, ventricular fibrillation; VT, ventricular tachycardia.
Note: The listed side effects are not comprehensive, and other adverse reactions to these drugs are known to occur.

Various degrees of heart block may develop after surgery, most frequently after valve replacement and congenital procedures that involve manipulations near the atrioventricular conduction system. First-degree block (PR interval > 200 milliseconds) is not uncommon, causes no symptoms, usually disappears spontaneously, and requires no treatment. In patients with first-degree heart block early after surgery we frequently leave a ventricular demand pacemaker in place as a backup, in case the degree of conduction disturbance worsens. Second-degree block occurs only when some atrial impulses are conducted to the ventricle. If this results in a significant bradycardia, treatment is sequential atrioventricular pacing via the temporary epicardial leads.

Third-degree (complete) heart block is a serious problem since, in the postoperative patient, the ventricular escape rate may be only 30 to 40 beats per minute. Complete heart block occurs much more frequently in valve surgery patients and following repeat operations (73–76). Secure placement and testing of the pacing wires at the time of surgery for these patients are important. For complete heart block, sequential atrioventricular pacing is the treatment of choice. If the pacing wires fail to capture, reversing the polarity of the wires may be successful. If not, pacing with a transcutaneous pacemaker via cutaneous electrodes applied to the skin is indicated for the patient with complete heart block or symptomatic bradycardia with signs of poor perfusion that cannot be paced otherwise. This technique is, however, uncomfortable for the awake patient and, in most cases, should be replaced by passage of a temporary transvenous pacing wire. Most of these patients with early postoperative third-degree heart block will regain normal atrioventricular conduction within hours to days after surgery, although some, particularly valve surgery patients, will require placement of a permanent pacemaker. No patient with surgically related complete heart block should be discharged from the hospital without pacemaker implantation.

Management of Temporary Cardiac Pacing Systems

Use of temporary pacing for bradycardia can be lifesaving for the postoperative patient. Since complete heart block is rare in CABG surgery patients, some authorities have recommended selective placement of epicardial temporary pacing leads in these patients (77,78). It is, however, our current standard to routinely attach temporary ventricular pacing electrodes to the heart in all patients at the time of surgery. In addition, atrial leads are placed in all valve surgery patients and any others thought to be at increased need for postoperative dual chamber pacing. Optimal placement involves good contact with the myocardium and avoidance of contact with coronary arteries, bypass grafts, and mediastinal drainage tubes. Bipolar pacing electrodes are used with the ventricular wire being attached to the RV and the atrial wire, if used, to the right atrium. Valve surgery patients receive both atrial and ventricular wires unless the patient is in permanent atrial fibrillation in which case only the ventricular electrode is placed. The pacing wires exit through the chest wall and are attached to an external pacemaker (pulse generator). A daily check of the patient's underlying rhythm, the minimum current that the pacemaker is able to sense (sensitivity), the pacing capture threshold, and the pacemaker battery indicator is performed (79).

Contemporary external pacemakers sense native myocardial depolarization and deliver current to the leads for pacing. They provide for both atrial and ventricular pacing and for adjusting the length of time between the atrial and ventricular impulses. The demand mode of pacing causes the pacemaker to deliver current to the heart only when the sensed rate is below the rate set by the operator. The asynchronous mode provides a pacing current to the heart irrespective of the native heart rate. Most frequently, the demand mode is used with the backup rate setting at 60 beats per minute for adults. The sensitivity of sensing is also adjustable. Failure of the device to sense appropriately may be due to a loose connection, too low a sensitivity setting, a failing lead, or early battery depletion. Failure of pacing (failure to capture) may be due to poor contact between the pacing electrode and the heart (due to the development of fibrosis at the lead/myocardium interface), myocardial ischemia, hyperkalemia, failure to turn on the pulse generator, battery failure, setting the pacer output too low, or poor contact between the pacing leads and the generator. If easily correctable causes of failure to capture are not apparent, reversing the polarity of the electrodes may result in pacing.

Pacing modes are coded by abbreviations. The first letter refers to the chamber being paced (A for atrium, V for ventricle, D for both). The second letter is the chamber being sensed (A, V, or D). The third letter denotes the response to the sensed event (I for inhibit, T for trigger, D for triggering of a ventricular complex in response to a sensed atrial complex). Typically, patients with intact conduction early after surgery will have their pacemaker set at the VVI mode with a backup rate of 60 beats per minute. Therefore, if the ventricular rate becomes <60, the ventricle will be paced automatically at 60, irrespective of the status of the atrium or atrioventricular conduction. In general, use of the VOO mode, in which pacing spikes are delivered to the ventricle irrespective of the native electrical activity, is not recommended for the postoperative patient. This is because delivery during the repolarization phase of the native beat might occur. This "R on T" phenomenon is known to cause VF (80). Patients with bradycardia are often paced using the DDD mode. When intact atrioventricular conduction is present, the DDD mode actually functions as the AAI mode in which the paced atrial complex is conducted naturally to the ventricle. But, if native conduction fails, the ventricle will be paced thus maintaining the programmed heart rate. This mode is advantageous in patients with variable native sinus node function and/or intermittent atrioventricular block.

Most patients have their epicardial pacing wires removed 1 or 2 days prior to anticipated discharge from the hospital, preferably in the morning. If the patient is receiving heparin, it should be discontinued sufficiently prior to wire removal to allow for normalization of the activated clotting time. Although serious bleeding related to wire removal is rare (<1/1,000), it may occur and can require emergency sternal re-entry for control. Thus, instruments for emergency reopening of the patient are available on all well-equipped cardiac surgery units. The wires are extracted by gentle continuous traction while the patient's rhythm is being monitored. If significant resistance to removal is encountered, the wires are pulled taut and cut at the skin level; the retained wire is allowed to retract into the patient. This technique is used routinely for patients that have been anticoagulated with warfarin (Coumadin). After removal, the patient is kept at bed rest for 2 hours, with continuous monitoring for the next 12 to 24 hours. Some patients may experience ventricular arrhythmias during wire removal although these are generally short lived and do not require treatment (81). Of note, magnetic resonance imaging of the patient with epicardial pacing wires exiting from the skin is not advised (79).

Postoperative Tachyarrhythmias

Approximately one third of patients who undergo open heart procedures suffer postoperative tachyarrhythmias. Most of these are supraventricular (atrial fibrillation and flutter) and are easily recognized as such. Occasionally, however, a wide QRS tachycardia occurs, and it may be difficult to determine the exact nature of the arrhythmia.

Wide QRS-Complex Tachycardia

Wide complex tachycardia is defined as being present when the QRS duration is 0.12 seconds or longer. Most instances of wide complex tachycardia are VT, supraventricular tachycardia (SVT) with aberrant conduction, or pre-excited tachycardias mediated by an accessory pathway [Wolff–Parkinson–White syndrome (WPW)]. *Generally, wide complex tachycardia should be considered to be VT and if the patient is unstable, electrical cardioversion is the initial treatment of choice* (72). If this is not successful, amiodarone administration should be considered for the empiric treatment of wide complex tachycardia of uncertain mechanism. The adult dose is 300 mg IV over 10 minutes with a repeat dose of 150 mg IV as needed.

If the wide complex tachycardia is *regular*, it is most likely to be VT or SVT.

If it is felt to be supraventricular, adenosine (6 mg rapid IV infusion, followed by 12 mg in 1 to 2 minutes if required) is recommended. While adenosine's action is very short lived, it will frequently terminate wide complex SVT without much effect in VT. Thus, adenosine may be useful both as a diagnostic and therapeutic agent. If these measures are not successful, procainamide should be considered, especially for wide complex tachycardia of unknown type in the patient with good LV function. Procainamide is administered at a rate of 20 mg per minute intravenously up to a total dose of 15 mg/kg. Careful monitoring of the blood pressure and ECG is performed during the loading procedure as it may cause prolongation of the QT interval and act as a negative inotropic agent. It may then be given by continuous infusion at 1 to 4 mg per minute (adult dose) with monitoring of blood levels and the patient's QT interval. Procainamide may convert atrial fibrillation to sinus rhythm and slows conduction in accessory bypass tracts if such are involved in the tachycardia. Amiodarone remains the drug of choice for the treatment of regular wide complex tachycardia. Consultation with an electrophysiologist is recommended when the exact nature of the patient's tachyarrhythmia is not clear or if it does not respond to first-line treatment.

If *irregular*, the wide complex tachycardia may be polymorphic VT (including torsades de pointes), atrial fibrillation with atrioventricular bypass tract conduction (WPW syndrome), or atrial fibrillation with aberrant conduction. Polymorphic (irregular) VT is the most dangerous because pulseless cardiac arrest may be imminent. If the patient is unstable, expeditious electrical cardioversion using 150 J with a biphasic defibrillator or 360 J if using a monophasic device is indicated. If the tachycardia is associated with a preceding long QT interval, torsades de pointes may be present. Treatment involves discontinuing precipitating drugs and the administration of magnesium, as discussed previously. Wide complex tachycardia due to atrial fibrillation in association with pre-excitation (WPW syndrome) in the postoperative patient is rare. Recognition and treatment of this arrhythmia may require expert consultation (82). If present, treatment is amiodarone. Drugs that block the atrioventricular node may worsen the situation when used to treat atrial fibrillation with pre-excitation. Drugs to avoid in this situation include adenosine, digoxin, diltiazem, and verapamil. If the irregular wide complex tachycardia is judged to be atrial fibrillation with aberrancy, the management is the same as for narrow complex tachycardia.

Narrow QRS-Complex Tachycardia

Determining the nature of narrow complex tachycardia may be difficult. Most often, *regular* narrow complex tachycardias are sinus tachycardia (ST), re-entry SVT (so-called paroxysmal tachycardia), atrial flutter, or junctional tachycardia. If the narrow complex tachycardia is *irregular*, it is most likely atrial fibrillation.

Sinus Tachycardia and Re-entry Supraventricular Tachycardia

ST may be the result of hypovolemia, anemia, fever, agitation, or inadequate pain relief. It may, however, be a compensatory response to compromised cardiac function and may indicate a serious problem such as ongoing myocardial ischemia or tamponade. When ST is present, evaluation should be undertaken to rule out the presence of a low cardiac output state. This would include physical examination, measurement of arterial pH, and echocardiogram to evaluate LV function. During the first few hours after surgery, occasional adult patients exhibit ST, often associated with hypertension. This hyperdynamic state is more common in younger male adults and may be related to a greater-than-normal catecholamine response to the stress of operation. ST in the intubated patient early after operation may suggest a patient who is awake and feeling pain but who cannot move because of continued muscle paralysis.

For patients with uncomplicated ST, the initial treatment is assurance of adequate cardiac filling pressures and adequate pain control. If correction of hypovolemia and pain does not alleviate the tachycardia and low cardiac output is not present, treatment with a β-adrenergic antagonist may be indicated. Esmolol is particularly well suited for this purpose because of its short half-life and rapid reversibility when discontinued. Caution must be exercised because hypotension or bradycardia may result, necessitating abrupt discontinuation of the drug.

It may difficult to differentiate ST from SVT that is due to a re-entrant mechanism (re-entry SVT). In both arrhythmias, P waves may be difficult to identify. In general, re-entry SVT is faster than ST with the rate being above 140 in adults, 180 in children, and 220 in infants. The onset and termination is usually abrupt whereas ST may develop and dissipate in a more gradual fashion. Also, SVT is more regular than ST with no beat-to-beat variability in the R-R interval. A bolus dose of adenosine will often convert re-entry SVT. The adult IV push dose is 3 mg if administered through a central line, 6 mg if administered via a peripheral IV site (70). If unsuccessful, a double bolus dose may be tried. If the tachyarrhythmia converts, it was most likely re-entry SVT. Long-term rate control may be achieved with diltiazem or a β-blocker.

Atrial Fibrillation and Flutter

In adults, postoperative atrial arrhythmias occur frequently; the incidence is much lower in children. The most common postoperative atrial arrhythmia is atrial fibrillation, which occurs in about 30% of patients. Postoperative atrial fibrillation is an event of significance as it is associated with increased rates of cognitive changes, renal dysfunction, infection, and longer hospital stay (83).

Risk factors associated with postoperative atrial fibrillation include older patient age, previous atrial fibrillation, chronic obstructive pulmonary disease, valve surgery, postoperative withdrawal of β-blocker or angiotensin-converting enzyme inhibitor medication, obesity, and perioperative red blood cell transfusions (84,85). It has been suggested that performing CABG surgery without the use of CPB ("off pump") may be associated with a lower incidence of postoperative atrial arrhythmias, although this result has not been consistently demonstrated (86). Although the cause of these arrhythmias is unknown, contributing factors may include manipulation and cannulation of the atrium, pericardial inflammation, intraoperative ischemia, autonomic imbalance, and the effects of endogenous and administered catecholamines.

Most commonly, atrial fibrillation develops on the second or third day after surgery, and the reason for this delay is not clear. For most patients, the ventricular rate response to atrial fibrillation is usually 110 to 150 beats per minute, and this rate is generally well tolerated. With the onset of tachycardia, however, the patient frequently feels warm, becomes diaphoretic, and may become anxious. Thus, it is useful to warn patients preoperatively about the possibility (and the generally benign nature) of postoperative atrial fibrillation. Algorithms useful for the prediction of patients most likely to experience atrial fibrillation following CABG have been developed (87,88).

Patients with marginal cardiac function who develop atrial fibrillation may suffer hemodynamic deterioration due to loss of the normal synchronized "atrial kick" that contributes about 10% to 15% to the cardiac output. Rare patients suffer extreme tachycardia (more than 200 beats per minute) with severe hypotension. Atrial fibrillation is usually recognized by the irregular nature of the ventricular response. Analysis of the patient's arterial blood pressure monitor tracing usually aids in the diagnosis. If the ventricular response is uniform, making the diagnosis more difficult, an atrial electrogram may be obtained by recordings from the atrial pacing wires that were implanted at surgery (Fig. 4.2) (79). This will reveal the atrial complexes that are irregular in rhythm, amplitude, and polarity. Intravenously administered adenosine, which blocks atrioventricular conduction, can be used to cause transient slowing of the ventricular rate so that atrial activity can be analyzed. Its action is rapid but evanescent; hence, it is useful only for diagnostic, not therapeutic, purposes.

A treatment strategy for perioperative atrial fibrillation is shown in Fig. 4.3.

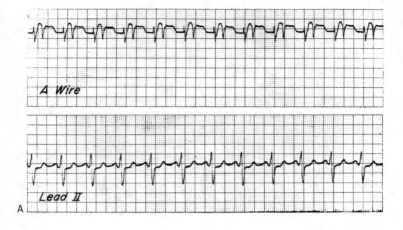

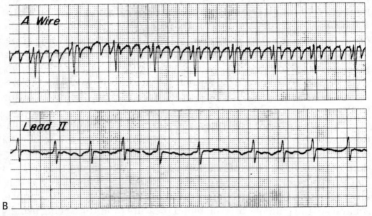

FIGURE 4.2 Atrial electrode tracings. Recordings made from atrial electrodes (*A wire*) and corresponding lead II for a patient with normal sinus rhythm **(A)** and a patient with atrial fibrillation/flutter **(B)**. Atrial activity is much more easily analyzed in the atrial wire tracing than in conventional leads.

Prevention of Postoperative Atrial Fibrillation. Because atrial arrhythmias are so common after cardiac surgery, a variety of drugs, administered prophylactically, have been investigated to attempt to reduce the incidence of their occurrence. These agents include various β-blockers, sotalol, amiodarone, digoxin, procainamide, propafenone, various calcium channel blockers, and magnesium. Many of the studies have

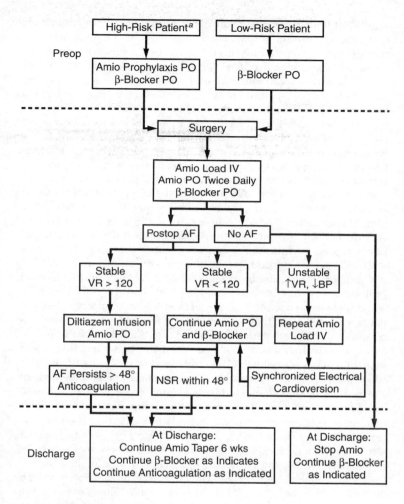

Amio = Amiodarone
VR = Ventricular Response
BP = Blood Pressure

FIGURE 4.3 Atrial fibrillation (AF) management algorithm. NOTE: This is only one of many potential algorithms that may be used to manage AF in cardiac surgery patients. No drug should be administered if contraindications are present. [a]High risk for AF valve surgery, age >70 years, history of paroxysmal AF. AMIO, amiodarone; BP, blood pressure; VR, ventricular response.

significant limitations, and many of the results have been conflicting. One consistent result of most studies, however, is the demonstration that the prophylactic administration of an oral β-blocker reduces the incidence of postoperative atrial fibrillation, by as much as 40% (89,90).

Preoperative treatment with oral *β-blocker* drugs has associated with improved postoperative results for CABG surgery patients and is a measured quality-of-care parameter. One of the major benefits of preoperative β-blockade in cardiac surgery patients is a reduction in the incidence of postoperative atrial fibrillation (91,92). Therefore, in the absence of contraindications such as severe bradycardia or bronchospastic lung disease, preoperative treatment with a β-blocker is standard care. A common dose regimen is metoprolol at 12.5 to 25 mg orally two to four times daily. Typically, the last preoperative dose is given the night before surgery for morning operations or early in the morning for patients undergoing surgery in the afternoon. After surgery, the oral administration of the β-blocker is begun as soon as the patient is able to take pills. Contraindications include heart rate <60 beats per minute and systolic blood pressure <90 mm Hg.

Amiodarone has also been demonstrated to reduce the incidence of postoperative atrial fibrillation and is widely used (92–96). Generally, we administer preoperative prophylactic amiodarone selectively to patients who are judged to be at increase risk for postoperative atrial fibrillation (97,98). Such patients include those undergoing valve procedures, those with a history of previous atrial fibrillation, and those older than 70 years. A common adult dosing schedule is 400 mg orally three times daily for 2 or 3 days prior to surgery or an IV loading dose of 150 mg followed by infusion of 1.0 mg per minute for 12 hours followed by 0.5 mg per minute for 24 hours or up until surgery, whichever comes first. Adverse effects of short-term amiodarone administration include bradycardia and hypotension. Amiodarone may be given to patients also receiving a β-blocker although the adverse effects are likely to be more common. Alternative dosing regiments involve loading the patient with amiodarone intravenously on the day after surgery with an oral dosing for several days after. If atrial fibrillation does not occur, the drug is discontinued at the time of discharge (99).

Many other interventions have been reported to reduce the incidence of postoperative atrial fibrillation. IV *magnesium* administration during surgery and during the early postoperative period has been associated with reduced atrial fibrillation incidence (100,101). Because of this, and the fact that postoperative hypomagnesemia is common after cardiac surgery, we routinely administer magnesium, 2 g IV, in the operating room after weaning the patient from CPB. Some patients also receive postoperative magnesium supplementation (2 g IV every 12 hours for two doses). At hospitals that administer intraoperative magnesium as a component of the cardioplegia solution, this further supplementation may not be advisable and the magnesium level should be measured. Preoperative statin administration has been demonstrated to significantly reduce postop atrial fibrillation, even in patients already receiving β-blocker and/or amiodarone (102,103). Statin administration should be instituted and continued until the time of surgery and restarted soon postoperatively in all patients with hyperlipidemia. Routine administration to all patients undergoing cardiac surgery has not become standard but this may change as further information becomes available.

Sotalol (a β-blocker with additional antiarrhythmic properties), administered prophylactically, has also been demonstrated to reduce postoperative atrial fibrillation (84,92).

Other therapies have been reported to reduce atrial fibrillation after heart surgery although consensus regarding their usefulness are lacking at this time. These include calcium channel blocker drugs, antiinflammatory agents, polyunsaturated fatty acids, postoperative atrial pacing, removal of the aortic fat pad at the time of surgery (ventral cardiac denervation), creation of an incision in the posterior pericardium to facilitate drainage of blood into the chest space, heparin-coated CPB tubing, thoracic epidural anesthesia, and mild hypothermia instead of moderate hypothermia (84,104). Of note, digoxin is not effective (92).

In our practices, all CABG surgery patients receive preoperative β-blocker treatment unless contraindications are present. A statin drug is administered preoperative to patients with hyperlipidemia and/or coronary artery disease. Amiodarone is used instead of the β-blocker in patients with contraindications. Patients at increased risk for atrial fibrillation (this includes most valve surgery patients) receive preoperative amiodarone prophylaxis. All patients receive magnesium in the operating room after the discontinuation of CPB. The β-blocker, amiodarone, and statin therapies are resumed as early after surgery as possible.

Treatment of Atrial Fibrillation. If atrial fibrillation develops, hypoxemia, acidosis, hypokalemia, and hypomagnesemia should be ruled out and, if present, corrected. The serum potassium level should be maintained at 4.2 mEq/L or even 4.5 mEq/L or greater. The method of management of atrial fibrillation depends on the status of the patient. If the patient is hemodynamically compromised, *electrical cardioversion* is the treatment of choice (105). This is especially useful for the patient who develops atrial fibrillation or flutter during the first few hours after surgery and is still intubated and under the effect of general anesthesia. R-wave synchronized cardioversion is performed with external paddles, placed a bit more cephalad across the chest wall than for ventricular defibrillation (to place the atria directly in the path of the delivered energy), and begun using 50 to 100 J (0.2 to 1.0 J/kg for infants). Biphasic shock waveforms are preferred because of greater efficacy with lower energy. It is important to ensure that the *synchronization circuit* of the cardioversion energy source is used to prevent discharge during the vulnerable T wave portion of the patient's ECG, as this may cause in VF. If the patient is awake, pretreatment with a short-acting sedative, such as midazolam, is desirable to prevent pain and memory of the event. If successful conversion is not achieved at the initial energy setting, a higher energy level should be tried.

If the patient has had atrial fibrillation for more than 48 hours and is stable and electrical cardioversion is desired, transesophageal echocardiography may be indicated to rule out the presence of thrombus in the left atrium or atrial appendage. If clot is present, delaying the cardioversion and anticoagulation of the patient is indicated.

Although frequently initially successful, electrical cardioversion of early postoperative atrial arrhythmias often provides only temporary restoration of sinus rhythm, likely because the underlying precipitating factors leading to the development of the arrhythmia remain unchanged. Drug treatment is therefore usually indicated.

When atrial fibrillation or flutter occurs several days after surgery, the patient is usually extubated, hemodynamically stable, and alert. In this situation, drug treatment is usually preferable to electrical cardioversion unless the patient is hemodynamically unstable.

For patients with atrial fibrillation who are hemodynamically relatively stable, the treatment involves *rate control, conversion to sinus rhythm*, and *anticoagulation* if the arrhythmia persists. If the patient's heart rate is <120 beats per minute, treatment to reduce it further is probably not indicated. For those with tachycardia >120 beats per minute, *rate control* may usually be achieved by the administration of β-adrenergic antagonist, a calcium channel blocking drug, or amiodarone (Table 4.4). IV diltiazem is a frequently a preferred choice for this setting

TABLE 4.4	Amiodarone Administration to Treat Postoperative Atrial Fibrillation (Adult Doses)

Loading dose (IV infusion)
- 150 mg over 10–20 min (monitor BP); may repeat in 3–5 min, then
- 1 mg/min for 6 h, then
- 0.5 mg/min until taking orally, then
- 200 mg PO t.i.d. for 1 wk, then
- 200 mg PO b.i.d. for 1 wk, then
- 200 mg PO q.d. for 2 wk, then
- Discontinue amiodarone

b.i.d., twice a day; BP, blood pressure; IV, intravenous; PO, oral; q.d., once daily; t.i.d., three times a day. *Note:* A variety of amiodarone dosing protocols exist. This is one example. The doses should be modified based on patient size. Caution should be used in patients with liver, renal, or pulmonary disease.

as it is quick acting (106). Alternatively, continuous esmolol infusion may be used although this may result in hypotension more often and may contribute to bronchospasm or congestive heart failure. For both drugs, the goal is to reduce the ventricular response to below 110 beats per minute while maintaining the systolic blood pressure above 90 mm Hg.

Multiple drugs are effective in the conversion of atrial fibrillation to sinus rhythm. These include including amiodarone, procainamide, propafenone, ibutilide, flecainide, and sotalol (90,101,107,108). Amiodarone is effective and widely used for the treatment of postoperative atrial fibrillation because it provides both rate control and conversion to sinus rhythm in most patients and it has a favorable side effect profile (109,110). Amiodarone is a complex drug with both α- and β-adrenergic inhibitory action in addition to effects on sodium, potassium, and calcium channels. It may be administered intravenously or orally. It is particularly useful for patients with poor LV function. Table 4.4 lists the typical adult dosing schedule. When given intravenously, the major acute side effects are hypotension and bradycardia, both of which are usually manageable with fluid infusion, pressor drug administration, and temporary pacing, if necessary.

When administered long-term, amiodarone is a potentially toxic drug with multiple side effects and drug interactions. Toxicities include corneal microdeposits, optic neuropathy, blue-gray skin discoloration, photosensitivity, hypothyroidism, pulmonary toxicity, peripheral neuropathy, and hepatotoxicity (111,112). In addition, amiodarone potentiates warfarin anticoagulation and patients receiving maintenance amiodarone doses will usually need a reduction of 25% to 33% in their warfarin dose (113). In general, the short-term use of amiodarone for postoperative arrhythmia treatment has been found to be safe and effective but treated patients should be closely observed, keeping the potential for pulmonary and other toxicities in mind (114,115). For the patient who develops atrial fibrillation after cardiac surgery and who is begun on amiodarone, the oral treatment is usually continued for 2 to 3 months and (assuming sinus rhythm is present) is then discontinued.

Ibutilide is used for conversion of atrial fibrillation to sinus rhythm. Use in the postoperative setting is relatively limited but efficacy has been demonstrated (116). It is, however, associated with ventricular proarrhythmia (specifically torsades de pointes), particularly in patients with very low EFs or heart failure (90). Other agents used to convert atrial fibrillation include propafenone, procainamide, sotalol, and flecainide. Their use for the management of postoperative atrial fibrillation is, however, limited (108).

It is important to note that atrial fibrillation in patients with preexcitation re-entry tachycardia (WPW syndrome) represent a special situation. Such patients are identified by the presence of a δ-wave on the normal sinus rhythm ECG. Treatment with a drug that blocks atrioventricular node conduction (including adenosine, digoxin, verapamil, diltiazem, and possibly β-blockers) is contraindicated and may precipitate serious ventricular arrhythmias, including VF (82,105).

In our practices for the management of acute postoperative atrial fibrillation, we generally administer diltiazem to reduce the ventricular rate to <120 beats per minute and simultaneously begin amiodarone intravenously to promote conversion to sinus rhythm.

Atrial Flutter. Atrial flutter is usually characterized by a regular ventricular response with a rate of about 150 beats per minute. This represents an atrial contraction rate of about 300 per minute with 2:1 atrioventricular block allowing for only every other atrial complex to be conducted and to result in ventricular contraction. The degree of block may, however, be variable resulting in an irregular ventricular response. In atrial flutter, the atrial electrogram will demonstrate regular atrial complexes, usually at 230 to 350 beats per minute, with uniform amplitude and polarity. These atrial "flutter waves" are usually recognizable on the standard ECG tracing and facilitate the diagnosis of atrial flutter. Occasional patients will have faster atrial flutter rates in the range of 340 to 430 beats per minute.

Atrial flutter (but not fibrillation) may be treated by rapid overdrive atrial pacing (80,117). This is performed by using a pacemaker mode that can deliver up to 800 electrical impulses per minute. The pacemaker is connected to the atrial pacing electrodes (not the ventricular, as this may result in VF) and the atrium is captured by pacing at a rate about 20% faster than the underlying atrial rate (which is usually either two or three times the ventricular rate). When monitoring lead II, evidence of atrial capture is seen when the atrial depolarization wave reverses polarity. Rapid atrial pacing is maintained for 10 to 15 seconds and then abruptly stopped. This often results in conversion of atrial flutter to atrial fibrillation, a rhythm generally more easily controlled by medications. Pharmacologic therapy of atrial flutter is the same as that for atrial fibrillation.

Persistent Postoperative Atrial Arrhythmias

Patients with postoperative atrial fibrillation and atrial flutter are at increased risk for thrombotic stroke. If the arrhythmia persists for more than 48 hours, anticoagulation with heparin and/or warfarin is indicated unless contraindications are present (90).

Junctional Ectopic Tachycardia

Postoperative *junctional ectopic tachycardia* is a potentially dangerous arrhythmia that occurs in up to 10% of congenital heart surgery patients. This topic is discussed in Chapter 7.

Ventricular Tachyarrhythmias

Premature ventricular contractions (PVCs) are impulses that arise in an ectopic ventricular focus. While common in adult heart disease patients, they are uncommon in children. When present after surgery, PVCs are usually not a problem in themselves but they may serve as an indicator of less obvious disturbances such as metabolic and electrolyte abnormalities such as hypokalemia, hypoxia, myocardial ischemia, acidosis, alkalosis, or digoxin toxicity. Thus, when new-onset PVCs occur early after surgery, especially at a frequency of >4 to 6 per minute, the patient's blood gases and serum potassium levels should be checked. A 12-lead ECG is indicated to rule out myocardial ischemia. If this is normal and the patient is otherwise stable, specific treatment is not usually required for unifocal, single PVCs. Because of the potential proarrhythmic side effect of most antiarrhythmic drugs, pharmacologic treatment of asymptomatic PVCs can lead to the development of more dangerous arrhythmias in up to 10% of patients. One safe way to eliminate PVCs is by overdrive pacing, in which the atrium is paced at a rate of 5 to 10 beats per minute faster than the native heart rate. When the heart rate increases in this way, there is less time for ectopic pacemakers to become depolarized to threshold levels and to initiate premature beats.

More serious ventricular tachyarrhythmias occur in about 1% of patients after cardiac surgery. Patients with LV hypertrophy and those undergoing ventricular aneurysm or endocardial resection are at greatest risk for this complication. Prophylactic administration of antiarrhythmic agents (such as lidocaine or procainamide) does not necessarily prevent the development of postoperative ventricular arrhythmias in this group of patients and because of their proarrhythmic effects (particularly procainamide), may be counterproductive.

Nonsustained ventricular tachycardia (NSVT) is defined as 3 or more ventricular beats occurring at a rate of more than 100 per minute lasting <30 seconds or without hemodynamic compromise. Occasional episodes of NSVT do not require treatment although it is prudent to rule out hypokalemia, hypomagnesemia, and hypoxia as contributing factors. For patients with NSVT in association with myocardial ischemia or infarction, β-blocker therapy is indicated and prophylactic lidocaine administration is not recommended (118). If episodes of NSVT persist, particularly in association with hemodynamic compromise, administration of amiodarone (loading dose followed by continuous infusion) may be considered.

Sustained VT, even if hemodynamically well tolerated, should be treated immediately because deterioration to VF may occur soon. In general, any wide QRS tachycardia should be treated as ventricular in origin until proven otherwise. If the patient is hemodynamically stable,

treatment of VT may be begun with amiodarone (preferred), procainamide, or lidocaine. If VT persists, synchronized electrical cardioversion is performed.

VF results in sudden total cessation of the cardiac output and must
be treated immediately by electrical defibrillation. See the discussion
regarding cardiac arrest earlier in this chapter for further details.

PERIOPERATIVE MYOCARDIAL ISCHEMIA AND INFARCTION

Myocardial ischemia, either transient or irreversible leading to infarction, may occur during and after cardiac surgery. Early recognition of
the presence of myocardial ischemia can lead to treatment to limit the
damage that occurs and to support the patient's hemodynamic status.
In the case of coronary spasm, prompt treatment can result in complete
reversal of the condition.

Perioperative Infarction

When rigorously searched for with frequent ECGs and enzyme determinations, the incidence of perioperative MI for first time (primary) coronary
bypass operations is as high as 10% (119). The incidence in repeat (redo)
coronary operations is even greater. There appears to be no difference in
the MI rate for CABG procedures performed "off pump" as compared with
those using CPB (120). While the perioperative MI rate is lower in valvular
and congenital procedures, the potential for MI due to coronary artery injury or embolism is present with all open heart surgeries. Unless extensive
ECG and enzymatic is performed, many perioperative MIs go unnoticed.
Not surprisingly, the operative mortality in those with perioperative in-
farcts is increased, as is the incidence of major adverse cardiovascular
events (121,122). Furthermore, both the patient's postoperative health-related quality of life and long-term survival are adversely affected (123,124).
Efforts to identify preoperative factors predictive of perioperative MI have
had conflicting results although patients with diabetes and those undergoing repeat operations consistently have a higher rate of MI.

The diagnosis of perioperative MI may be difficult as there is a con-
tinuum of myocardial injury ranging from a small degree of injury to full-
blown transmural infarction with the development of classic (new Q-
wave) electrocardiography changes. Release of myocardial creatine
kinase-myocardial band (CK-MB) isoenzyme is the most studied method
to detect perioperative myocardial ischemia and correlation with long-
term outcome. The usual pattern of CK-MB release results in a peak of
serum enzyme concentrations at 12 to 16 hours after surgery; some release occurs in nearly all patients who undergo cardiac surgery of any type.
A significantly greater peak serum level and a more prolonged period of
enzyme elevation, however, are observed in those patients who, by other

tests, are found to suffer perioperative infarction. In general, for adult coronary bypass surgery patients, peak postoperative CK-MB activity of <20 U/L (with no ECG changes) suggests no significant myocardial injury while CK-MB activity of more than 50 U/L suggests perioperative infarction (125). Various other CK-MB "cutoff" levels have been suggested to make the diagnosis of perioperative MI. Large infarctions are associated with peak CK-MB more than ten times the upper limit of normal. Following CABG, CK-MB release of more than five to eight times the upper limit of the reference range is associated with reduced 40-month survival (126).

Troponin I is a cardiac-specific regulatory protein that is released as a result of cardiac, but not skeletal, muscle injury. Following MI, troponin I peaks later (36 hours), and elevated levels persist longer than CK-MB. Troponin measurement in CABG surgery patients with impaired renal function must be interpreted with caution (127). Experience has demonstrated that the troponin level can be used to identify myocardial damage with the magnitude of the enzyme rise correlating with the amount of injury and elevated levels are generally associated with poorer outcomes (123,128–131).

Significant transmural MI is usually (but not always) associated with ECG changes. The patterns of ECG changes according to the location of the infarct are summarized in Table 4.5. The postoperative ECG is not as sensitive as cardiac enzyme analysis for the diagnosis of

 TABLE 4.5 Electrocardiographic (ECG) Identification of Acute Myocardial Infarction (MI) Location

ECG changes associated with transmural MI
1. Hyperacute or inverted T waves
2. ST-segment elevation
3. New Q wave (longer than 0.04 second duration or >1/3 height of QRS complex)

ECG changes associated with non–Q wave (subendocardial) MI
1. ST-segment depression
2. Inverted T waves

Location of Infarction	ECG Leads Demonstrating ECG Changes Listed Above
Anteroseptal	V_1, V_2
Anteroapical	V_2, V_3
Anterolateral	V_4–V_6, aVL
Large anterior	V_1–V_6
Lateral	I, aVL, V_5, V_6
Inferior	II, III, aVF
Posterior[a]	V_1, V_2, V_3

[a]The changes in a posterior MI are mirror images of those in anterior infarctions, i.e., inverted hyperacute T-waves and ST-segment depression.

perioperative infarction, and even the presence of new Q waves may not be 100% diagnostic (132). A significant number of patients will have "diagnostic" elevations of CK-MB but will not demonstrate new Q waves.

A recent consensus panel has defined perioperative MI as increase in cardiac enzymes (preferably troponin) greater than five times the 99th percentile of the upper limit of normal in addition to either new pathologic Q waves or new left bundle branch block, or angiographically documented new graft or native coronary artery occlusion, or imaging evidence of new loss of viable myocardium (133).

Perioperative MI may occur during surgery (due to injury to a coronary artery or intracoronary embolism) or may occur early after the operation (due to closure of a bypass graft). Grafts that suffer early closure are often grafts that have been placed to small, diffusely diseased arteries. The amount of myocardium at risk may be limited and graft closure may not be clinically recognized. On the other hand, closure of a graft to a major artery that is perfusing a large amount of myocardium may be quite serious. In general, however, early postoperative graft patency cannot be predicted on the basis of elevated postoperative cardiac enzymes alone. Electrocardiographic correlation improves the ability to make the diagnosis of closure of a graft. Even so, the diagnosis of perioperative MI does not correlate well with the presence of bypass graft closure. Many patients with a closed graft will not have an MI and patients with a perioperative MI may have no closed grafts.

Patients suspected to have suffered an uncomplicated perioperative MI are treated the same as those who experience a non–surgery-related infarction with early institution of aspirin and β-blocker therapies. Antithrombotic treatment with heparin is usually contraindicated during the early postoperative period. Complications such as low cardiac output and arrhythmias are managed as described elsewhere in this chapter. Prophylactic antiarrhythmia drug administration is not indicated. After recovery, it is useful to measure the patient's EF by echocardiography to determine the extent of damage incurred. Not uncommonly, it is found that no significant decrease in the EF has occurred, a finding that can be reassuring for the patient and the surgeon alike.

Coronary Artery Spasm

Coronary artery spasm during the early postoperative period after cardiac surgery (most commonly CABG procedures) can be an unrecognized cause of sudden, severe cardiovascular collapse that may be fatal (134,135). This complication often presents as acute hypotension with the ECG demonstrating ST-segment elevation, although VT, fibrillation, or atrioventricular block also may occur as initial manifestations. When this happens in the operating room, nitroglycerin may be injected directly into vein grafts for relief of the spasm. When it occurs in the postoperative patient, treatment with IV nitroglycerin, diltiazem, and/or isosorbide dinitrate is begun. The ability to administer these agents may be limited, however, by the development of hypotension. Emergency coronary arteriography to confirm the diagnosis of coronary spasm and for direct injection of vasodilator drugs into the affected coronary artery or vein graft grafts is likely the most effective management strategy. If this fails, successful stenting of coronary spasm has been reported (136). If the patient is severely hypotensive or suffers cardiac arrest, emergency sternotomy should be performed for open cardiac massage and direct injection of vasodilator drugs into the saphenous vein grafts (e.g., nitroglycerin in 0.2-mg increments).

The radial artery is also used as bypass conduit for coronary artery bypass grafting and is susceptible to spasm. This complication, with resultant myocardial ischemia, may occur in up to 5% to 10% of patients who receive radial artery grafts. Prophylactic treatment with various agents, including nitrates, calcium channel blockers, phosphodiesterase inhibitors, α-blockers, and combinations of these, have been described in an effort to prevent postoperative radial artery spasm (137). Consensus regarding the optimal treatment has not yet been reached. In our practices, patients are frequently treated early postoperatively with IV nitroglycerin and then switched to oral isosorbide mononitrate or diltiazem for a period of 1 month following surgery.

PULMONARY COMPLICATIONS

Abnormalities of gas exchange or ventilation are not unusual after cardiac surgery. In fact, nearly all patients develop atelectasis to various degrees. Preoperative identification of patients at risk for pulmonary complications and proper attention to postoperative pulmonary care will help minimize the incidence and severity of these complications. Adults with acquired heart disease may have been heavy cigarette smokers and may suffer significant chronic obstructive lung disease. Despite the preoperative presence of significantly abnormal pulmonary function test results, however, successful surgery may usually be achieved in these patients (138). Thus, even severe preoperative pulmonary dysfunction is not usually a contraindication to cardiac surgery when the benefits of the planned operation are judged to outweigh the risk. Preoperative pulmonary (spirometric) function testing and blood gas determination will aid in determining the patient's risk of postoperative pulmonary complications and will provide baseline information for postoperative comparison (139).

Atelectasis

Radiographic evidence of atelectasis is present during the early postoperative period in most patients who have undergone heart surgery. Most commonly, the left lower lobe is affected, the degree of atelectasis is subsegmental, and the radiographic appearance is exacerbated after the patient is extubated. Examination of the patient usually reveals crackles (rales), even though congestive heart failure is not present.

Although the sternotomy incision is less painful and less debilitating than lateral thoracotomy incisions, a significant decrease in pulmonary function still occurs after cardiac surgery via this approach. CPB increases lung water content thus resulting in further abnormalities of ventilation and gas exchange early after surgery. In adults undergoing coronary bypass procedures, there is a reduction of at least 25% to 50% in forced vital capacity and forced expiratory volume in 1 second postoperatively. This decrease may be larger in patients who have undergone mobilization of the internal mammary artery than those who have not (140). Vigorous pulmonary toilet, with frequent use of the incentive spirometer and early ambulation, is generally effective treatment for postoperative atelectasis. As the patient becomes more active, the atelectasis clears although some may remain radiographically evident on the predischarge chest x-ray. Continuous positive airway pressure (CPAP) in the form of nasal CPAP may be useful in reducing postoperative atelectasis and pulmonary complications (141). Bronchoscopy is rarely necessary to remove secretions.

Bronchospasm

Bronchospasm is occasionally encountered either intra- or postoperatively. Patients at increased risk are those with pre-existing asthma and those who suffer chronic obstructive lung disease with a reactive component. When present during closure of the sternum, hyperinflation of the lungs may cause hypotension due to compression of the heart as the sternal halves are being brought together. If present during the early postoperative period in the ventilated patient, severe bronchospasm may result in hypoxemia and high-ventilatory pressures.

Acute bronchospasm is treated by the administration of β-adrenergic bronchodilators, most commonly by the inhalation route. For the patient suffering acute bronchospasm inhalation administration of epinephrine may also be performed and is effective. Drugs with more selective β-2 action, such as albuterol and metaproterenol will have less cardiovascular effects (predominantly tachycardia) and a longer duration of action. These may be administered via the endotracheal tube from a nebulizer or from a metered-dose inhaler. Low-dose epinephrine infusion (0.5 to 1.0 μg per minute) may also be effective for reducing bronchospasm. Corticosteroids, although slower to act, are also effective and do not result in wound-healing problems when used as a short course during the perioperative period (142). For patients with known severe reactive airway disease, we frequently administer steroids several hours preoperatively and for a few days postoperatively. Chronic bronchospasm may be treated with inhaled corticosteroids, the nonsteroidal anti-inflammatory agent cromolyn sodium, and/or theophylline. These agents are not, however, generally used for acute management of bronchospasm following cardiac surgery.

It should be remembered that bronchospasm might be a manifestation of pulmonary edema. Thus, for the postoperative patient with new-onset dyspnea and wheezing, a chest x-ray is indicated. If pulmonary edema is present, diuresis is the mainstay of the treatment although bronchodilator therapy may still be of use.

Phrenic Nerve Injury

Temporary or permanent injury to one or both phrenic nerves may occur during cardiac surgery. In some patients, this occurs as the result of direct trauma such as during mobilization of the internal mammary artery or during a difficult dissection in a patient undergoing reoperation. In others, it may be the result of cold injury if ice-saline slush was placed within the pericardial sac during aortic crossclamping for the purpose of myocardial protection.

In adults undergoing surgery using topical ice slush, radiographic evidence of phrenic nerve dysfunction may occur in up to 25% of patients. This is associated with an increased incidence of postoperative atelectasis and the appearance of an elevated (usually left) hemidiaphragm on postoperative chest radiographs (143). While many adult patients with unilateral phrenic nerve dysfunction may not be severely compromised, if both phrenic nerves are injured, severe morbidity may result (144). Use of a foam pad placed between the ice and the pericardium to insulate the left phrenic nerve from the slush can effectively lower the incidence of this complication. Thus, some use an insulating pad routinely and others use cold saline irrigation instead of slush. In most adults, postoperative phrenic nerve dysfunction does not result in serious consequences and diaphragmatic function returns with time, although up to 25% of those affected do not fully recover diaphragmatic function, which may be particularly debilitating for patients with preoperative chronic obstructive pulmonary disease (145).

In children, diaphragmatic paralysis occurs in up to 5% of patients and can be a serious problem (146,147). Infants do not tolerate loss of hemidiaphragmatic function as well as adults and may not be able to be weaned from mechanical ventilation as the result of the injury.

Definitive diagnosis of diaphragmatic paralysis is based on the demonstration of paradoxical movement of the diaphragm during fluoroscopic or ultrasound examination. In the patient who is receiving positive-pressure ventilation, the paralyzed diaphragm may appear normal on the chest x-ray; thus, one of these tests is necessary to confirm the diagnosis of phrenic nerve paralysis. Diaphragmatic paralysis should be suspected in the pediatric patient who cannot be weaned from the ventilator as expected. In some children, diaphragmatic function will return, but if ventilatory dependency continues, early consideration should be given to performing a diaphragmatic plication procedure (142,148).

Phrenic nerve dysfunction following heart–lung and lung transplantation is an important clinical problem that results in prolonged need for ventilator support and intensive care unit stay (149).

Prolonged Respiratory Insufficiency

Most patients are extubated within 6 hours of surgery. Some patients, particularly the elderly ones or those who have had long operations, may be too somnolent for early extubation. In these patients, ventilator support is continued and repeated efforts to wean are made; extubation is usually achieved within 24 hours.

Postoperative respiratory failure occurs in nearly 10% of adult patients. This complication is more common in patients undergoing complicated procedures (e.g., valve and CABG combined), patients with advanced age, current smoking, poor LV function, renal failure, intraoperative instability, and the need for intra-aortic balloon pump (150,151). After 24 hours, failure to wean is usually due to oxygenation failure [characterized by low partial pressure of oxygen (Po_2) levels], ventilatory failure [with high partial pressure of carbon dioxide (Pco_2) levels], or both.

When weaning failure occurs, efforts are directed at optimization of the patient's cardiac performance and volume status, correction of ongoing metabolic abnormalities, reduction in narcotic and sedative drug administration, and provision of sufficient nutrition. Bronchoscopy may be indicated, particularly if bronchial mucus plugging is suspected to be present.

Patients who need prolonged positive-pressure ventilation require careful management. No patient dependent on a respirator for his or her life should be left unattended. Ventilator alarm systems must remain activated at all times. Periods off the respirator (required for tracheal care, x-ray films, etc.) must be limited to 1 or 2 minutes at a time, and the patient's cutaneous pulse oximetry saturation monitor should be watched closely. Whenever a patient appears to be ventilated improperly or if there is any question of ventilator malfunction, the nurse, respiratory therapist, or physician in attendance should immediately begin hand ventilation while the problem is being resolved.

Determining the adequacy of mechanical ventilation is based on both physical examination, pulse oximetric measurement of the arterial oxygen saturation, and arterial blood gas analysis. The patient who "looks comfortable" may be surprisingly hypoxic; thus the use of pulse oximetry to continuously measure the patient's arterial oxygen saturation is standard. The pulse oximeter, however, does not provide information regarding Pco_2 and acid–base status and should not be relied on as the sole method of monitoring the ventilator-dependent patient. Periodic blood gas determinations are essential.

A useful method of quantitating the lung's ability to transfer oxygenate to the blood is to determine the alveolar–arterial (A–a) gradient:

$$\text{A–a gradient} = [713(F_{IO_2}) - (Pa_{CO_2}/0.8)] - Pa_{O_2}$$

The A–a gradient is an estimate of the degree of intrapulmonary shunting. The normal value for a young patient is approximately 10, rising to 25 for the elderly patient. The A–a gradient can be measured periodically to provide a valuable objective index of progress in patients who cannot undergo extubation early after surgery.

An early goal of prolonged ventilatory management is to reduce the patient's inspired oxygen concentration [fractional inspired oxygen (F_{IO_2})] to below 50%. Prolonged exposure to concentrations above this level is associated with detrimental changes in the lungs. Thus, we use the lowest F_{IO_2} that will yield an arterial oxygen saturation of 92% to 94%. The addition of PEEP will frequently allow for improved oxygenation at lower F_{IO_2}. Patients who are fluid-overloaded (as are many cardiac surgery patients early after operation) should undergo vigorous diuresis as long as adequate cardiac function is maintained. For some patients, especially those with concomitant renal insufficiency, venovenous hemofiltration can be very useful. This technique provides for the removal of excess fluid in addition to the elimination of cardiopulmonary toxic substances that may be contributing to the respiratory failure.

The patient undergoing prolonged ventilatory support must not be allowed to starve. Failure to maintain nutrition may impair respiratory muscle function and further hamper efforts at weaning the patient from the ventilator. If it is anticipated that extubation and normal feeding are more than a few days away (or if a few days have already passed), then nutrition must begin. If bowel activity is present, a soft small-bore nasogastric tube is used for enteral feedings; if not, central venous hyperalimentation is begun.

Preferences for the route of endotracheal intubation differ among institutions. In general, the oral route is preferred when the period of intubation is expected to be short. This route of intubation is often easier to perform but can cause trauma to the mouth and is uncomfortable for the awake patient. The nasal route is more comfortable but is associated with sinusitis and pressure necrosis of the skin of the nares (contributed to, in some patients, by low cardiac output).

Prolonged endotracheal intubation is uncomfortable and has the potential for local complications such as vocal cord ulceration and posterior commissure stenosis. Performance of a tracheostomy provides for better patient comfort, lower airway resistance, reduced bacterial contamination of the lower airway, and is useful during a slow weaning protocol. This latter feature is particularly valuable as the patient may be disconnected from the ventilator (or placed on a positive-pressure support system) for increasingly longer periods of time as the ability to breathe on his or her own improves. This avoids the trials of extubation and, sometimes, reintubation, which are traumatic and dangerous for the patient and may be required to wean the patient from prolonged endotracheal intubation. In the past, it has been suspected that tracheostomy early after sternotomy incision may be a risk factor for the subsequent development of a deep sternal wound infection although recently this proposition has been challenged (152,153). Because tracheostomy is frequently very useful in weaning the patient with postoperative respiratory failure from the ventilator, we generally consider tracheostomy after 7 to 10 days of ventilator dependency or repeated failures at extubation. Use of the percutaneous dilatational tracheostomy technique may be preferable for surgeons who have experience with this method (154,155).

Acute Respiratory Distress Syndrome

Acute respiratory distress syndrome (ARDS) is a form of severe respiratory insufficiency that may occur in the presence of relatively normal cardiac function. It is characterized by injury to both the alveolar vascular endothelial and the alveolar epithelial cells resulting in increased capillary permeability, alveolar flooding, impaired removal of edema fluid from the alveolar space, and reduced surfactant production (156). This results in extravasation of protein-containing fluid in the alveolar space, hypoxemia, decreased lung compliance, increased work of breathing, diffuse pulmonary infiltrates on chest radiograph, and pulmonary hypertension (157). Although the cause is not known, ARDS appears to result from, at least in part, a florid inflammatory process that has been termed *systemic inflammatory response syndrome*, which may be contributed to the use of CPB (158). ARDS after cardiac surgery is rare, occurring in <1% of patients, but has a high mortality rate (159,160).

Treatment of postoperative ARDS is largely supportive. Prevention and treatment of infections and nutritional supplementation (preferably by the enteral route) are important. Diuresis to reduce preload while maintaining adequate cardiac output may be helpful in reducing extravascular lung water. The optimal method of ventilator management for patients with ARDS is not clear. However, the use of smaller tidal volumes (6 mL/kg body weight) to avoid alveolar distension and maintaining plateau pressure (airway pressure after a 0.5-second pause at the end of inspiration) below 30 cm H_2O has been associated with lower ARDS mortality (161,162). A moderate level of PEEP (5 to 8 cm H_2O) is used to lower the FIO_2 to below 60% while maintaining the arterial saturation above 90%, if possible. A relatively high ventilatory rate may be needed to prevent severe hypercarbia. At present, there are no medications currently used for the specific early treatment of ARDS; routine use of steroids is not recommended.

Transfusion-related acute lung injury is an immune-mediated, underrecognized, complication that is reported to occur following approximately 1 of 2,000 red blood cell transfusions, although it may also occur after the transfusion of other blood products (163). Characterized by the presence of noncardiogenic pulmonary edema, the patient experiences dyspnea, cough, fever, pulmonary infiltrates, and hypoxia (164–166). Most reactions occur within 6 hours of the transfusion. Management is essentially the same as for other forms of ARDS.

Pneumothorax

Pneumothorax may occur in patients after open heart surgery, especially when they are receiving positive-pressure ventilation. It is more common in those with pre-existing obstructive or bullous disease and those requiring significant levels of PEEP. Tension pneumothorax may develop quickly in the mechanically ventilated patient; this possibility should be kept in mind during the evaluation of a patient who has suddenly decompensated. Although breath sounds may be diminished on the affected side, the noise produced by the ventilator and other noise in the intensive care unit may cause the breath sounds to appear equal despite the presence of a large pneumothorax. Other clues to the presence of tension pneumothorax include distended neck veins and tracheal deviation away from the involved hemithorax. If the patient is severely hypotensive and a pneumothorax is strongly suspected, treatment is begun by inserting a 16-gauge IV catheter (cannula-over-needle type) into the pleural space. A rush of air exiting from the chest through the cannula, associated with hemodynamic improvement of the patient, confirms the diagnosis. If the patient is sufficiently stable, then a chest x-ray may be obtained before definitive therapy (167). This will reveal collapse of the lung and, if tension is present, shifting of the mediastinal structures away from the affected side.

Definitive therapy is the placement of a chest tube (Fig. 4.4). The insertion site is usually at the fourth or fifth interspace in the anterior axillary line. For pneumothorax, the tube is directed superiorly. For adequate drainage of blood or fluid, the tube should be directed either posteriorly or along the diaphragm. The anterior axillary line is preferred because more posteriorly located tubes are more uncomfortable.

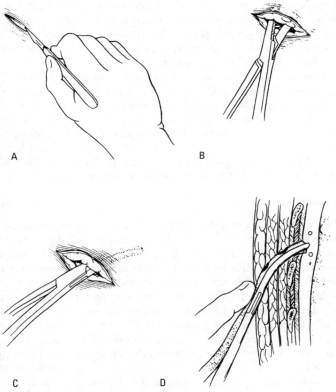

FIGURE 4.4 Insertion of a chest tube. A chest tube may be inserted safely, even in patients with coagulopathy who are on ventilators, if proper technique is used. Under local anesthesia, a small incision is made and a tunnel dissected bluntly through the subcutaneous tissues to the rib (**A**). A tract through the intercostal muscles is created bluntly *over* the superior surface of the rib selected to avoid trauma to the intercostal vessels that follow the inferior edge (**B** and **C**). A gloved finger may be inserted into the pleural space to verify that the lung is not adherent, if in doubt. A pleural tube of adequate caliber (*not* a Foley catheter) is guided into the pleural space with a clamp (**D**), attached to a water seal drainage system, and sutured securely.

The diaphragm rises as high as the sixth intercostal space laterally; therefore, the insertion site should not be lower than this interspace.

Pleural Effusions

Postoperative pleural effusions are very common in cardiac surgery patients, occurring in 40% to 90% of patients depending on the modality used to make the diagnosis (168). Typically, the effusions become evident after the second postoperative day, are usually small in size, and are most often on the left side. They may be more common in patients who have had the internal mammary artery mobilized for use as coronary artery bypass conduit. The use of ice slush for cooling of the heart may also be a contributing factor. Patients with chronic congestive heart failure frequently have pleural effusions before surgery and although these may be drained during surgery, it is not unusual for the effusions to recur. Thus, for these patients we often place separate, laterally located, soft (Blake) drains that remain in place postoperatively until the daily drainage is <100 to 150 mL on each side. These are place in addition to the larger bore chest tubes placed anteriorly to drain the mediastinum.

Most postoperative effusions, particularly smaller ones, will resolve with diuresis and time. Larger effusions, particularly in patients with impaired lung function, will result in dyspnea and will require drainage. Most often, in our practices, drainage is achieved by ultrasound-guided thoracentesis performed by the radiologist. In a few patients, significant effusions will recur and require repeat thoracentesis or chest tube placement. Rarely, the effusion is difficult to drain (often due to loculations) and causes compression and entrapment of the lung. For these patients, decortication may be indicated (169).

Chylothorax, due to injury to the thoracic duct, is a rare complication that may occur especially in children who undergo surgery for congenital lesions. Continued drainage of the protein-rich fluid may result in malnutrition. Conservative management includes closed drainage, total parenteral nutrition, and a diet of medium chain triglycerides. In some patients, chylothorax is a major problem and may require treatment by thoracic duct ligation, application of fibrin glue, talc pleurodesis, and/or pleuroperitoneal shunt (170). For adults with chylothorax, the use of video-assisted thoracoscopy has been advocated (171).

References

1. Reynolds HR, Hochman JS. Cardiogenic shock: current concepts and improving outcomes. *Circulation* 2008;117:686–697.
2. Rao V, Ivanov J, Weisel RD, et al. Predictors of low cardiac output syndrome after coronary artery bypass. *J Thorac Cardiovasc Surg* 1996;112:38–51.

3. Beattie S. Heart failure with preserved LV function: pathophysiology, clinical presentation, treatment, and nursing implications. *J Cardiovasc Nurs* 2000; 14(4):24–37.

4. Dietl CA, Berkheimer MD, Woods EL, et al. Efficacy and cost-effectiveness of preoperative IABP in patients with ejection fraction of 0.25 or less. *Ann Thorac Surg* 1996;62:401–409.

5. Dyub Am, Whitlock RP, Abouzahr LL, et al. Preoperative intra-aortic balloon pump in patients undergoing coronary bypass surgery: a systematic review and meta-analysis. *J Card Surg* 2008;23:79–86.

6. Doty DB. The surgeon's response to a low-output state after cardiopulmonary bypass: etiologies and remedies. *J Cardiac Surg* 1990;5:256–262.

7. Reichert SL, Visser CA, Koolen JJ, et al. Transesophageal echocardiography in hypotensive patients after cardiac surgery. Comparison with hemodynamic parameters. *J Thorac Cardiovasc Surg* 1992;104:321–326.

8. Little WC, Freeman GL. Pericardial disease. *Circulation* 2006;113:1622–1632.

9. Hosokawa K, Nakajima Y. An evaluation of acute cardiac tamponade by trans-esophageal echocardiography. *Anesth Analg* 2008;106:61–62.

10. Hartzler GO, Maloney JD, Curtis JJ, et al. Hemodynamic benefits of atrioven-tricular sequential pacing after cardiac surgery. *Am J Cardiol* 1977;40:232–236.

11. Eichorn EJ, Diehl JT, Konstam, MA, et al. Left ventricular inotropic effect of atrial pacing after coronary artery bypass grafting. *Am J Cardiol* 1989;632: 687–692.

12. Insler SR, O'Connor MS, Leventhal MJ, et al. Association between postopera-tive hypothermia and adverse outcome after coronary artery bypass surgery. *Ann Thorac Surg* 2000;70:175–181.

13. Kim YD, Katz NM, Ng L, et al. Effects of hypothermia and hemodilution on oxygen metabolism and hemodynamics in patients recovering from coronary artery bypass operations. *J Thorac Cardiovasc Surg* 1989;97:36–42.

14. Kranke P, Eberhart LH, Roewer N, et al. Pharmacologic treatment of postoper-ative shivering: a quantitative systematic review of randomized controlled tri-als. *Anesth Analg* 2002;94:453–460.

15. Kastrup M, Markewitz A, Spies C, et al. Current practice of hemodynamic monitoring and vasopressor and inotropic therapy in post-operative cardiac surgery patients in Germany: results from a postal survey. *Acta Anesthesiol Scand* 2007;51:347–358.

16. Holmes CL. Vasoactive drugs in the intensive care unit. *Curr Opin Crit Care* 2005;11:413–417.

17. DiSesa VJ. The rational selection of inotropic drugs in cardiac surgery. *J Car-diac Surg* 1987;2:385–391.

18. Doyle AR, Dhir AK, Moors AH, et al. Treatment of perioperative low cardiac output syndrome. *Ann Thorac Surg* 1995;59:S3–S11.

19. Dunning J, Khasati N, Barnard J. Low dose (renal dose) dopamine in the criti-cally ill patient. *Interact Cardiovasc Thorac Surg* 2004;3:114–117.

20. Schenarts PJ, Sagrafves SG, Bard MR, et al. Low-dose dopamine: a physiologi-cally based review. *Curr Surg* 2006;63:219–215.

21. Gillies M, Bellomo R, Doolan L, et al. Bench-to-bedside review: inotropic drug therapy after adult cardiac surgery—a systematic literature review. *Crit Care* 2005; 9:266–279.

22. Fowler MB, Alderman EL, Oesterle SN, et al. Dobutamine and dopamine after cardiac surgery: greater augmentation of myocardial blood flow with dobuta-mine. *Circulation* 1984;70:1103–1111.

23. Disesa VJ, Brown E, Mudge GH, et al. Hemodynamic comparison of dopamine and dobutamine in the postoperative volume-loaded, pressure-loaded and normal ventricle. *J Thorac Cardiovasc Surg* 1982;83:256–263.
24. Totaro RJ, Raper RF. Epinephrine-induced lactic acidosis following cardiopulmonary bypass. *Crit Care Med* 1997;25:1693–1699.
25. Heringlake M, Wernerus M, Grunefeld J, et al. The metabolic and renal effect of adrenaline and milrinone in patients with myocardial dysfunction after coronary artery bypass grafting. *Crit. Care* 2007;11:R51. http://ccforum.com/content/11/2/R51.
26. Butterworth JF IV, Prielipp RC, Royster RL, et al. Dobutamine increases heart rate more than epinephrine in patients recovering from aortocoronary bypass surgery. *J Cardiothorac Vasc Anesth* 1992;6:535–541.
27. Balderman SC, Aldridge J. Pharmacologic support of the myocardium following aortocoronary bypass surgery: a comparative study. *J Clin Pharmacol* 1986;26:175–183.
28. Lathi KG, Shulman MS, Diehl JT, et al. The use of amrinone and norepinephrine for inotropic support during emergence from cardiopulmonary bypass. *J Cardiothorac Vasc Anesth* 1991;5:250–254.
29. Levy JH, Bailey JM, Deeb GM. Intravenous milrinone in cardiac surgery. *Ann Thorac Surg* 2002;73:325–330.
30. Lobato EB, Urdaneta F, Martin TD, et al. Effects of milrinone versus epinephrine on grafted internal mammary artery flow after cardiopulmonary bypass. *J Cardiothorac Vasc Anesth* 2000;14:9–11.
31. Kikura M, Levy JH, Michelsen LG, et al. The effect of milrinone on hemodynamics and left ventricular function after emergence from cardiopulmonary bypass. *Anesth Analg* 1997;85:16–22.
32. Yamada T, Takeda J, Katori N, et al. Hemodynamic effects of milrinone during weaning from cardiopulmonary bypass: comparison of patients with a low and high prebypass cardiac index. *J Cardiothorac Vasc Anesth* 2000;14:367–373.
33. Feneck RO, Sherry KM, Withington PS, et al. Comparison of the hemodynamic effects of milrinone with dobutamine in patients after cardiac surgery. *J Cardiothorac Vasc Anesth* 2001;15:306–315.
34. Kikura M, Sato S. The efficacy of preemptive milrinone or amrinone therapy in patients undergoing coronary artery bypass grafting. *Anesth Analg* 2002;94:22–30.
35. Hauptman PJ, Kelly RA. Digitalis. *Circulation* 1999;99:1265–1270.
36. Mullis-Jansson SL, Argenziano M, Corwin S, et al. A randomized double-blind study of the effect of triiodothyronine on cardiac function and morbidity after coronary bypass surgery. *J Thorac Cardiovasc Surg* 1999;117:1128–1135.
37. Klemperer JD, Klein I, Gomez M, et al. Thyroid hormone treatment after coronary-artery bypass surgery. *N Engl J Med* 1995;333:522–1527.
38. Lazar HL, Philippides G, Fitgerald C, et al. Glucose-insulin-potassium solutions enhance recovery after urgent coronary artery bypass grafting. *J Thorac Cardiovasc Surg* 1997;113:354–362.
39. Bothe W, Olschewski M, Beyersdorf F, et al. Glucose-insulin-potassium in cardiac surgery: a meta-analysis. *Ann Thorac Surg* 2004;78:1650–1658.
40. Burger AJ. A review of the renal and neurohormonal effects of B-type natriuretic peptide. *Congest Heart Fail* 2005;11:30–38.
41. Mentzer RM, Oz MC, Sladen RN, et al. Effects of perioperative nesiritide in patients with left ventricular dysfunction undergoing cardiac surgery. *J Am Coll Cardiol* 2007;49:716–726.

42. Salzberg SP, Filsoufi F, Anyanwu A, et al. High-risk mitral valve surgery: perioperative hemodynamic optimization with nesiritide (BNP). *Ann Thorac Surg* 2005;80:502–506.
43. Gordon GR, Schumann R, Rastegar H, et al. Nesiritide for treatment of perioperative low cardiac output syndromes in cardiac surgical patients: an initial experience. *J Anesth* 2006;20:307–311.
44. Brackbill ML, Stam MD, Schuller-Williams RV, et al. Perioperative nesiritide versus milrinone in high-risk coronary artery bypass graft patients. *Ann Pharmacother* 2007;41:427–432.
45. Sackner-Bernstein JD, Kowalski M, Fox M, et al. Short-term risk of death after treatment with nesiritide for decompensated heart failure: a pooled analysis of randomized controlled trials. *JAMA* 2005;293:1900–1905.
46. Simsic JM, Scheurer M, Tobias JD, et al. Perioperative effects and safety of nesiritide following cardiac surgery in children. *J Intensive Med* 2006;21:22–26.
47. Trost JC, Hillis LD. Intra-aortic balloon counterpulsation. *Am J Cardiol* 2006;97:1391–1398.
48. Vlahakes GJ. Management of pulmonary hypertension and right ventricular failure: another step forward. *Ann Thorac Surg* 1996;61:1051–1052.
49. Alsaddique AA. Recognition of diastolic heart failure in the postoperative heart. *Eur J Cardiothorac Surg* 2008;34:1141–1148.
50. Alsaddique AA, Royse AG, Royse CF, et al. Management of diastolic heart failure following cardiac surgery. *Eur J Cardiothorac Surg* 2009;35:241–249.
51. Robitaille A, Denault AY, Couture P, et al. Importance of relative pulmonary hypertension in cardiac surgery: the mean systemic-to-pulmonary artery pressure ratio. *J Cardiothorac Vasc Surg* 2006;20:331–339.
52. Piazza G, Goldhaver SZ. The acutely decompensated right ventricle: pathways for diagnosis and management. *Chest* 2005;128:1836–1852.
53. Fullerton DA, Jaggers J, Wollmering MM, et al. Variable response to inhaled nitric oxide after cardiac surgery. *Ann Thorac Surg* 1997;63:1251–1256.
54. George I, Xydas S, Topkara VK, et al. Clinical indication for use and outcomes after inhaled nitric oxide therapy. *Ann Thorac Surg* 2006;82:2161–2169.
55. Shim JK, Choi YS, Oh YJ, et al. Effect of oral sildenafil citrate on intraoperative hemodynamics in patients with pulmonary hypertension undergoing valvular heart surgery. *J Thorac Cardiovasc Surg* 2006;132:1420–1425.
56. Trachte AL, Lobato EB, Urdaneta F, et al. Oral sildenafil reduces pulmonary hypertension after cardiac surgery. *Ann Thorac Surg* 2005;79:194–197.
57. Fattouch K, Sbraga F, Bianco G, et al. Inhaled prostacyclin, nitric oxide, and nitroprusside in pulmonary hypertension after mitral valve replacement. *J Card Surg* 2005;20:171–176.
58. Griffiths MJD, Evans TW. Inhaled nitric oxide therapy in adults. *N Engl J Med* 2005;353:2683–2695.
59. Fullerton DA, McIntyre RC, Kirson LE, et al. Impact of respiratory acid-base status in patients with pulmonary hypertension. *J Thorac Cardiovasc Surg* 1996;61:696–701.
60. El-Banayosy, Brehm C, Kizner L, et al. Cardiopulmonary resuscitation after cardiac surgery: a two-year study. *J Cardiothoracic Vasc Anesth* 1998;12:390–392.
61. Suominen P, Palo R, Sairanen H, et al. Perioperative determinants and outcome of cardiopulmonary arrest in children after heart surgery. *Eur J Cardiothorac Surg* 2001;19:127–134.
62. American Heart Association. Guidelines 2005 for cardiopulmonary resuscitation and emergency cardiovascular care. *Circulation* 2005;112:IV-1– IV-211.

63. American Heart Association. Guidelines 2005 for cardiopulmonary resuscitation and emergency cardiovascular care: pediatric advanced life support. *Circulation* 2005;112:IV-167–IV-187.

64. Eisenberg MS, Mengert TJ. Cardiac resuscitation. *N Engl J Med* 2001;344: 1304–1313.

65. Torres NE, White RD. Current concepts in cardiopulmonary resuscitation. *J Cardiothorac Vasc Anesth* 1997;11:391–407.

66. American Heart Association. Guidelines 2005 for cardiopulmonary resuscitation and emergency cardiovascular care: neonatal resuscitation guidelines. *Circulation* 2005;112:IV-188–IV-195.

67. Fiser SM, Tribble CG, Kern JA, et al. Cardiac reoperation in the intensive care unit. *Ann Thorac Surg* 2001;71:1888–1893.

68. Aung K, Htay T. Vasopressin for cardiac arrest: a systematic review and meta-analysis. *Arch Intern Med* 2005;165:17–24.

69. American Heart Association. Guidelines 2005 for cardiopulmonary resuscitation and emergency cardiovascular care: monitoring and medications. *Circulation* 2005;112:IV-78–IV-83.

70. Kette F, Weil MH, Gazmuri RJ. Buffer solutions may compromise cardiac resuscitation by reducing coronary perfusion. *JAMA* 1991;266:2121–2126.

71. American Heart Association. Guidelines 2005 for cardiopulmonary resuscitation and emergency cardiovascular care: management of cardiac arrest. *Circulation* 2005;112:IV-58–IV-66.

72. American Heart Association. Guidelines 2005 for cardiopulmonary resuscitation and emergency cardiovascular care: management of symptomatic bradycardia and tachycardia. *Circulation* 2005;112:IV-67–IV-77.

73. Cook DJ, Bailon JM, Douglas TT, et al. Changing incidence, type, and natural history of conduction defects after coronary artery bypass grafting. *Ann Thorac Surg* 2005;80:1732–1737.

74. Dawkins S, Hobson AR, Kalra PR, et al. Permanent pacemaker implantation after isolated aortic valve replacement: incidence, indications, and predictors. *Ann Thorac Surg* 2008;85:108–112.

75. Gordon RS, Ivanov J, Cohen G, et al. Permanent cardiac pacing after a cardiac operation: predicting the use of permanent pacemakers. *Ann Thorac Surg* 1998;66:1698–1704.

76. Lewis JW, Webb CR, Pickard SD, et al. The increased need for a permanent pacemaker after reoperative cardiac surgery. *J Thorac Cardiovasc Surg* 1998;116:74–78.

77. Imren Y, Benson AA, Oktar GL, et al. Is use of temporary pacing wires following coronary bypass surgery really necessary? *J Cardiovasc Surg (Torino)* 2008;49:261–267.

78. Bethea BT, Salazar JD, Grega MA, et al. Determining the utility of temporary pacing wires after coronary artery bypass surgery. *Ann Thorac Surg* 2005;79: 104–107.

79. Reade MC. Temporary epicardial pacing after cardiac surgery: a practical review. Part 1: general considerations in the management of epicardial pacing. *Anaesthesia* 2007;62:264–271.

80. Reade MC. Temporary epicardial pacing after cardiac surgery: a practical review. Part 2: selection of epicardial pacing modes and troubleshooting. *Anaesthesia* 2007;62:364–373.

81. Carroll KC, Reeves LM, Anderson G, et al. Risks associated with removal of ventricular epicardial pacing wires after cardiac surgery. *Am J Crit Care* 1998;7:444–449.

82. Wendt DJ, Lemmer JH, Kienzle MG. Rapidly conducting atrial fibrillation complicating surgical coronary revascularization in a patient with intermittent pre-excitation. *J Electrophys* 1989;3:152–155.

83. Mathew JP, Fontes ML, Tudor IC, et al. A multicenter risk index for atrial fibrillation after cardiac surgery. *JAMA* 2004;291:1720–1729.

84. Echahidi N, Pibarot P, O'Hara G, et al. Mechanisms, prevention and treatment of atrial fibrillation after cardiac surgery. *J Am Coll Cardiol* 2008;51:793–801.

85. Koch CG, Li L, Van Wagoner DR, et al. Red cell transfusion is associated with an increased risk for postoperative atrial fibrillation. *Ann Thorac Surg* 2006; 82:1747–1757.

86. van Dijk D, Nierich AP, Jansen EWL, et al. Early outcome after off-pump versus on-pump coronary bypass surgery: results from a randomized study. *Circulation* 2001;104:1761–1766.

87. Magee MJ, Herbert MA, Dewey TM, et al. Atrial fibrillation after coronary artery bypass grafting: development of predictive risk algorithm. *Ann Thorac Surg* 2007;83:1707–1712.

88. Shi AD, Hogue CW, Zhang H, et al. Clinical prediction rule for atrial fibrillation after coronary artery bypass grafting. *J Am Coll Cardiol* 2004;44:1248–1253.

89. Crystal E, Connolly SJ, Sleik K, et al. Interventions on prevention of postoperative atrial fibrillation in patients undergoing heart surgery: a meta-analysis. *Circulation* 2002;106:75–80.

90. Fuster V, Ryden LE, Cannom DS, et al. ACC/AHA/ESC 2006 guidelines for the management of patients with atrial fibrillation–executive summary: a report of the American College of Cardiology/American Heart Association Task Force on Practice Guidelines (Writing Committee to Revise the 2001 Guidelines for the Management of Patients with Atrial fibrillation). *J Am Coll Cardiol* 2006;48:854–906.

91. Crystal E, Garfinkle MS, Connolly SS, et al. Interventions for preventing postoperative atrial fibrillation in patients undergoing cardiac surgery. *Cochrane Database Syst Rev* 2004;(4):CD003611.

92. Burgess DC, Kilborn MJ, Keech AC. Interventions for prevention of post-operative atrial fibrillation and its complications after cardiac surgery: a meta-analysis. *Eur Heart J* 2006;27:2846–2857.

93. Daoud EG, Strickberger SA, Man KC, et al. Preoperative amiodarone as prophylaxis against atrial fibrillation after heart surgery. *N Engl J Med* 1997;33:1785–1790.

94. Bagshaw SM, Galbraith D, Mitchell LB, et al. Prophylactic amiodarone for prevention of atrial fibrillation after cardiac surgery: a meta-analysis. *Ann Thorac Surg* 2006;82: 1927–1937.

95. Wurdeman RL, Mooss AN, Mohiuddin SM, et al. Amiodarone vs sotalol as prophylaxis against atrial fibrillation/flutter after heart surgery: a meta-analysis. *Chest* 2002;121:1203–1210.

96. Haan CK, Geraci SA. Role of amiodarone in reducing atrial fibrillation after cardiac surgery in adults. *Ann Thorac Surg* 2002;73:1665–1669.

97. DiDomenico RJ, Massad MG. Pharmacologic strategies for prevention of atrial fibrillation after open heart surgery. *Ann Thorac Surg* 2005;79:728–740.

98. Barnes BJ, Kirkland EA, Howard PA, et al. Risk-stratified evaluation of amiodarone to prevent atrial fibrillation after cardiac surgery. *Ann Thorac Surg* 2006;82:1332–1337.

99. Zebis LR, Christensen TD, Thomsen HF, et al. Practical regimen for amiodarone use in preventing postoperative atrial fibrillation. *Ann Thorac Surg* 2007;83:1326–1331.

100. Miller S, Crystal E, Garfinkle M, et al. Effects of magnesium on atrial fibrillation after cardiac surgery: a meta-analysis. *Heart* 2005;91:618–623.

101. Dunning J, Treasure T, Versteegh M, et al. Guidelines and management of de novo atrial fibrillation after cardiac and thoracic surgery. *Eur J Cardiothorac Surg* 2006;30:852–872.

102. Kourliouros A, De Souza A, Roberts N, et al. Dose-related effect of statins on atrial fibrillation after cardiac surgery. *Ann Thorac Surg* 2008;85:1515–1520.

103. Lertsburapa K, White CM, Kluger J, et al. Preoperative statins for the prevention of atrial fibrillation after cardiothoracic surgery. *J Thorac Cardiovasc Surg* 2008;135:405–411.

104. Creswell LL, Alexander JC, Ferguson TB, et al. Intraoperative interventions: American College of Chest Physicians guidelines for the prevention and management of postoperative atrial fibrillation after cardiac surgery. *Chest* 2005;128:28–35.

105. Mann CJ, Kendall S, Lip GYH, et al. Acute management of atrial fibrillation with acute hemodynamic instability and in the postoperative setting. *Heart* 2007;93:45–47.

106. Tisdale JE, Padhi ID, Goldberg AD, et al. A randomized, double-blind comparison of intravenous diltiazem and digoxin for atrial fibrillation after coronary artery bypass surgery. *Am Heart J* 1998;135:739–747.

107. Kochiadakis GE, Igoumenidis NE, Hamilos ME, et al. A comparative study of the efficacy and safety of procainamide versus propafenone versus amiodarone for the conversion of recent-onset atrial fibrillation. *Am J Cardiol* 2007;99:1721–1725.

108. Martinez-Marcos FJ, Garcia-Garmendia JL, Ortega-Carpio A, et al. Comparison of intravenous flecainide, propafenone, and amiodarone for conversion of acute atrial fibrillation to sinus rhythm. *Am J Cardiol* 2000;86:950–953.

109. Vardos PE, Kochiadakis, Igoumenidis NE, et al. Amiodarone as a first-choice drug for restoring sinus rhythm in patients with atrial fibrillation. *Chest* 2000;117:1538–1545.

110. Martinex EA, Bass EB, Zimetbaum P. Pharmacologic control of rhythm: American College of Chest Physicians Guidelines for the prevention and management of postoperative atria fibrillation after cardiac surgery. *Chest* 2005;128:48S–55S.

111. Vassallo P, Trohman RG. Prescribing amiodarone: an evidence-based review of clinical indications. *JAMA* 2007;298:1312–1322.

112. Zimetbaum P. Amiodarone for atrial fibrillation. *N Engl J Med* 2007;356:935–941.

113. Sanoski CA, Bauman JL. Clinical observations with the amiodarone/warfarin interaction. *Chest* 2002;121:19–23.

114. Ashrafian H, Davey P. Is amiodarone an underrecognized cause of acute respiratory failure in the ICU? *Chest* 2001;120:275–282.

115. Dimopoulou I, Marathias K, Daganou M, et al. Low-dose amiodarone-related complications after cardiac operations. *J Thorac Cardiovasc Surg* 1997;114:31–37.

116. VanderLugt JT, Mattioni T, Denker S, et al. Efficacy and safety of ibutilide fumarate for the conversion of atrial arrhythmias after cardiac surgery. *Circulation* 1999;100:369–375.

117. Peters RW, Weiss DN, Carliner NH, et al. Overdrive pacing for atrial flutter. *Am J Cardiol* 1994;74:1021–1023.

118. Antman EM, Anbe DT, Armstrong PW, et al. ACC/AHA guidelines for the management of patients with ST-elevation myocardial infarction. *Circulation* 2004;110:e82–e293.

119. Yau JM, Alexander JH, Hafley G, et al. Impact of perioperative myocardial infarction on angiographic and clinical outcomes following coronary artery bypass grafting (from Project of Ex-vivo Vein graft Engineering via Transfection [PREVENT] IV). *Am J Cardiol* 2008;102:546–551.

120. Alamanni F, Dainese L, Naliato M, et al. On- and off-pump coronary surgery and perioperative myocardial infarction: an issue between incomplete and extensive revascularization. *Eur J Cardiothorac Surg* 2008;118–126.

121. Adabag AS, Rector T, Mithani S, et al. Prognostic significance of elevated cardiac troponin I after heart surgery. *Ann Thorac Surg* 2007;83:1744–1750.

122. Klatte K, Chaitman BR, Theroux P, et al. Increased mortality after coronary artery bypass graft surgery is associated with increased levels of postoperative creatinine kinase-myocardial band isoenzyme release. *J Am Coll Cardiol* 2001;38:1070–1077.

123. Jarvinen O, Julkunen J, Saarinen T, et al. Perioperative myocardial infarction s negative impact on health-related quality of life following coronary artery bypass graft surgery. *Eur J Cardiothorac Surg* 2004;26:621–627.

124. Brenner SJ, Lytle BW, Schneider JP. Association between CK-MB elevation after percutaneous coronary intervention or surgical revascularization and three-year mortality. *J Am Coll Cardiol* 2002;40:1961–1967.

125. Birdi I, Angelini GD, Bryan AJ. Biochemical markers of myocardial injury during cardiac operations. *Ann Thorac Surg* 1997;63:879–884.

126. Petäjä L, Salmenperä, Pulkki K, et al. Biochemical injury markers and mortality after coronary bypass grafting: a systematic review. *Ann Thorac Surg* 2009;87:1981–1992.

127. Wiessner R, Hannemann-Pohl K, Ziebig R, et al. Impact of kidney function on plasma troponin concentrations after coronary artery bypass grafting. *Nephrol Dial Transplant* 2008;23:231–238.

128. Nesher N, Alghamdi AA, Singh SK, et al. Troponin after cardiac surgery: a predictor or a phenomenon? *Ann Thorac Surg* 2008;85:1348–1354.

129. Botha P, Nagarajan DV, Lewis PS, et al. Can cardiac troponins be used to diagnose a perioperative myocardial infarction post cardiac surgery? *Interactive Cardiovasc Thorac Surg* 2004;3:442–449.

130. Muehlschlegel JD, Perry TV, Liu K-Y, et al. Troponin is superior to electrocardiogram and creatinine kinase MB for predicting clinically significant myocardial injury after coronary artery bypass grafting. *Eur Heart J* 2009;30:1574–1583.

131. Greenson N, Macoviak J, Krishnasway P, et al. Usefulness of cardiac troponin I in patients undergoing open heart surgery. *Am Heart J* 2001;141:447–455.

132. Crescenzi G, Bove T, Pappalrdo F, et al. Clinical significance of a new Q wave after cardiac surgery. *Eur J Cardiothorac Surg* 2004;25:1001–1005.

133. Thygesen K, Alpert JS, White HD. Joint ESC/ACCF/AHA/WHF Task Force for the redefinition of Myocardial Infarction. Universal definition of myocardial infarction. *J Am Coll Cardiol* 2007;50:2173–2195.

134. Paterson HS, Jones MW, Baird DK, et al. Lethal postoperative coronary artery spasm. *Ann Thorac Surg* 1998;65:1571–1573.

135. Lemmer JH Jr, Kirsh MM. Coronary artery spasm following coronary artery surgery. *Ann Thorac Surg* 1988;46:108–115.

136. Schena S, Wildes T, Beardslee MA, et al. Successful management of unremitting spasm of the nongrafted right coronary artery after off-pump coronary artery bypass grafting. *J Thorac Cardiovasc Surg* 2007;133:1649–1650.

137. Attran S, John L, El-Gamel A. Clinical and potential use of pharmacological agents to reduce radial artery spasm in coronary artery surgery. *Ann Thorac Surg* 2008;85:1483–1489.
138. Samuels LE, Kaufman MS, Morris RJ, et al. Coronary artery bypass grafting in patients with COPD. *Chest* 1998;113:878–882.
139. Fuster RG, Argudo JA, Albarova OG, et al. Prognostic value of chronic obstructive pulmonary disease in coronary artery bypass grafting. *Eur J Cardiothorac Surg* 2006;29:202–209.
140. Wahl GW, Swinburne AJ, Fedullo AJ, et al. Effect of age and preoperative airway obstruction on lung function after coronary artery bypass grafting. *Ann Thorac Surg* 1993;56:104–107.
141. Zarbock A, Mueller E, Netzer S, et al. Prophylactic nasal continuous positive airway pressure following cardiac surgery protects from postoperative pulmonary complications: a prospective, randomized, controlled trial in 500 patients. *Chest* 2009;135:1252–1259.
142. Matthay MA, Wiener-Kronish JP. Respiratory management after cardiac surgery. *Chest* 1989;95:424–434.
143. Curtis JJ, Nawarawong W, Walls JT, et al. Elevated hemidiaphragm after cardiac operations: incidence, prognosis, and relationship to the use of topical ice slush. *Ann Thorac Surg* 1989;48:764–768.
144. Chandler KW, Rozas CJ, Kory RC, et al. Bilateral diaphragmatic paralysis complicating local cardiac hypothermia during open heart surgery. *Am J Med* 1984;77:243–249.
145. Katz MG, Katz R, Schachner A, et al. Phrenic nerve injury after coronary artery bypass grafting: will it go away? *Ann Thorac Surg* 1998;65:32–35.
146. Akay TH, Ozkan S, Gultekin B, et al. Diaphragmatic paralysis after cardiac surgery in children: incidence, prognosis, and surgical management. *Pediatr Surg Int* 2006;22:341–346.
147. Joho-Arreola AL, Bauersfeld U, Stauffer UG, et al. Incidence and treatment of diaphragmatic paralysis after cardiac surgery in children. *Eur J Cardiothoracic Surg* 2005;27:53–57.
148. Watanabe T, Trusler GA, Williams WG, et al. Phrenic nerve paralysis after pediatric cardiac surgery. *J Thorac Cardiovasc Surg* 1987;94:383–388.
149. Ferdinande PG, Bruyninck F, Van Raemdonck D, et al. Phrenic nerve dysfunction after heart-lung and lung transplantation. *J Heart Lung Transplant* 2002;21:142–145.
150. Filsoufi F, Rahmanian PB, Castillo JG, et al. Predictors and late outcomes of respiratory failure in contemporary cardiac surgery. *Chest* 2008;133:713–721.
151. Reddy SLC, Grayson AD, Griffiths EM, et al. Logistic model for prolonged ventilation after adult cardiac surgery. *Ann Thorac Surg* 2007;84:528–536.
152. Stamenkovic SA, Morgan IS, Pontefract DR, et al. Is early tracheostomy safe in cardiac patients with median sternotomy incisions? *Ann Thorac Surg* 2000;69:1152–1154.
153. Rahmanian B, Adams DH, Castillo JG, et al. Tracheostomy is not a risk factor for deep sterna wound infection after cardiac surgery. *Ann Thorac Surg* 2007;84:1984–1992.
154. Byhahn C, Rinne T, Halbig S, et al. Early percutaneous tracheostomy after median sternotomy. *J Thorac Cardiovasc Surg* 2000;120:329–334.
155. Melloni G, Muttini S, Gallioli G, et al. Surgical tracheostomy versus percutaneous dilatational tracheostomy. A prospective-randomized study with long-term follow-up. *J Cardiovasc Surg (Torino)* 2002;43:113–121.

156. Ware LB, Matthay MA. The acute respiratory distress syndrome. *N Engl J Med* 2000;342:1334–1349.
157. Peruzzi WT, Franklin ML, Shapiro BA. New concepts and therapies of adult respiratory distress syndrome. *J Cardiothoracic Vasc Anesth* 1997;11:771–786.
158. Asimakiopoulos G, Smith PLC, Ratnatunga CP, et al. Lung injury and acute respiratory distress syndrome after cardiopulmonary bypass. *Ann Thorac Surg* 1999;68:1107–1115.
159. Milot J, Perron J, Lacasse Y, et al. Incidence and predictors of ARDS after cardiac surgery. *Chest* 2001;119:884–888.
160. Christenson JT, Aeberhardt J-M, Badel P, et al. Adult respiratory distress syndrome after cardiac surgery. *Cardiovasc Surg* 1995;4:15–21.
161. The Acute Respiratory Distress Syndrome Network. Ventilation with lower tidal volumes as compared with traditional tidal volumes for acute lung injury and the acute respiratory distress syndrome. *N Engl J Med* 2000;342:1301–1308.
162. Malhotra A. Low-tidal-volume ventilation in the acute respiratory distress syndrome. *N Engl J Med* 2007;357:1113–1120.
163. The Society of Thoracic Surgeons Blood Conservation Guideline Task Force and The Society of Cardiovascular Anesthesiologists Special Task Force on Blood Transfusion. Perioperative blood transfusion and blood conservation in cardiac surgery: the Society of Thoracic Surgeons and The Society of Cardiovascular Anesthesiologists clinical practice guideline. *Ann Thorac Surg* 2007;83:S27–S86.
164. Looney MR, Gropper MA, Matthay MA. Transfusion-related acute lung injury—a review. *Chest* 2004;126:249–258.
165. Jawa RS, Aillo S, Kulaylat MN. Transfusion-related acute lung injury. *J Intensive Care Med* 2008;23:109–121.
166. Toy P, Popovsky MA, Abraham E, et al. Transfusion-related acute lung injury: definition and review. *Crit Care Med* 2005;33:721–726.
167. O'Connor AR, Morgan WE. Radiological review of pneumothorax. *Br Med J* 2005;330:1493–1497.
168. Cohen M, Sahn SA. Resolution of pleural effusions. *Chest* 2001;119:1547–1562.
169. Heidecker J, Sahn SA. The spectrum of pleural effusions after coronary artery bypass grafting surgery. *Clin Chest Med* 2006;27:267–283.
170. Bond SJ, Guzzetta PC, Snyder ML, et al. Management of pediatric postoperative chylothorax. *Ann Thorac Surg* 1993;56:469–472.
171. Fahimi H, Casselman FP, Mariani MA, et al. Current management of postoperative chylothorax. *Ann Thorac Surg* 2001;71:448–451.

Postoperative Complications Involving Other Organ Systems

BLEEDING AFTER HEART SURGERY

Management of early postoperative bleeding is a familiar task for those who care for patients who undergo cardiac surgery. Some bleeding occurs after all cardiac operations and it is significant enough to require early re-exploration to control hemorrhage in 2% to 6% of patients (1–4). In adults, excessive postoperative bleeding occurs in association with repeat operations, emergency procedures, preoperative cardiogenic shock, combined procedures, female gender, small body mass index, older age, peripheral vascular disease, renal insufficiency (creatinine above 1.8 g/dL), poor nutrition (albumin level <4 g/dL), and in patients who have experienced prolonged cardiopulmonary bypass (CPB) durations (5,6). Preoperative treatment with antithrombotic and antiplatelet drugs is also a major contributor. Risk models have been developed that aid in predicting a specific patient's anticipated need for perioperative blood product transfusion (7–9).

Extensive preoperative laboratory testing of hemostasis parameters is not necessary; careful medical history of bleeding tendencies usually suffices with further testing performed in patients with the history of bleeding problems. A simple screening question is to ask the patient if he or she previously had tooth extractions and, if so, if excessive bleeding occurred with the procedure; patients who have had teeth pulled without difficulty are unlikely to have a serious congenital bleeding abnormality. Certainly, the history taking should include a careful review of the patient's medications with particular emphasis on recent ingestion of aspirin, clopidogrel, and nonsteroidal anti-inflammatory drugs (NSAIDs). For patients without a history of bleeding or easy bruising, we routinely measure only the platelet count prior to surgery. If the patient does have bleeding tendencies or has been on warfarin, the preoperative prothrombin time (PT), international normalized ratio (INR), and activated partial thromboplastin time (aPTT) are also determined. Patients who are receiving warfarin prior to surgery may not, however, have increased bleeding. Thus, urgently needed surgery should not be postponed, and it is not always required to totally reverse the warfarin effect prior to operation (10,11).

In children, the determinants of excessive postoperative bleeding are not well defined but preoperative cyanosis is a risk factor. Because of their smaller blood volume, children are more affected by hemodilution from the bypass circuit volume, with a larger reduction in platelets and soluble coagulation factors occurring as a result. Furthermore, neonates may be relatively deficient in various coagulation factors (such as factors XII and II) and coagulation inhibitors (such as antithrombin III) (12). Prostaglandin E_1 inhibits platelet function and preoperative treatment with this agent may result in more bleeding. Polycythemic cyanotic children have lower levels of fibrinogen and other clotting factors with increased fibrin split products that contribute to postoperative bleeding.

Excessive bleeding after open-heart surgery may be due to one or several of many factors including inadequate surgical hemostasis (surgical bleeding), platelet depletion, platelet dysfunction, plasma clotting factor deficiency, residual heparin effect (incomplete reversal by protamine), excessive protamine administration, hypothermia, increased fibrinolytic activity, and consumption coagulopathy (13). For the patient suffering excessive bleeding early after heart surgery, the major problem is determining whether the bleeding is secondary to a reversible coagulation abnormality or whether it is due to a surgical cause such as a leaking suture line.

Mediastinal drainage tubes are routinely placed at the completion of the operation and are attached to suction collection receptacles. These allow for frequent measurements of the rate of bleeding. Although there is no strict definition of "excessive" postoperative bleeding, concern is raised when the mediastinal tube output exceeds 4 to 5 mL/kg per hour during the first few hours after operation. Typically, postoperative bleeding decreases significantly during the first 3 to 4 hours after surgery and becomes relatively minimal (<0.5 to 1.0 mL/kg per hour) by 6 hours. When the bleeding exceeds these general guidelines, efforts must be made to determine the presence or absence of treatable conditions (e.g., coagulopathy) and whether to return the patient to the operating room for surgical exploration. When the rate of bleeding is massive (i.e., more than 8 to 10 mL/kg per hour), the prompt return of the patient to the operating room for exploration is nearly always indicated. Clues to the presence of surgical bleeding include the continuous excessive chest tube output in a patient with relatively normal coagulation studies and the sudden development of significant drainage in the patient who was previously not bleeding, especially in conjunction with hemodynamic instability.

Nonsurgical (microvascular) bleeding after cardiac surgery using CPB is a multifactorial problem. Contributors include reduced platelet number and function, hemodilution from the extracorporeal circuit solution, activation of the hemostatic system caused by the interaction of blood with the bypass circuit surfaces (which are not covered by endothelium), activation of the extrinsic clotting system due to tissue trauma and fibrinolysis. The central mediator in the process of clot formation is the generation of thrombin that acts to convert fibrinogen to fibrin, the basic building block of clot. To prevent thrombosis during CPB heparin, acting to catalyze endogenous antithrombin III, is administered, although some degree of thrombin formation and subclinical clot formation does occur, even in the presence of "adequate" heparinization. This subclinical thrombin production and clot formation results in consumption of clotting factors during CPB. Other effects of thrombin include the release of tissue plasminogen factor (with subsequent plasmin generation and fibrinolysis), activation of protein C, and release of tissue factor inhibitor. CPB also induces a complex series of reactions involving both enzyme cascades and cellular elements collectively termed the "systemic inflammatory response." This phenomenon is the result of the activation of complement, kallikrein, bradykinin, leukocytes, platelets, endothelium, and other mediators of inflammation, and is due to contact of the blood elements with the nonendothelialized surface of the bypass tubing and oxygenator, surgical trauma, and reperfusion of transiently ischemic tissue (especially lung) (14).

Coronary artery bypass procedures performed without the use of CPB result in less activation of the inflammatory responses and are generally associated with less postoperative bleeding and transfusions (15,16). "Off-pump" operations are not practical for valve procedures or all coronary bypass operations, but they do have an important role in the management of patients with coronary disease, especially those at higher risk for neurologic complications due to aortic atherosclerosis.

Platelets and Bleeding in Cardiac Surgery Patients

Platelet abnormalities, either in quantity or quality, are a major contributor to nonsurgical postoperative bleeding following procedures using CPB.

Thrombocytopenia

Postoperative thrombocytopenia may result from hemodilution due to the priming volume of the CPB circuit. In patients with a normal preoperative platelet count, this usually does not, however, result in a platelet count below 100,000 platelets/mm^3. Long CPB durations will result in a greater decrease in the platelet count due to consumption. Postoperative thrombocytopenia is likely to be more frequent in patients who required intra-aortic balloon pump or ventricular assist device placement before surgery.

Patients who have been treated with heparin may develop *heparin-induced thrombocytopenia* (HIT). This acquired syndrome of thrombocytopenia that may occur with or without thrombosis is discussed in Chapter 3.

Platelet Dysfunction

An important cause of postoperative microvascular bleeding is the variable and temporary decrease in platelet function that accompanies surgery using CPB. Post-bypass platelet dysfunction is likely related to platelet activation and degranulation (depletion of active intracellular mediators) during bypass as the result of contact with the nonendothelialized surfaces of the bypass circuit (tubing and oxygenator) and/or to direct trauma to the platelet glycoprotein (GP) membrane receptors, in particular the GP Ib receptor. In addition, heparin itself activates platelets to some degree. Hypothermia also contributes to platelet dysfunction. HAs a result of these influences, prolongation of the patient's bleeding time early after cardiac surgery is common; this abnormality usually disappears within 2 to 4 hours after the procedure. Coronary artery bypass graft (CABG) procedures performed without CPB may have less bleeding, at least in part, because the platelets are not subjected to the effects of the extracorporeal circulation circuit.

Drugs that Cause Platelet Dysfunction

Drug-induced platelet dysfunction is a major concern for cardiac surgeons. The use of various antiplatelet agents by cardiologists to treat acute coronary syndromes (unstable angina and myocardial infarction) or as adjuncts to percutaneous coronary interventions (angioplasty and stent placement) has become routine (17–19). Table 5.1 lists the commonly administered platelet inhibitors.

Aspirin. Aspirin is administered routinely to patients with coronary artery disease both as chronic treatment and for acute coronary syndromes and percutaneous coronary interventions. Aspirin permanently inhibits platelet cyclo-oxygenase activity within 1 hour of ingestion of a single dose. This induces a defect in thromboxane A_2-dependent function, thereby inhibiting platelet activation leading to impaired platelet aggregation and clot formation. Efficacy of aspirin treatment, in a variety of cardiovascular settings, has been well demonstrated (18). After receiving a single aspirin dose, all platelets that are present in the patient become inhibited within 1 hour; free aspirin is rapidly cleared from the plasma. The anucleate platelets cannot manufacture more cyclo-oxygenase and therefore the platelets are affected for the remainder of their existence. Platelets have a lifespan of about 10 days, so after about 5 days <50% of the platelets present in the patient are aspirin-inhibited, assuming no further aspirin ingestion. Some, but not all, aspirin-treated patients (hyperresponders) who undergo cardiac surgery bleed more and require more transfusions (especially of platelets)

TABLE 5.1

Commonly Used Platelet-Inhibiting Drugs

	Aspirin	Clopidogrel	Abciximab	Eptifibatide	Tirofiban
Mechanism of action	Cyclooxygenase inhibitor	Inhibits ADP-mediated aggregation	Inhibits platelet membrane IIb/IIIa receptor	Inhibits platelet membrane IIb/IIIa receptor	Inhibits platelet membrane IIb/IIIa receptor
Onset of action	<1 h	<2 h (with loading dose)	<1 h	<1 h	<1 h
Effective duration of action	Irreversible (lasts for life of platelet; 7 to 10 d	Irreversible (lasts for life of platelet; 7 to 10 d	Biologic effect for 12 to 24 h	4 to 6 h	4 to 6 h
Implications for surgery	Not clear; may be desirable to discontinue if possible, but not necessary; may cause more bleeding, but may have advantageous effects	If elective, discontinue drug for 5 to 7 d before operation	May cause more bleeding, but effect is reversible with platelet transfusion; not a contraindication to emergency surgery	Effect wears off relatively quickly; emergency surgery not associated with bleeding problems	Effect wears off relatively quickly; emergency surgery not associated with bleeding problems

than patients who have not received aspirin with several days of operation (20–23). The majority, however, do not experience excessive postoperative bleeding (14).

Most patients coming for CABG surgery are being treated with aspirin. Aspirin treatment prior to CABG is associated with improved postoperative outcomes, including reduced mortality (24,25). In our practices, we do not delay surgery for the aspirin-treated CABG patient nor do we routinely discontinue the aspirin prior to CABG. We do, however, hold the drug for several days prior to elective valve procedures. Early treatment with aspirin following CABG improves the patency rates of the bypass grafts and may also be associated to reduced incidences of other complications (26,27). When used for this purpose, aspirin should be given within 6 hours of the surgery. It is our custom to administer aspirin (325 mg) by rectal suppository to patients who have undergone coronary bypass within 6 hours after arrival in the intensive care unit as long as excessive bleeding is not present.

Clopidogrel. Clopidogrel (Plavix®) is a thienopyridines with platelet inhibitory properties that is clearly effective when used to treat patients with coronary and vascular disease (18,28). Clopidogrel inhibits, via a liver-transformed metabolite, adenosine diphosphate (ADP)-induced platelet aggregation. Given orally only, clopidogrel is frequently administered at 75 mg per day and with this dose it requires several days before a steady state of approximately 50% inhibition of ADP-induced platelet aggregation is achieved. Large loading doses, commonly 300 to 600 mg, are frequently administered to patients before undergoing percutaneous coronary stent placement. Following this dose, significant platelet inhibition and prolongation of the bleeding time is achieved within hours (29). Like aspirin, the clopidogrel platelet inhibitory effect is permanent for the affected platelets and it requires 5 to 7 days for the effect to wear off. When given for these purposes, clopidogrel is usually administered in conjunction with aspirin, resulting in an additive effect. Patients who have received clopidogrel within 5 days of cardiac surgery (usually CABG) have significantly increased rates of bleeding, blood product transfusion, and need for early reoperation for bleeding (30–33). When a patient taking clopidogrel is considered for surgery, the increased risk of bleeding must be weighed against the risk of postponing the procedure (34–36). For totally elective patients, we discontinue the patient's clopidogrel for 4 to 6 days before operation while aspirin therapy (if indicated) is continued. If the operation is urgent, we delay surgery for 3 to 5 days often administering heparin or a platelet GP IIb/IIIa inhibitor (such as eptifibatide) during the waiting period. If the operation is an emergency that cannot be postponed, we proceed with the procedure but expect to transfuse platelets, often in large quantity.

Platelet Glycoprotein IIb/IIIa Receptor Inhibitors. Platelet aggregation, essential for clot formation, is mediated by the platelet membrane GP receptor denoted GP IIb/IIIa. Inhibition of this receptor results in powerful interference with platelet function and thrombosis. Administration is associated with improved outcomes in patients with acute coronary syndromes or who are undergoing percutaneous coronary intervention procedures (18). Drugs that specifically inhibit the GP IIb/IIIa receptor include abciximab, eptifibatide, and tirofiban. All three drugs are administered by the intravenous route only. Occasionally, patients treated with GP IIb/IIIa inhibitors require emergency cardiac surgery (most often CABG) while under the effect of the GP IIb/IIIa inhibitor. Because of the increased risk of bleeding complications, an understanding of the GP IIb/IIIa inhibitors is important for those who participate in the care of patients treated with these agents.

Abciximab (ReoPro®) is an antibody directed against the GP IIb/IIIa receptor. Abciximab has a very strong affinity for the platelet GP IIb/IIIa receptor. After administration of a bolus dose of abciximab, the GP IIb/IIIa receptors are quickly bound by the antibody and inhibited while free drug is rapidly cleared. Since no free drug remains in the patient's plasma, subsequent platelet transfusions effectively reverse the abciximab effect by diluting the abciximab that has become platelet bound. When called upon to operate on a patient recently treated with abciximab, the drug should be immediately discontinued but protamine and platelets should not be administered prior to surgery unless serious ongoing bleeding is present. Postponing surgery for 12 to 48 hours, often while maintaining the patient on heparin, will result in improved platelet aggregation and may be practical for stable patients. If necessary for ongoing ischemia, however, abciximab-treated patients should not be denied emergency surgery that is otherwise indicated, although they are likely to require platelet transfusions (37–40). Unless required for uncontrollable bleeding, platelets should not be given preoperatively as this might precipitate closure of a critically stenotic major coronary artery and will subject the transfused platelets to the adverse effects of CPB.

Eptifibatide (Integrilin®) and *tirofiban* (Aggrastat®) are molecules smaller than abciximab that have lesser degrees of affinity for the platelet GP IIb/IIIa receptor and shorter durations of action. They are generally not associated with increased bleeding in patients who require urgent coronary bypass surgery soon after discontinuation of the drug (41–43).

The use of potent platelet inhibiting drugs has improved the care of coronary artery disease patients but has complicated the life of surgeons. Most often, patients requiring emergency bypass surgery for failed coronary interventions and/or ongoing acute myocardial infarction have received multiple antiplatelet agents and these drugs have additive effects. While these patients can be successfully operated upon, there may be an associated increased incidence of transfusion and complications. Surgery, if otherwise indicated due to ongoing ischemia or critical anatomy, should *not*, however, be withheld because of the drug-induced platelet defect that is present. Recognition of the problem and discussion with the patient and his or her family members preoperatively is advised.

Clotting Factors and Fibrinogen

CPB, because of hemodilution and consumption, results in decrease in plasma clotting factor concentrations, especially factors V and VIII (44). Generally, however, the postoperative levels usually remain well above the level (25% to 30% of normal) required for normal hemostatic function. Thus, clotting factor deficiency is not a frequent cause of postoperative bleeding. It may, however, play a role in patients who have received massive transfusions of packed red blood cells (RBCs), due to further dilution of the clotting factors, and in very polycythemic patients whose plasma volume is reduced. Assessment of plasma clotting factor function is done by measurement of the PT and the INR. These parameters reflect activity of the extrinsic portion of the clotting system. While the INR has a normal upper-limit value of 1.2, values of up to 1.5 indicate sufficient clotting factor concentration to effect normal clotting under most circumstances. For the bleeding patient with prolongation of the INR (above 1.5), treatment of clotting factor deficiency consists of the administration of a sufficient quantity of fresh frozen plasma (FFP) (14). Thus, 15 mL/kg of FFP (3 to 4 units for the average-size adult) is administered while monitoring the patient's filling pressures (central venous and pulmonary artery diastolic or wedge pressure) to avoid fluid overload. If the INR is prolonged but the patient is not bleeding, plasma transfusion is not indicated and the patient is closely observed. Likewise, if the PT and INR are normal, FFP is not indicated.

Fibrinogen is necessary for clot formation but hypofibrinogenemia is not a frequent contributor to postoperative bleeding. Although reductions in fibrinogen levels occur following CPB, a significant deficiency is not present unless the fibrinogen level falls below 70 mg/dL. Causes of hypofibrinogenemia in postoperative patients include consumptive coagulopathy, major hemorrhage, fibrinolytic therapy, excessive fibrinolysis, and uncommon hereditary disorders. If the patient is bleeding and a low fibrinogen level (below 100 mg/dL) is confirmed, treatment with cryoprecipitate is indicated. In general, however, hypofibrinogenemia is an uncommon cause of postoperative bleeding and usually occurs in conjunction with other indicators of an ongoing coagulopathy. If the patient is not bleeding significantly, transfusion of cryoprecipitate is not indicated.

Heparin

To prevent thrombosis within the CPB circuit during surgery, large doses of heparin are administered to the patient. Heparin, a negatively charged polysaccharide, catalyzes the naturally occurring coagulation inhibitor, antithrombin III and its action is dependent upon adequate antithrombin III levels (45,46). Heparin sensitivity is variable among individuals and is lower in pediatric patients. At the end of the CPB period, heparin is reversed by the administration of protamine. Protamine, a positively charged polypeptide, binds with heparin, removing it from antithrombin III, and the ability of the blood to coagulate is restored. During CPB, the adequacy of heparinization is most commonly measured by the activated clotting time (ACT). Intraoperative management of anticoagulation for CPB is discussed in Chapter 2.

After completion of bypass and the administration of protamine, the reappearance of circulating heparin in the blood from the extravascular to the intravascular space with resultant bleeding (so-called heparin rebound) has been described proposed. The incidence of heparin rebound and its contribution to postoperative bleeding is uncertain. In any event, incomplete reversal of heparin by protamine is suggested by a prolongation of the ACT or the aPTT, although these tests are not specific for heparin. Performance of the thrombin time (TT) using blood drawn directly from the patient's vein (to avoid contamination by heparin flush solution) will confirm the presence or absence of residual heparin. Treatment of demonstrated residual heparin effect is by the administration of protamine, which should be given slowly to avoid hypotension. The empiric administration of protamine to the patient with normalized ACT and/or aPTT is not advised; protamine excess can result in greater perioperative blood losses as protamine itself is a weak anticoagulant.

Low-molecular-weight heparin (LMWH) preparations, derived by depolymerization of unfractionated heparin, are effective for the treatment of acute coronary syndromes and deep venous thrombosis (DVT). Because of ease of administration by subcutaneous injection and the lack of need for laboratory monitoring, LMWH is frequently used in heart disease patients. Occasionally surgeons are called upon to operate on patients who have recently received LMWH and the presence of recently administered LMWH is associated with increased postoperative bleeding, transfusion requirements, and the need for re-exploration for postoperative bleeding (47,48). LMWH activity, in contrast to unfractionated heparin, is not accurately measurable by tests such as the ACT or aPTT and is not effectively reversed by protamine (49). We therefore suggest that patients who are scheduled to undergo cardiac surgery and are being treated with LMWH be switched over to continuous unfractionated heparin infusions at least 24 hours prior to the surgical procedure to allow time for the LMWH activity to wear off.

Early following surgery, some patients require anticoagulation for the presence of a mechanical valve, atrial fibrillation, or other reasons. When treated with heparin (either unfractionated or low molecular weight), these patients are at increased risk of hemorrhagic complications, including postoperative bleeding requiring re-exploration (50).

Fibrinolysis

The tissue trauma of surgery, particularly in conjunction with the use of extracorporeal circulation, causes increased release of tissue plasminogen activator with a resultant increase in the breakdown of fibrin, namely the process of fibrinolysis. Fibrinolysis occurs to some degree in all patients after cardiac surgery, probably to a greater degree in those who underwent procedures using CPB and likely more in those with cyanotic heart disease. Excessive fibrinolysis is associated with increased postoperative bleeding and drugs that inhibit fibrinolysis are administered to reduce bleeding. Laboratory studies suggestive of fibrinolysis include a shortened euglobulin clot lysis time, decreased fibrinogen level, and elevated level of D-dimers and elevated level fibrinogen degradation products (FDPs). A positive D-dimer result is indicative of fibrinolysis, although not necessarily to a pathologic extent. Elevation of both the D-dimers and FDPs may indicate the presence of disseminated intravascular coagulation. The relative contribution of fibrinolysis to postoperative bleeding is unclear, although drugs with antifibrinolytic activity are associated with reduced postoperative bleeding when administered during cardiac surgery (see Chapter 3).

Disseminated Intravascular Coagulation

Serious consumption coagulopathy (or disseminated intravascular coagulation; DIC) is an unlikely cause of early postoperative bleeding following cardiac surgery. The condition is characterized by the enhanced and abnormally sustained generation of thrombin with resultant decreases in fibrinogen, clotting factors, and platelet levels in association with increased PT, aPTT, and D-dimers (51). These perturbations are also common following open-heart surgery using CPB but rarely in association with pathologic clotting. Typically, the abnormalities return toward normal after 12 to 24 hours. If the presence of DIC is suspected, however, treatment of the patient with an antifibrinolytic drug (such as tranexamic acid or aminocaproic acid) is contraindicated.

MANAGEMENT OF THE BLEEDING PATIENT

When excessive bleeding is present, replacement of the blood loss at a rate sufficient to maintain the patient's red cell volume and intravascular volume at desired levels is required. Although blood conservation and avoidance of blood product transfusion are important, overzealous application of these principles may result in dangerous anemia or hypovolemia, particularly if the rate of blood loss suddenly increases. Although lower hematocrit levels may be acceptable for the nonbleeding patient, if the patient is bleeding excessively, it is wise to provide a margin of safety and transfuse blood so as to maintain the hematocrit level in the 24% to 28% range. Control of hypertension, if present, will help reduce the rate of bleeding. For this purpose, an intravenous infusion of a short-acting agent such as nitroglycerin, nitroprusside, or esmolol is administered (see Chapter 3).

Massive bleeding mandates prompt reoperation. There are no definite criteria to assist in the recognition of patients with surgically correctable causes of excessive mediastinal bleeding. Surgical bleeding is, however, more likely to be present if the patient has high mediastinal tube output with relatively normal coagulation test parameters or if the patient, who was not bleeding initially, develops sudden excessive output. If the patient is sufficiently stable for transport, re-entry may be performed in the operating room. This is preferable, as recannulation and CPB support may be required to correct a difficult-to-reach bleeding site. If the patient is unstable, however, re-exploration may be performed in the intensive care unit. It is important for every cardiac surgical intensive care unit to have a sterile set of instruments (including wire cutters and sternal retractor) and a good light source ready at all times for this purpose. Often the bleeding site can be repaired in the intensive care unit. If not, it is usually possible to control the bleeding with digital pressure and transfuse the patient until he or she is sufficiently stable for transfer to the operating room for definitive repair. Open resuscitation in the intensive care unit results in surprisingly few infections if sterile technique is used and antibiotics are administered (52).

When the rate of bleeding is excessive, but not massive, the decision whether to reoperate may be a difficult one. The approach to this situation is to correct the hemostatic abnormalities as best as possible and, if bleeding continues, then to proceed with exploration. It is best to have a low threshold for early return of the bleeding patient to the operating room for exploration. Delay in returning the bleeding patient to the operating room for re-exploration is associated with adverse outcomes as compared to earlier return (53,54). A common criterion for reoperation is when the patient bleeds 300 mL per hour over two or three consecutive hours or 500 mL in 1 hour.

A useful algorithm for the management of the bleeding patient is shown in Fig. 5.1. Examination of the patient may provide clues to the nature of the patient's bleeding. Diffuse oozing from the skin incision and intravenous catheter sites suggests a platelet abnormality; failure

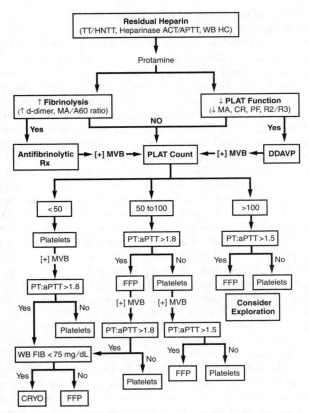

FIGURE 5.1 Treatment algorithm for patients with excessive post cardiopulmonary bypass microvascular bleeding. TT/HNTT, whole-blood TT/heparin-neutralized TT test (Hemochron); heparinase ACT, heparinase kaolin-activated clotting time test (ACT); heparinase aPTT, heparinase-aPTT test (CoaguCheck Plus); WB HC, whole-blood heparin concentration cartridge (Hepcon instrument); D-dimers, whole-blood D-dimer assay (SimpleRED test); MA, maximum amplitude (thromboelastograph); MA/A60 ratio, maximum amplitude/amplitude at 60 minutes (thromboelastograph); CR, clot ratio values (hemoSTATUS cartridge; Hepcon); PF, platelet force measurements (Hemodyne); R2/R3, R2, and R3 slope values (Sonoclot); WB FIB, whole-blood fibrinogen test (Hemochron); platelets, platelet transfusion (6 U of random donor or apheresis unit equivalent); DDAVP, desmopressin acetate; antifibrinolytic Rx, antifibrinolytic therapy (e.g., ϵ-aminocaproic acid, tranexamic acid, aprotinin); FFP, plasma therapy (2 U of fresh frozen plasma); (+) MVB, continued microvascular bleeding; PT:aPTT, prothrombin time and aPTT control values (values/mean values from a normal reference population); PLAT count, platelet count (1,000/µL). (From Despotis GJ, Levine V, Saleem R, et al. DDAVP reduces blood loss and transfusion in cardiac surgical patients with impaired platelet function identified using a point-of-care test: a double-blind, placebo-controlled trial. *Lancet* 1999;354:106–110, with permission).

of blood within the mediastinal tubes to clot suggests a platelet or co-agulation factor abnormality or both; and the presence of clotted blood in the patient's tubes suggests relatively normal hemostatic function and the presence of surgical bleeding.

Laboratory studies regarding the patient's clotting status are essential. When the patient is bleeding excessively, the following studies should be drawn, preferably by a new venipuncture: platelet count, PT and INR, aPTT, and fibrinogen level.

Platelet dysfunction is the most common cause of microvascular (nonsurgical) postoperative bleeding following CPB, particularly in patients who have been treated with platelet inhibitors prior to surgery. Therefore, for the patient presumably suffering microvascular bleeding, transfusion of platelets is a common first step, even if the platelet count has not been determined or if it is in the relatively normal range (55). Although the patient's platelet count may be relatively normal, the platelets may be dysfunctional and may not provide for adequate clot formation. Apheresis platelet units are used. One apheresis platelet unit provides the approximate platelet volume of six random donors but is obtained from a single volunteer, thus limiting the exposure to the recipient. Children receive 5 to 10 mL/kg of platelet concentrate, whereas adults receive 1 apheresis platelet unit (equal in volume to about six random donor platelet units).

After transfusion, the platelet count should be repeated. If bleeding continues and the count is <75,000/mm^3, a repeat platelet transfusion should be performed.

If the patient's PT is >17 to 18 seconds or the INR is >1.5, a plasma clotting factor deficiency is likely present and treatment with FFP (2 to 3 units for an adult or 15 mL/kg) is indicated. Plasma is not indicated for an INR of <1.6 seconds and other causes for the ongoing bleeding should be sought. If the INR is abnormal but the patient is not bleeding, plasma is not indicated.

For the bleeding patient, if the INR is normal but the aPTT is significantly prolonged (1.5 times control value), consideration should be given to the possibility of a continued heparin effect and to the administration of more protamine. The presence of unneutralized heparin may also be confirmed by use of the ACT, the TT, or heparin concentration measurement (Hepcon®). Treatment is the administration of more protamine (usually 25 to 50 mg, slowly, for an adult). If the patient is not bleeding, transfusion of plasma or cryoprecipitate is not necessary, despite a longer-than-normal aPTT.

If the patient is bleeding and the fibrinogen level is <100 mg/dL, transfusion of cryoprecipitate is indicated. The usual adult dose is 10 units, which will increase the serum fibrinogen level by about 100 mg/dL. The pediatric dose is 1 unit of cryoprecipitate per 5 kg of body weight. It should be noted that FFP also contains fibrinogen with each FFP unit having the approximate fibrinogen equivalent of 2 units of cryoprecipitate.

Excessive postoperative bleeding results in the need for RBC transfusion, sometimes in large volumes. In the past, blood that was shed into the patient's chest tube drainage collection receptacle might be filtered and transfused back to the patient in an effort to reduce the need for RBC transfusion. It has subsequently been realized that this practice is associated with risks of activation of the extrinsic clotting pathway, lipid and thrombus emboli, and increased postoperative infections. For these reasons, this practice is no longer recommended (22).

Desmopressin (DDAVP) is not generally used to treat excessive postoperative bleeding. It may, however, have a role for certain patients who demonstrated platelet function defects (by thromboelastography or platelet function testing), although this remains an off-label use with mixed published results (14).

Cardiac Tamponade

The most serious acute result of excessive postoperative mediastinal bleeding is the development of cardiac tamponade, a potentially fatal complication that may develop slowly or rapidly and may be difficult to diagnose (56,57). Tamponade should be suspected in the unstable patient who was bleeding initially, but then suddenly slows as coagulation defects have been corrected. Blood within the chest tubes begins to clot and the tubes no longer drain well; blood collects within the mediastinum putting pressure on the heart, resulting in tamponade. The classic physical examination signs of tamponade (muffled heart sounds, jugular venous distention, Kussmaul's sign, and pulsus paradoxus) may be difficult to discern or may be absent in the intubated patient in the noisy intensive care unit environment. Hypotension, narrowed pulse pressure, tachycardia, low mixed venous oxygen saturation, and elevated venous pressures are nonspecific and may be present as the result of either tamponade or ventricular dysfunction. Hemodynamic measurements will demonstrate elevation of the central venous pressure to the level of the left heart filling pressure (left atrial, pulmonary artery capillary wedge, or pulmonary artery diastolic pressure), referred to as "equalization of filling pressures." In many patients, the chest x-ray may reveal a widened mediastinal shadow, although this is also common in postoperative patients without tamponade.

Echocardiography is a generally accurate method to determine the presence of cardiac tamponade. The finding of diastolic collapse of the right atrium is a sign of increased intrapericardial pressure or of hypovolemia, while diastolic collapse of the right ventricle is more specific for tamponade (58,59). Occasional patients, especially with regional tamponade with a loculated blood collection located posterior or lateral to the heart, may not be easily diagnosed by transthoracic echocardiography. In this instance, transesophageal echocardiography (TEE) is superior to transthoracic echocardiography for making the diagnosis. Strong consideration of TEE should be made when faced with a patient has an inappropriately low cardiac output and high filling pressures, even if the transthoracic echo is not diagnostic.

Even if echocardiography does not demonstrate tamponade, a high index of suspicion still must be maintained; immediate decompression may be lifesaving for the patient who has acutely decompensated for uncertain reasons. In some instances, the degree of suspicion may be high, the patient is acutely unstable, and echocardiography is not readily available. In such cases, it is best to err on the side of unnecessary reopening of the patient as compared to dangerous deterioration of the patient's hemodynamic status. Frequently, if urgent decompression is needed, it may be accomplished by opening the inferior portion of the patient's wound and introducing a gloved finger into the mediastinal space. If the diagnosis of tamponade is correct, the surgeon (and patient) will be rewarded by an outpouring of bloody fluid and rapid improvement in the patient's hemodynamic status. If this does not produce relief, the surgeon should proceed with sternotomy in the intensive care unit; this may be accomplished with considerable success (52,60). Patients with tamponade who are stable may be transferred to the operating room for a re-entry sternotomy and clot removal, generally with minimal complications and little or no increase in the length of hospital stay. *The greatest danger is that cardiac tamponade may go unrecognized and untreated.* Thus, a high level of suspicion should be maintained and there should be little hesitancy to re-explore the patient who may be suffering postoperative tamponade.

Tamponade may also develop later in the patient's postoperative course, even after discharge from the hospital (61,62). In this setting, the presentation is usually not obvious and the patient may appear to be suffering from congestive heart failure or myocardial insufficiency. Frequently, patients with delayed cardiac tamponade have been treated with warfarin. General malaise, lack of appetite, exertional dyspnea, and rising creatinine are clues to the diagnosis; echocardiography will confirm or rule out the condition. Treatment is drainage, either by percutaneous catheter placed by echocardiographic guidance or by limited sternotomy and placement of pericardial tubes (63).

Intractable Hemorrhage

Intractable life-threatening bleeding following cardiac surgery is rare but may occur as the result of coagulopathy not correctable with standard therapies including platelet, FFP and cryoprecipitate transfusion, and surgical re-exploration. In such cases, treatment with recombinant-activated factor VII (rFVIIa), an "off-label" (not FDA-approved) use, may be of value. While the mechanism of action of rFVIIa in this setting is not entirely understood, reports of efficacy are multiple. Definitive evidence from randomized controlled trials regarding the use of rFVIIa in cardiac surgery patients as "rescue therapy" is currently lacking, safety information is incomplete, and optimal dosing recommendations are not well defined (14,64–67). Concern regarding an increase in thrombotic complications (such as myocardial infarction and stroke) has been raised and therefore generalized use of rFVIIa to prevent or control bleeding is not recommended by some authorities (68). The patient's past history of thrombotic events such as DVT and/or pulmonary embolism (PE) or known hypercoagulopathy should be considered, as such patients might be at increased risk for thrombotic complications related to rFVIIa treatment. FVIIa should not be given to patients who are considered to have ongoing disseminated intravascular coagulation.

Prior to the administration of rFVIIa, it should be reasonably well assured that the patient is not bleeding from a surgical cause. Full reversal of the heparin effect with protamine should have been achieved. Correction of abnormal laboratory clotting studies (by transfusion of appropriate hemostatic blood products), correction of acidosis and hypothermia, and maintenance of adequate platelet count prior to administration will improve the effectiveness of rFVIIa treatment.

Common dosing recommendations of rFVIIa range from 40 to 100 mcg/kg body weight. Smaller doses have been recommended by some because of the high cost of rFVIIa and the potential for thrombotic complications (69). Our current dose is 50 mcg/kg, rounding to the nearest drug vial size (currently 1,200 mcg, 2,400 mcg, or 4,800 mcg). If ineffective, a second dose may be considered.

The use of rFVIIa should be considered only in cases of continued life-threatening postoperative bleeding where standard therapy has failed. It is important to be sure that a surgically correctable cause for the bleeding has been excluded. In most cases, this requires reoperation prior to rFVIIa treatment.

RENAL FAILURE

Postoperative renal insufficiency of some degree develops in 5% to 30% of patients undergoing cardiac surgery with approximately 1% requiring postoperative dialysis (71,72). Preoperative renal dysfunction is clearly associated with postoperative renal failure and increased operative mortality and complication rates (73,74). In fact, even mild elevation of the patient's preoperative serum creatinine level is associated with poorer postoperative outcomes, including higher mortality (75,76). Other preoperative risk factors associated with postoperative renal failure include advanced age, the presence of cardiogenic shock, pre-existing congestive heart failure, peripheral arterial disease, diabetes mellitus, female gender, and chronic obstructive pulmonary disease. In general, valve and complex procedures have a higher rate of this complication. Intraoperative variables associated with postoperative renal failure include the length of time on CPB, insertion of an intra-aortic balloon pump, and severe during anemia requiring RBC transfusion (77,78). The use of CPB for CABG may result in more postoperative renal impairment as compared to conventional "of pump" procedures, although this finding has not been universal (79–81).

A number of postoperative renal failure scoring systems have been devised. By assigning weight to preoperative risk factors, the likelihood of postoperative renal failure requiring dialysis may be estimated (82–84). One useful clinical score system is shown in Fig. 5.2.

Renal failure after cardiac surgery is often due to acute tubular necrosis that is due, at least in part, to impaired kidney perfusion (85). Factors that may contribute to this include hypotension, the use of vasoactive agents, and cholesterol emboli. Perioperative administration of nephrotoxic drugs, including NSAIDs, angiotensin-converting enzyme inhibitors, angiotensin receptor blockers, antibiotics, and contrast media are other potential contributors to postoperative renal dysfunction (67,86,87). Acute tubular necrosis is a reversible process, although proper management is required to prevent secondary complications (hyperkalemia, fluid overload, and uremia) until renal function returns.

Efforts to reduce the incidence of postoperative renal failure by the administration (before, during, or after surgery) of a variety of pharmacologic agents have been made. These include diuretics, dopamine, fenoldopam, mannitol, N-acetylcysteine, diltiazem, and others. Unfortunately, at this time, no drug has proven to conclusively protect the kidneys from injury during or after open-heart surgery (88–91). Potentially modifiable contributors to postoperative renal failure include preoperative anemia, perioperative RBC transfusions, and surgical re-exploration (92).

In the early postoperative period, the presence of renal insufficiency should be suspected in the patient with reduced urinary output (<0.5 mL/kg per hour for two to three consecutive hours) and rising creatinine levels. To be sure that the patient's bladder catheter is not obstructed, it is irrigated with a small volume of sterile saline (30 to 60 mL for adults). Bedside ultrasound, examination of the bladder is also a convenient method of ruling out a distended bladder that cannot empty. Ultrasound of the kidneys is performed to exclude ureteral

Last Creatinine	0.5	1.0	1.5	2.0	2.5	3.0	3.5	4.0 and higher
Points (Creatinine * 10)	5	10	15	20	25	30	35	40

Age	<55	55-59	60-64	65-69	70-74	75-79	80-84	85-89	90-94	95-99	100+
Points	0	1	2	3	4	5	6	7	8	9	10

Surgery	CABG Only	AV Only	AV + CABG	MV Only	MV + CABG
Points	0	2	5	4	7

Diabetes	No Diabetes	Controlled Orally	Insulin Dependent
Points	0	2	5

MI Recent	No Recent MI	Within Last 3 weeks
Points	0	3

Race	White	Non-White
Points	0	2

Chronic Lung Disease	No	Yes
Points	0	3

Reoperation	No Prior CV Surgery	Prior CAB or Other CV Surgery
Points	0	3

NYHA Class	I,II,III	IV
Points	0	3

Cardiogenic Shock	No	Yes
Points	0	7

Score

Total Score:

Total Score	0	2	4	6	8	10	12	14	16	18	20	22	24	26	28	30	32	34	36	38	40	42	44	46	48	50	52	54	56	58	60	62	64	66	68+
Risk of Dialysis, %	0.1	0.1	0.1	0.1	0.2	0.2	0.2	0.3	0.4	0.5	0.7	0.9	1.1	1.3	1.5	1.8	2.1	2.5	3	3.4	4.7	5.4	6.2	7.1	8.1	9.2	10	11	13	14	15	16	18	19	20

	21	22	24	25	28	31	33	35	40	42	44	48	55	56	59	59	62	64	66	70	80	85

FIGURE 5.2 Nomogram to predict postoperative renal dysfunction needing dialysis. (Reprinted with permission from Mehta RH, Grab JD, O'Brien SM, et al. Bedside tool for predicting the risk of postoperative dialysis in patients undergoing cardiac surgery. *Circulation* 2006;114:2208–2216.)

obstruction and evaluate kidney size (small kidneys suggest chronic renal insufficiency). Any medications that may contribute to renal insufficiency, including NSAIDs (such as ketorolac and ibuprofen) or angiotensin-converting enzyme inhibitors (such as lisinopril and captopril), should be discontinued.

Hypovolemia, low cardiac output, and hypotension will contribute significantly to kidney injury. If filling pressures are low or normal (central venous or pulmonary capillary wedge pressure <15 to 18 mm Hg), a fluid challenge should be given. If the hematocrit level is low (<21% to 23%), the transfusion of RBCs may be indicated as volume loading with crystalloid or colloid fluid will further lower the hematocrit level. Otherwise, a bolus infusion of 500 to 1,000 mL of crystalloid solution or 5% albumin may be administered over 30 to 60 minutes or 10 mL/kg for pediatric patients. If the cardiac output is suboptimal, appropriate inotropic drug support may be indicated. If the heart rate is <80 beats per minute, a trial of pacing may improve both cardiac output and renal blood flow. If the patient's blood pressure is on the lower end of the normal range, any antihypertensive medications should be discontinued. If the blood pressure is below normal, volume loading and vasoactive drug treatment is indicated (see Chapter 3). Elderly patients with new onset renal insufficiency may benefit from increasing the blood pressure to high-normal ranges (140 to 150 mm Hg), particularly if they have long-standing preoperative hypertension.

If there is little or no response to the fluid challenge, a dose of furosemide (40 to 80 mg IV for adults; 1 to 2 mg/kg IV for infants) with or without a concomitant dose of chlorothiazide (0.5 to 1.0 g IV) is sometimes successful in initiating urine flow. Alternatively, a continuous infusion of furosemide may be effective in maintaining satisfactory urine output in the patient who has sufficient preload (93). There is no conclusive evidence that furosemide in this setting reduces renal dysfunction and side effects such as ototoxicity may occur (94,95). The evidence for using low-dose dopamine (2 to 3 mg/kg/min IV) to improve urine flow is also not conclusive. Side effects such as tachyarrhythmias and pulmonary shunting may occur. Therefore, the routine use of dopamine to prevent or treat acute renal failure is not recommended (96–98).

Despite these measures, oliguric renal failure may develop and, in this setting, consultation with a nephrologist is appropriate. The management of the patient centers on preventing complications of the oliguric state. Fluid intake should be closely monitored and may be estimated as the daily output plus about 500 mL in adults. Frequent physical examination will help to follow the state of hydration of the patient. Potassium should not be administered unless the serum level falls below 3.5 mEq/L. Replacement should be done cautiously, in small amounts, and frequent determinations of the serum potassium level are required to recognize hyperkalemia early. Magnesium-containing antacids should be discontinued and replaced with aluminum or calcium antacids to prevent hypermagnesemia and to decrease intestinal absorption of phosphate. Patients on drugs eliminated by renal excretion must be monitored carefully, and dosages should be changed as indicated. Examples would include cimetidine and cefazolin. Consultation with the hospital-based pharmacist is of considerable value in this situation. Careful attention to the renal failure patient's nutrient requirements, with low protein and low phosphate diet, is also important (99).

For most oliguric patients, intervention will be likely be required to treat hyperkalemia, acidemia, fluid overload (often manifesting as respiratory insufficiency), or complications of uremia, such as lethargy and pericarditis. There is no consensus among nephrologists on when to begin renal replacement therapy (RRT) for acute onset renal failure. Early and intensive institution RRT appears, however, to be associated with improved outcomes as compared to more conservative treatment (100). Conventional intermittent hemodialysis may not be well tolerated by patients with recent cardiac surgery because of the possibility of hypotension and cardiovascular collapse. For adult patients, continuous renal replacement (venovenous hemofiltration) therapies have proven to be very successful for the management of acute renal failure (101). In this technique, gradual filtration of the blood is accomplished at a rate slower than intermittent hemodialysis and filtrate removal is by hydrostatic pressure. Solutes (such as potassium, urea, and creatinine) accompany the fluid, and the removed fluid is replaced with physiologic (potassium-free) solution as needed. Larger molecules such as heparin, insulin, and vancomycin are also removed by hemofiltration. Up to 500 mL per hour of fluid may be removed. Continuous RRT allows for better control of fluid and metabolic parameters, particularly in hemodynamically unstable patients. Venovenous hemofiltration employs a pump to remove venous blood (from a femoral or subclavian vein), does not rely on arterial pressure, provides good control of the blood flow and filtration rate, and has become the technique of choice in most intensive care units.

Nonoliguric renal failure after cardiac surgery is generally easier to manage and requires RRT infrequently. When the patient urinates in satisfactory or even excessive amounts, it is important to accurately monitor urine output, daily weight, and serum electrolyte concentrations. Volume replacement should be provided as indicated to prevent hypovolemia and electrolyte abnormalities, usually by matching the urine output with administration of one-half normal saline.

For infants with renal failure, peritoneal dialysis can be performed conveniently at the bedside and has been the usual form of RRT for these patients, although experience with continuous veno-venous hemofiltration has been described (102,103).

Acute renal failure requiring dialysis after cardiac surgery is a complication associated with high mortality, but most of the patients who die also suffer failure of other organ systems. Contemporary management improves the prognosis of patients who suffer this postoperative complication (104).

INFECTIOUS COMPLICATIONS

Major infections occur in approximately 3.5% of adult cardiac surgery patients. They occur most frequently in patients with obesity, diabetes mellitus, previous myocardial infarction, urgent operative status, cardiogenic hock, dialysis-dependent renal failure, long CPB durations, and immunosuppressive therapy (105). Perioperative transfusion of RBCs is also associated with postoperative bacterial infection (106). Vein harvest site infections, mediastinitis, and septicemia are the most common infectious complications.

Wound Infections and Mediastinitis

Wound infections after a sternotomy incision may be superficial, involving only the skin and subcutaneous fat, or they may be deep, involving the sternum and underlying mediastinal structures. They are clearly an important contributor to postoperative morbidity and mortality in patients undergoing cardiac surgery (107,108).

Superficial infections are characterized by drainage from the wound and local inflammation while the underlying sternum remains stable. In this instance, removal of the overlying skin sutures, culture of the drainage, administration of antibiotics, and local dressings are often successful treatment.

Bacterial mediastinitis (deep sternal wound infection) occurs in about 0.25 to 4% of adult patients undergoing open-heart surgery and is associated with increased short- and long-term mortality rates (109–111). In our experience, the incidence in children is much lower. The reported incidence in heart transplantation patients is, however, higher (112). In various published reports, the risk factors identified for the development of serious postoperative sternal wound complications include obesity, smoking, repeat operations, prolonged operative time, early chest re-exploration for postoperative bleeding, RBC blood transfusion, prolonged postoperative mechanical ventilation, and prolonged postoperative low cardiac output (105,113,114). CABG patients with preoperative glycosylated hemoglobin (HbA_{1c}) levels above 6% are at increased risk for both superficial and deep sternal wound infections (115). While the use of a single internal mammary (internal thoracic) artery for coronary bypass conduit is not considered a risk factor, the use of both internal mammary arteries is associated with an increased

TABLE 5.2	Infection Risk Scores for Major Infection After Coronary Artery Bypass Graft	
	Preop Only	**Combined**
Preoperative variables		
Age (for each 5 years over 55)	1 point	1 point
BMI 30 to 40 kg/m^2	4 points	3 points
BMI 40 + kg/m^2	9 points	8 points
Diabetes	3 points	3 points
Renal failure	4 points	4 points
Congestive heart failure	3 points	3 points
Peripheral vascular disease	2 points	2 points
Female gender	2 points	2 points
Chronic lung disease	2 points	3 points
Cardiogenic shock	6 points	N/A
Myocardial infarction	2 points	N/A
Concomitant surgery	4 points	N/A
Intraoperative variables		
Perfusion time 100 to 200 min	N/A	3 points
Perfusion time 200 to 300 min	N/A	7 points
Intra-aortic balloon pump	N/A	5 points

Note: A patient's total risk score is calculated by adding the total points for all risk factors present. Use Table 5.3 to determine the infection risk associated with that total risk score.
Adapted from Fowler VG, O'Brien SM, Muhlbaier LW, et al. Clinical predictors of major infections after cardiac surgery. *Circulation* 2005;112(suppl I):I-358–I-365.

incidence of sternal wound complications, particularly in diabetic patients (116,117). Using a technique of "skeletonization," in which the internal mammary artery is dissected from the chest wall without an attached pedicle of chest wall tissue, may lower this risk (118). The decision to use bilateral internal mammary arteries should weigh both the benefit of increased long-term graft patency (as compared to vein grafts) and the potential risk of sternal wound problems. Such decisions are individualized based on the age of the patient and the presence of other medical problems. Generally we avoid the use of both internal mammary arteries in patients with advanced age, diabetes mellitus, severe obesity, and chronic obstructive pulmonary disease, current smoking, and previous radiation therapy to the sternal area.

Risk scores used to predict surgical site infections have been developed. A useful scoring system for CABG patients is shown in Tables 5.2 and 5.3 (105,119).

In general, patients with tracheostomies are considered to be at increased risk for sternal incision infections due to the close proximity of the incision to the tracheal stoma, which is colonized by bacteria. If the tracheostomy is present before the sternotomy, all efforts should be

TABLE 5.3 Estimated Probability of Infection by Risk Score Category

Risk Score	Probability of Infection (%)	
	Preop Only	**Combined**
0	0.9	0.8
1	1.0	0.9
2	1.1	1.0
3	1.3	1.2
4	1.5	1.3
5	1.6	1.5
6	1.9	1.8
7	2.1	2.0
8	2.4	2.3
9	2.7	2.7
10	3.1	3.0
11	3.5	3.5
12	4.0	4.0
13	4.5	4.5
14	5.1	5.2
15	5.8	6.0
16	6.6	6.7
17	7.4	7.6
18	8.2	8.5
19	9.1	9.4
20	9.9	10.2
21	10.7	11.1
22	11.4	11.8
23	12.1	12.5
24	12.9	13.4
25	13.6	14.0
26+	16.0	16.2

Note: A patient's total risk score calculated from Table 5.2 may be used to estimate probability of major infection.
Adapted from Fowler VG, O'Brien SM, Muhlbaier LW, et al. Clinical predictors of major infections after cardiac surgery. *Circulation* 2005;112(suppl I):I-358–I-365.

made to isolate the stoma from the incision during the procedure and to avoid connecting the mediastinal dissection with the plane of the pretracheal fascia. If the tracheostomy is required postoperatively, the skin incision should be placed as high as possible, taking care to limit the dissection so that it does not communicate with the previous substernal dissection. The sternal wound should be protected from the tracheostomy by dressings. With such precautions, the risk of postoperative mediastinitis associated with tracheostomy can be minimized, although reports in this regard differ (120,121). In our practices, this risk appears to be low and the benefit of early tracheostomy for the patient with postoperative respiratory failure is generally great. Therefore, the trend has been to perform tracheostomy earlier (perhaps after 6 to 7 days on the ventilator) in these patients.

The use of electrical clippers to remove chest hair, rather than manual shaving, is associated with a lower incidence of mediastinitis and is standard (122). Other nonpharmacologic measures to reduce postoperative sternal wound infections include preoperative smoking cessation, avoidance of applying bone wax to the sternal edges, double-gloving, judicious use of cautery to minimize tissue damage, and aggressive postoperative serum glucose management in both diabetic and nondiabetic patients (see Chapter 3).

Patients undergoing cardiac surgery should receive prophylactic antibiotics. The antibiotic should be administered within 60 minutes prior to the skin incision (123). The most common organism associated with sternal wound infections is *Staphylococcus species*, either *Staphylococcus epidermidis or Staphylococcus aureus.* Methicillin-resistant isolates of *S. aureus* are becoming increasingly prevalent (124,125). The prophylactic antibiotic of choice is cefazolin. At institutions where methicillin-resistant *Staphylococcus* is an important pathogen, vancomycin should administered in addition to, but not used in place of, cefazolin. Vancomycin should not, however, be used routinely as it promotes the emergence of vancomycin-resistant organisms. The adult cefazolin dose is 1 to 2 g and the pediatric dose is 15.0 mg/kg of body weight. Often a second 1 g cefazolin dose (for adults) is given to the patient after weaning from CPB. Postoperatively, the patient receives the same dose of cefazolin every 8 hours for 24 to 48 hours, but for no longer (109). Patients who have definite and significant cephalosporin or penicillin allergy should receive vancomycin preoperatively and for no more than 48 hours after surgery; an aminoglycoside, usually gentamicin or levofloxacin, may be added to improve gram-negative organism coverage (117).

Most *S. aureus* infections are due to organisms that colonize the patient's own hands and/or nose. Preoperative self-administration of the topical antibiotic mupirocin has been demonstrated to be highly effective in reducing nasal *S. aureus* and the incidence of associated infections. Short-term therapy with intranasal mupirocin has been demonstrated to be effective in reducing sternal wound infections and routine administration is recommended (117,126). Mupirocin ointment is applied to the nares in the evening before and the morning of surgery and twice daily for 5 days afterward.

The early diagnosis of sternal infection and mediastinitis after cardiac surgery can be difficult. At least 50% of the infections are not evident until after the patient has been discharged from the hospital. Those due to coagulase-negative *Staphylococci* may be difficult to recognize as they often present late and have less apparent signs and symptoms (127,128). The standard chest radiograph is of little value in predicting infection or sternal dehiscence. A vertical sternal lucency (the so-called sternal stripe) is frequently seen on early postoperative chest x-ray but is not a sensitive indicator of infection or dehiscence in the absence of other findings. In some patients, fever, leukocytosis, and a positive blood culture will be the first manifestations of a hidden infection that only later becomes obvious. The most common early sign is fluid drainage from the wound; sternal instability usually develops subsequently. Sterile sternal dehiscence with instability but without drainage sometimes occurs. These will require rewiring, but are infectious complications.

In some patients, the diagnosis of sternal infection and mediastinitis is not clear-cut and chest computed tomography (CT) might be of value (129). If infection is present, there is often a mediastinal soft tissue mass with bilateral pleural effusions, an excessive mediastinal fluid with air-fluid levels, bone destruction, and separation of the sternum. Needle aspiration of the mediastinum under CT scan guidance for Gram stain and culture of the fluid obtained may aid in the diagnosis of mediastinitis.

Treatment of serious sternotomy wound infections depends on the stage of the process at the time of diagnosis. If early, when the sternum is not destroyed, success may be achieved by prompt reoperation, debridement of the sternal edges, copious irrigation of the mediastinum, placement of retrosternal irrigation and drainage catheters, rewiring of the sternum, and closure of the fascia and skin (130,131). A dilute antibiotic solution, chosen according to Gram-stain results, is infused slowly through the irrigating catheters with the fluid exiting via the drainage catheters until the drainage fluid is sterile by culture (usually 3 to 5 days). Although often successful, this method has potential serious complications such as erosion of the catheters into mediastinal structures and systemic toxicity from absorption of the irrigating antibiotic. For these reasons, this technique is usually reserved for particular patients and is not used in our practices.

Our most frequent approach to treating serious deep sternal wound infections involves removal of the sternal wires, debridement of the sternum and cartilage, and placement of a wound vacuum-assisted closure dressing. In this method, nonviable appearing soft tissues are excised and the sternum is debrided to the point where healthy-appearing bleeding bone is encountered. A polyurethane foam pad is placed in the anterior mediastinum and between the remaining sternal edges and covered with an airtight dressing. Continuous local negative pressure is applied to the mediastinal tissues, in conjunction with appropriate systemic antibiotic administration. The foam dressing is performed every

48 hours. When the tissues appear clean with visible granulation tissue ingrowth, typically in 4 to 8 days, the patient is returned to the operating room for closure. Depending on the degree of sternal resection required, the remaining bone may or may not be rewired together. If the sternum cannot be reapproximated, pedicled muscle flaps, using the pectoralis major and/or rectus muscles, are used to fill the resulting empty space. Soft silastic drains are placed beneath the muscle flaps and placed to gentle suction. This technique, often performed in conjunction with a plastic surgeon, is associated with low mortality and morbidity and reduces the length of hospital stay as the patient may be discharged with the drains in place with planned removal in the office when the daily drainage volume becomes sufficiently small. In some patients, sufficient sternal bone remains and closure sternum is possible. For these, the use of rigid transverse plate fixation to facilitate approximation of the sternal halves can be advantageous (132). Our experience with the early aggressive use of sternal wound debridement, vacuum-assisted closure wound dressing, and subsequent muscle flap closure of the seriously infected mediastinum has been excellent and considerable success, both in adults and in children, has been reported in the literature (133–135).

In all instances, attention to the patient's nutritional state is of prime importance. Consultation with the hospital-based dietician, daily calorie counts, and vitamin supplementation are necessary for patients with wound infection. If oral intake is insufficient, early enteral tube or parenteral feeding should be administered to avoid malnutrition and to augment healing.

Infections at the site of *saphenous vein harvest site* are not rare and are more likely to occur in obese patients and patients with severe peripheral arterial disease. Spontaneous drainage of small-to-moderate amounts of noninfected serosanguineous fluid from leg incisions is common. For this, the application of dry dressings and leg elevation usually results in resolution. Often this drainage is the result of an underlying hematoma that has liquefied and the fluid drains out the neighboring skin incision. True leg wound infections are manifested by erythema, induration, and undue tenderness to palpation. If underlying fluctuance is present, incision and drainage, followed by open packing and secondary healing, in addition to treatment with appropriate antibiotics is indicated. Major infections can lead to the need for skin grafts, vascular procedures, and even amputations (136).

The use of endoscopic techniques for harvesting of the saphenous vein for CABG procedures has become commonplace and is associated with a reduced rate of leg wound infections and other complications (137,138). Concern has been raised that potential trauma to the endoscopically removed vein may compromise graft patency. Reported results in this regard have shown mixed outcomes (139,140).

Pneumonia

Pneumonia is the most frequent postoperative infectious complication in patients undergoing cardiac surgery, occurring in about 3.5% (141). It occurs most frequently in patients who are ventilator supported and is associated with high mortality, morbidity, and cost of hospitalization. Such ventilator-associated pneumonia (VAP) is most frequently caused by aspiration of contaminated oropharyngeal secretions and/or enteral tube feedings (142,143). Postoperative pneumonia is associated with preoperative smoking and chronic obstructive pulmonary disease, the need for reintubation or mechanical ventilation for more than 48 hours, the transfusion of than 4 units of blood, the presence of an nasogastric tube, and prolonged intensive care unit stay (144). Efforts to prevent VAP include reducing the duration of mechanical ventilation, position-ing patients in the semirecumbent position with the head of the bed el-evated 30° to 45°, the use of specially designed endotracheal tubes that provide for continuous aspiration of subglottic secretions, aggressive oral hygiene, and careful attention to enteral tube feedings to prevent high gastric residual collections (145).

The diagnosis of pneumonia is based on the presence of fever, leukocytosis, the development of an infiltrate on chest x-ray, and puru-lent sputum culture that grows a predominant organism. Suctioning the patient via the endotracheal tube to obtain a culture of the lower respiratory tract can be useful. The most common organisms in VAP are aerobic gram-negative bacilli, although considerable variability be-tween hospitals exists. For patients with hospital-acquired pneumonia, treatment antibiotic therapy should be begun immediately. Initial empiric antibiotic therapy for VAP is based on suspected potential pathogens, which is influenced by the result of gram stain examination of the patient's sputum and whether the patent is at risk for multidrug-resistant bacteria (146) or not. Once the results of culture and antibiotic susceptibility testing are available, specific therapy can be instituted. Treatment of confirmed pneumonia is by administration of specific an-tibiotics, aggressive pulmonary toilet, and ventilator support as required.

Catheter Sepsis

Most frequently, central venous catheters for monitoring and fluid ad-ministration purposes are placed in the patient's internal jugular vein. The rate of infection for this access site is low while use of the femoral and/or the subclavian vein is associated with a higher rate of infectious complications (147). Infection of an intravenous catheter can lead to fever, bacteremia, toxicity, shock, endocarditis, and bacterial seeding of the patient's fresh sternotomy incision. Patients who have been hospi-talized for a period of time before surgery or who have been transferred from an outside institution should be closely inspected to rule out the presence of phlebitis. Catheters or sheaths placed via the groin into the femoral artery or vein at the time of cardiac catheterization should be removed preoperatively if other access sites are possible, the patient is not heparinized, and surgery will not be performed for 12 to 24 hours. If surgery is imminent, we remove these groin cannulas postoperatively as soon as hemostatic function has returned, usually within 12 to 24 hours. In particular, femoral vein catheters are associated with an increased incidence of venous thrombosis and infection (148). If an infected peripheral intravenous catheter site is found preoperatively and the patient is stable, it is best to postpone the surgery and treat the patient with antibiotics (and vein excision if required) for several days. Sterile technique (including gloves, mask gown, and drapes) is mandatory when central venous catheters are being inserted. The use of catheters impregnated with chlorhexidine and silver sulfadiazine or minocycline is associated with a reduced infection rate (149).

When a postoperative patient develops a fever early after surgery, atelectasis is the most likely cause. Catheter infection, however, can also occur very early after surgery and can lead to severe sepsis. Infected central lines are usually not associated with redness or drainage at the insertion site. Thus, if the fever persists, blood cultures should be drawn, the catheter should be removed, and its tip should be cultured. In general, if central venous access is still needed for the care of the patient, this should be achieved through a new site rather than by exchanging the suspect catheter with a new one over a guidewire. For patients requiring prolonged central venous access, we usually insert a peripheral intravenous central catheter (PICC line) at the antecubital location and remove the jugular vein and/or femoral catheters.

GASTROINTESTINAL COMPLICATIONS

Gastrointestinal (GI) complications occur in about 1% to 4% of patients who undergo cardiac surgery. They are often insidious in onset, difficult to diagnose, and severe in their consequences. The most likely cause of these complications is visceral hypoperfusion in surgery or during the early postoperative (150–152). Risk factors for postoperative GI complications include older age, peripheral vascular disease, congestive heart failure, preoperative renal failure, chronic steroid use, long periods of CPB, blood transfusions, the use of an intra-aortic balloon pump, vasopressor support, and re-exploration for postoperative bleeding. Overall, the serious GI complications have a high mortality rate, up to 50%. Clinical manifestations of these problems may be subtle in the patient who has recently undergone open-heart surgery and a high index of suspicion is required to make the diagnosis. The most common complications encountered are ileus, bleeding, intestinal ischemia, cholecystitis, pancreatitis, and colonic pseudo-obstruction.

Intestinal Ileus

Failure of the intestinal contents to progress normally is not uncommon following major surgery and narcotic administration. To some degree, intestinal ileus is present in all patients following cardiac surgery but when prolonged, it will lengthen the time of hospital stay and may lead to the need for parenteral alimentation. Severe ileus occurs in <1% of patients. Clinically, the patient may be nauseated but severe abdominal pain is absent. The abdomen is usually distended and bowel sounds absent. Signs of peritoneal irritation are not generally present. An abdominal radiograph reveals mildly dilated bowel loops but without signs of bowel obstruction such as severe dilatation of the proximal small bowel and absence of air in the colon and rectum. Treatment of paralytic ileus is conservative with avoidance of narcotics as well as possible placement of a nasogastric suction tube and support with intravenous fluids and calories as indicated. A trial of metoclopramide (10 mg IV every 6 to 8 hours) may be of value, although the results of this treatment have been mixed (153,154). Having the alert patient try chewing gum may also help to promote GI motility (155). We have found this intervention to appear to be of benefit in occasional patients with postoperative ileus. Patients with postoperative ileus should be followed closely as differentiation between ileus and bowel ischemia may be difficult. With time, resolution of ileus occurs.

Gastrointestinal Tract Bleeding

Significant (GI) tract bleeding occurs in 0.5% to 1% of cardiac surgery patients, most commonly due to stress ulcer formation. Risk factors for this complication include patients who require ventilator support for more than 48 hours, history of previous GI bleeding, and impaired blood clotting (156). Prophylactic treatment with drugs to reduce the probability of GI bleeding has become widespread with the most common agents being the *histamine₂* receptor agonists (e.g., famotidine, ranitidine, or cimetidine) or *proton pump inhibitors* (e.g., omeprazole). These drugs do have significant potential side effects and drug interactions. The histamine₂ receptor agonists have potential neuropsychiatric effects that can contribute to the development of postoperative delirium. Omeprazole has been shown to significantly reduce the effectiveness of clopidogrel, an interaction of importance particularly for patients with coronary artery stents, and/or acute coronary syndromes (157,158). One suggested regimen for the prophylactic treatment of stress-related mucosal damage is famotidine, which is administered intravenously early after surgery (20 mg twice daily for adults). When taking the patient is able, the same dose is given by mouth or by nasogastric tube. Alternatively, omeprazole may be administered, keeping in mind the interaction with clopidogrel.

GI bleeding will be manifest by hematemesis, the appearance of blood in the nasogastric tube drainage, and/or by the passage of melanotic stool. When a significant amount of bleeding has occurred, the patient may become hypovolemic and hemodynamically unstable. Management involves placement of secure intravenous access, determination of the patient's hematocrit and coagulation status, gastric lavage, and consultation with a gastroenterologist and/or GI surgeon. For the hemodynamically unstable patient, a central venous catheter should be placed for volume and blood administration and central venous pressure should be measured to guide fluid therapy. Blood should be typed and crossmatched for transfusion as indicated, and other preparations for a possible emergency laparotomy should be made. Endoscopy is performed to determine the source of GI bleeding and to obtain cultures for *Heliobacter pylori*. In most patients, localized upper GI tract bleeding sites (duodenal or gastric ulcers) may be treated endoscopically by electrocoagulation and/or placement of clips, in conjunction with epinephrine injection at the site of the bleeding vessel. Treatment with an intravenous proton-pump inhibitor, omeprazole, or pantoprazole is begun (80 mg bolus dose plus continuous IV infusion at 8 mg per hour) for 72 hours, followed by transition to oral administration (159). Persistent or recurrent bleeding may require a second attempt at endoscopic hemostasis. Patients who fail this, who develop hypotension with rebleeding, or who have very large ulcers will require surgical treatment.

For patients with documented *H. pylori* infection and duodenal ulcer disease, omeprazole (or lansoprazole) is administered in conjunction with antibiotics (often clarithromycin and amoxicillin) for a 2-week course.

If the patient has experienced melena or bloody diarrhea but upper endoscopy is negative, lower GI tract bleeding is present and colonoscopy should be performed. Etiologies include mesenteric ischemia, bleeding from a polyp or diverticulum, or antibiotic-associated colitis secondary to *Clostridium difficile*. Treatment is specific to the cause.

Perforation of a duodenal (or gastric) ulcer is now a rare occurrence after cardiac operations. The patient, if awake, experiences sudden and severe abdominal pain that often radiates to the shoulder. No bowel sounds are heard on examination, and there is rigidity with signs of peritoneal irritation. An upright portable chest or cross-table lateral abdominal x-ray usually shows free air underneath the diaphragm, although this finding is not always present. Management of GI perforation requires gastric tube suction, fluid resuscitation as indicated, and antibiotic coverage. General surgical consultation should be obtained promptly, as surgical closure of the perforation (with or without a definitive peptic ulcer disease procedure) is often required.

Intestinal Ischemia

Mesenteric ischemia may be occlusive (due to an embolus) or nonocclusive due to impaired perfusion as may occur during or following cardiac surgery, especially in patients with mesenteric arterial stenoses or diffuse atherosclerosis. It may also occur after repair of aortic dissections in which successful perfusion of the mesenteric circulation is not achieved. Diagnosis of intestinal ischemia is often difficult, as it may not become evident until several days after surgery. Some patients may have a preoperative history of postprandial abdominal pain, anorexia, and weight loss indicative of chronic mesenteric arterial obstruction. Most often, however, the affected postoperative patient complains of diffuse abdominal pain and bloating. Upon palpation signs of peritoneal irritation are often present. An elevated serum lipase level, although nonspecific, may be a clue to the presence of bowel infarction. Fluid resuscitation and nasogastric suction should be implemented and the patient should be frequently examined. Colonoscopy, although difficult due to the unprepared colon, may be useful to diagnose ischemic or infracted bowel. Abdominal CT angiography or mesenteric arteriography may be of value (160). If deterioration occurs (increasing pain, tachycardia, fever), laparotomy should be performed to rule out or treat intestinal infarction. The mortality rate of intestinal ischemia requiring surgical exploration is very high (161,162).

Systemic cholesterol emboli can cause multisystem complications, including renal or GI complications. While frank bowel ischemia leading to an acute picture can occur, lesser degrees of involvement can produce delayed perforation or late intestinal stenosis.

Acute Cholecystitis

Acute cholecystitis (most frequently acalculous) occurs rarely of cardiac surgery patients but, even so, should be kept in mind when a patient complains of abdominal discomfort. It is often associated with multiorgan failure in critically ill patients and therefore has a high mortality rate (163). The patient often complains of right upper quadrant pain, may be febrile and often has leukocytosis. A septic hemodynamic pattern may develop and a variable degree of hyperbilirubinemia and abnormal liver enzyme levels may be present. Physical examination is often difficult because the patient will frequently guard when palpated because of the nearby sternotomy incision. Abdominal ultrasonography is the first diagnostic test and is very helpful if an enlarged gallbladder with a thickened wall is demonstrated or if there is fluid around the gallbladder. Hepatobiliary scans are also useful, but they have a significant incidence of false-positive results in patients who have recently undergone major surgery. The diagnosis, however, should be pursued since untreated cholecystitis can result in gangrene of the gallbladder. Laparoscopy can lead to definitive diagnosis and treatment (cholecystectomy), if indicated (164). In critically ill patients, a percutaneous cholecystostomy tube can palliate this condition. When the patient has recovered, if cholelithiasis and duct obstruction is ruled out by contrast cholecystography, the percutaneously placed tube may be removed 4 to 6 weeks following insertion. Of note is the observation that ongoing bile drainage can cause marked sensitivity to warfarin.

Acute Pancreatitis

Clinically evident pancreatitis following heart surgery is now rare (165). It is speculated that the relative hypoperfusion of the pancreas during the period of CPB, calcium administration, high-dose narcotic anesthesia, and vasoconstriction secondary to vasopressors may contribute to pancreatic injury. Clinically evident pancreatitis in the postoperative patient often becomes apparent on the fourth or fifth postoperative day when the patient complains of abdominal pain and nausea, vomiting, or anorexia. An elevated serum amylase level will suggest the diagnosis. Although asymptomatic elevation of the amylase level may occur and not require treatment.

The treatment of documented pancreatitis consists of withholding oral feedings and, if an ileus is present, placement of a nasogastric tube for suction drainage of the stomach. Postoperative pancreatitis is usually self-limiting, and most patients are able to restart a clear liquid diet within a few days. Severe hemorrhagic pancreatitis necessitating surgical drainage and pancreatic debridement is now very rare.

Acute Hepatic Failure

Acute hepatic failure most often accompanies prolonged low cardiac output and multiorgan failure in adult patients receiving maximum supportive therapy such as catecholamines, intra-aortic balloon pumping, and dialysis. It occurs rarely in children. Along with profound jaundice, hypoglycemia and coagulopathy may develop. Management consists mainly in general measures to support the circulation and provide nutrition and close monitoring of blood chemical constituents. Vitamin K and FFP should be administered if bleeding occurs. The mortality rate of fulminant hepatic failure following open-heart surgery is very high.

Nausea, Dysphagia, Diarrhea, and Hiccups

Some degree of postoperative nausea, occasionally with vomiting, is not unusual in patients who undergo cardiac surgery, likely the result of reduced GI motility and narcotic administration (166). In most patients, this may be successfully treated with intravenous ondansetron (2 to 4 mg, adult dose). Prochlorperazine may be given by rectal suppository (25 mg) or intramuscular injection (5 to 10 mg). For some patients, metoclopramide is successful in improving GI motility and relieving nausea.

Difficulty swallowing may occur after cardiac operations, especially in older patients in association with neurologic complications. In some affected patients, no cause for the swallowing difficulty is identified, although prolonged ventilation is a risk factor (167,168). Treatment is maintenance of nutrition with enteral or parenteral feeding, precautions to avoid aspiration, and consultation with a speech/swallowing therapist for modification of eating behavior and swallowing technique. Recovery of swallowing may be protracted but usually occurs.

Painful swallowing after cardiac surgery is not uncommon. Irritation from previously placed endotracheal and nasogastric tubes may be causative but, in some patients, the odynophagia may be due to overgrowth of *Candida albicans* in the oropharynx or esophagus (169). Simple oropharyngeal candida (thrush) is treated with oral nystatin. All antibiotics are discontinued unless absolutely needed to treat a documented infection. This is nearly always successful. Serious esophageal infections are diagnosed by barium swallow and/or endoscopy and may require intravenous or oral antifungal treatment for control.

Causes of postoperative diarrhea include excessive laxative/stool softener administration, tube feedings, intestinal ischemia (see earlier), and infection with the *C. difficile* bacterium. The latter is a serious, potentially fatal, disease that is associated with antibiotic administration. It is easily transmitted from one patient to another by the health care workers and therefore isolation of the patient with suspect *C. difficile* disease is indicated until the diagnosis is ruled out by stool sample culture. Treatment is with metronidazole or vancomycin, although the incidence of metronidazole-resistant disease is increasing (170).

Postoperative hiccups are a troublesome problem in occasional patients. Often thought to be due to diaphragmatic irritation that occurred during the procedure, the cause of hiccups is not really known and may be related to drugs (especially benzodiazepines and corticosteroids), esophageal distension, gastroesophageal reflux, or it may be of central nervous system origin (171). Suggested treatments are many and varied; chlorpromazine may be administered for the disorder (172). The starting adult dose is 25 to 50 mg by mouth three or

four times per day. The course of chlorpromazine treatment should be short as side effects may develop with prolonged treatment. Placement of a nasogastric tube may also result in termination of the hiccups (173).

NEUROLOGIC COMPLICATIONS

Cerebral dysfunction after cardiac surgery is an increasingly common and difficult problem in cardiac surgery as the patient population becomes older and patients have more complicating medical problems and undergo increasingly complex operations. For adults, the incidence of transient or permanent adverse cerebral outcomes (including stroke, encephalopathy, and/or delirium) may be as high as 10% to 50% (174–177). Not surprisingly, postoperative cerebral dysfunction is associated with increases in mortality, length, and cost of hospital stay, and the need for long-term care facilities.

Commonly recognized clinical risk factors for postoperative neurologic dysfunction are advanced age, previous neurologic events, cerebrovascular disease, diabetes mellitus, hypertension, previous cardiac surgery, preoperative infection, and urgent operation Other factors associated with postoperative strokes in adults include atherosclerosis of the ascending aorta, prolonged CPB time, intraoperative hemofiltration, and high blood transfusion requirement (178–181). Valve operations and complex operations, such as combined CABG and valve procedures, have increased stroke risk. Operations on the ascending aorta and procedures requiring hypothermic circulatory arrest are more likely to be associated with adverse cerebral outcomes, especially for elderly patients (182).

Postoperative neurologic events include stroke, transient ischemic attacks (TIAs), delirium, and cognitive decline.

Stroke

A perioperative stroke is the result of irreversible ischemic death of brain matter resulting in a gross neurologic deficit such as hemiparesis, caused by a disturbance in cerebral blood supply. Although often considered a "postoperative" complication, many strokes begin during the operative procedure. It is not until several hours after surgery, when the patient's anesthetic has worn off, that the deficit can be appreciated. Ischemia of the brain may occur secondary to global hypoperfusion due to inadequate blood flow and perfusion pressure during surgery, and this may be exacerbated by the presence of occlusive lesions in the patient's cerebral vessels. More commonly, however, strokes are the result of emboli to the cerebral circulation (183,184). Emboli to the brain during surgery may be composed of atherosclerotic debris, thrombus, fat,

Risk factor	Score
Age	(Age–25) x 1.43
Unstable angina	14
Diabetes mellitus	17
Neurological disease	18
Prior CABS	15
Vascular disease	18
Pulmonary disease	15

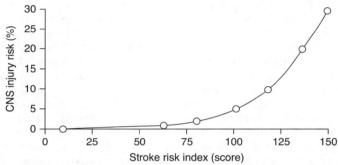

FIGURE 5.3 Multicenter preoperative stroke risk index for patients undergoing coronary artery bypass graft surgery. Definitions: diabetes mellitus–history of either type I or type II diabetes or insulin use on admission or before operation; neurologic disease–revious strok or trnsient ischemic attack; vascular disease–peripheral vascular disease, known carotid vascular disease, claudication or vascular surgery; pulmonary disease–emphysema, chronic bronchitis, asthma, restrictive lung disease. CABS = coronary artery bypass surgery, CNS = central nervous system. (From Arrowsmith JE, et al. Central nervous system complications of cardiac surgery. *Br J Anaesth* 2000;84:378–393, with permission.)

or air. Generally, recognized risk factors for stroke occurring with CABG include advanced age (over 70 years), previous stroke, hypertension, diabetes, cigarette smoking, and carotid bruit.

Risk prediction models for patients undergoing CABG surgery has been developed that may be used to predict an individual patient's preoperative risk of stroke (177,185). An example is shown in Fig. 5.3.

Patients with carotid artery occlusive disease have an increased risk of perioperative stroke and preoperative identification of these patients by carotid ultrasound examination is of value (186). If severe disease is present, either preoperative or concomitant carotid endarterectomy may be indicated. Chapter 1 discusses this issue in further. In our practices, preoperative ultrasound examinations are performed in patients over 70, patients with bruits or heart murmurs that could mask the auscultation of bruits, patients with previous strokes, patients with significant left main coronary artery obstruction, and patients with known peripheral vascular disease.

Efforts to prevent neurologic injury in cardiac surgery patients center largely on modifications of intraoperative technique. For coronary artery bypass procedures, it has been suggested that performing the operation without the use of CPB ("off-pump") may be associated with fewer strokes, but this has not been well proven (175,177,187,188).

Patients with atherosclerosis of the ascending aorta have an increased risk of adverse cerebral outcomes with cardiac surgery. Intraoperative TEE may be useful in identifying patients at increased risk for embolic stroke by revealing the presence of atherosclerotic plaque in the descending thoracic aorta, which is a marker for the increased likelihood of plaque being present in the ascending aorta. Examination of the ascending aorta is not usually feasible with this technique. The ascending aorta is, however, easily examined using a handheld (epiaortic) ultrasound transducer is also a useful technique. When plaque is found to be present, it is usually possible to modify the locations of aortic cannulation and cross-clamp application so as to avoid the plaque and thereby reducing the chance of plaque material embolism. In some patients, the degree of calcification present may require significant alterations in the operative plan. For coronary artery bypass procedures, this could mean performing the grafts with the patient on bypass but without cross-clamping the diseased aorta, the use of arterial grafts only so as to avoid the manipulation associated with sewing vein grafts to the ascending aorta, or avoiding CPB altogether and performing the procedure "off-pump" (beating heart technique). For the very severely diseased aorta, replacement may be indicated. In our practices, intraoperative epiaortic ultrasound has been found to be quick and simple to perform and is used in patients over 70 years of age, patients found to have plaque in the descending aorta by TEE, and those with palpable plaque in the ascending aorta. The use of intraoperative TEE and epiaortic ultrasound in efforts to reduce perioperative stroke has widely described (189–192).

Small lipid emboli may be associated with cerebral dysfunction following the use of CPB. The source of the fat appears to be from the re-infusion of blood suctioned from the pericardial sac during the procedure and the microemboli may be detected in the brain as lipid deposits that create small capillary and arteriolar dilatations that are associated with ischemic injury and neuronal dysfunction. Reducing the volume of blood returned directly to the patient through the arterial circuit (through the use of a cell saving device) may be associated with a lower burden of lipid microembolization (193).

Avoidance of cerebral hyperthermia (while rewarming the patient on CPB) may also help reduce the magnitude of neurologic dysfunction following CPB (194,195).

Large thrombus emboli are less common than microemboli. Patients with chronic atrial fibrillation, left atrial enlargement, left ventricular aneurysms, or large recent left ventricular infarctions may have mural thrombi attached to the affected chamber. In these patients, manipulation of the heart during surgery can lead to thrombus embolism and stroke. Thus, patients with left-side intracardiac thrombi identified by preoperative or intraoperative echocardiography are at increased risk for perioperative stroke.

Air emboli can damage the brain; thus, careful deairing of the heart is required whenever procedures on the left side of the heart are performed. Use of intraoperative TEE allows the surgeon to visualize air in the heart and to pursue deairing maneuvers before weaning the patient from CPB. The insufflation of carbon dioxide into the pericardial space results in displacement of air because carbon dioxide is heavier than air. Since carbon dioxide is more soluble than air, it dissipates more quickly and is less likely to cause vessel occlusion and resultant tissue damage. We routinely flood the thoracic cavity with carbon dioxide, delivered via a Jackson-Pratt drain, during procedures in which the heart is open to reduce the trapping of air in the cardiac chambers in an effort to reduce air embolism to the brain (196,197).

Massive air embolism can occur from a variety of intraoperative mishaps. It may be prevented to some degree by bubble sensor devices, arterial line filters, and careful deairing of the heart before resumption of contractions. If a massive air embolism does occur during CPB, immediate treatment by Trendelenburg positioning of the patient, placement of a stab wound in the ascending aorta for air escape, and retrograde perfusion through the superior vena cava is recommended (198). One form of therapy specific for the treatment of air embolism to the brain is the hyperbaric oxygen chamber. If available, hyperbaric oxygen therapy should be employed without delay after completion of the operation, as there is a clear relationship between outcome and treatment delay (199). This form of therapy can result in dramatic reversal of neurologic deficits that have occurred in some patients who have suffered large air emboli.

Symptomatic visual abnormalities occur occasionally after open-heart surgery (200). Potential etiologies include retinal emboli, anterior ischemic optic neuropathy, and occipital lobe infarction (cortical blindness). Embolism or hypoperfusion are causes; severe anemia during the operation and pre-existing glaucoma can contribute (201).

Postoperative atrial fibrillation that persists for more than 48 hours is associated with an increased incidence of stroke and is an indication for anticoagulation of the affected patient to prevent thromboembolism (202,203).

Treatment of the patient who has suffered a perioperative stroke is largely supportive and expectant. Maintenance of adequate oxygenation, oxygen carrying capacity, and acid–base status is of prime importance. Metabolic causes of encephalopathy (such as medications, narcotic or alcohol withdrawal, endocrinologic disorders, and renal or hepatic failure) and psychiatric etiologies should be considered and treated as well as possible. As soon as it is realized that the patient is definitely not awakening from anesthesia normally or that there is a focal neurologic deficit present, discussion with the family should be undertaken so as to alert them to the presence of the complication. When the patient is sufficiently stable to be transported, a CT scan of the head should be obtained. Although the CT scan is often normal early in the course of a stroke, the scan will rule out large intracerebral hemorrhages and cerebral edema. Having ruled out intracerebral hemorrhage, anticoagulation of the patient may be in order, especially if the stroke is thought to be due to thrombotic embolus. Early management of the acute stroke patient includes bed rest for at least 24 hours, keeping the head of the bed elevated at 20° to 30° (but not higher), adequate hydration, avoidance of hyperthermia (above 37.5°), and treatment of hyperglycemia. Consultation by a qualified and empathetic neurologist will assist both in management of the patient and in helping to address the questions raised by the naturally concerned family members.

Postoperative TIAs are defined as neurologic defects that are abrupt in onset and resolve within 24 hours. Less common than strokes, TIAs may herald an upcoming stroke or myocardial infarction. Investigation with carotid ultrasonography (if not done previously) and echocardiography (to rule out new intracardiac thrombus) may be indicated.

Delirium

Acute delirium is a transient syndrome characterized by impaired cognitive function, reduced consciousness, and ability to maintain attention. Patients suffering delirium may be hyperactive with agitated, combative, and loud behavior or hypoactive with withdrawn and quiet behavior. Delirium is a frequent postoperative problem, occurring in up to 3% to 50% of adult patients who have undergone cardiac surgery, depending on the diagnostic definition used and is associated with increased mortality, and poorer cognitive and functional outcomes (204). Factors associated with the development of postoperative delirium include prior stroke or TIA, cerebrovascular disease, age over 65, preoperative cardiogenic shock, atrial fibrillation, diabetes mellitus, urgent operation, postoperative blood transfusion, and low cardiac output (205–208). Avoiding the use of CPB and, interestingly, the preoperative administration of statin therapy may be associated with reduced incidence of postoperative delirium (209).

Management of delirium may be difficult and is centered on efforts to prevent the patient from harming himself. The presence of drug and/or alcohol withdrawal should be considered and, if likely, treated appropriately. Other metabolic and/or toxic conditions (such as sepsis) should be ruled out. Of note, the H_2-receptor antagonist drugs, such as famotidine, may contribute to delirium and should be discontinued and replaced with a proton-pump inhibitor such as omeprazole (210). The treatment of acute delirium is supportive. The patient should be provided a quiet environment and, if appropriate, given his or her eyeglasses and hearing aids. Catheters, including the bladder catheter should be removed as soon as possible. Delirious patients may not report pain and empiric scheduled treatment with a nonnarcotic such as acetaminophen can be instituted if no contraindications are present. Efforts to restore the patient's normal sleep cycle should be made. For hyperactive patients, a sitter may be necessary to closely watch the patient. For acute agitation, especially if the patient is a danger to him- or herself, treatment with haloperidol may be required but should be minimized. Haloperidol does have the potential for prolongation of the QT interval and should be used in care in patients who are receiving antiarrhythmics or other drugs that may potentiate this potential problem. Newer antipsychotic agents such as risperidone may also be of value. Benzodiazepines should be avoided as they may cause a worsening of the patient's condition (211,212). Properly applied physical restraints with appropriate documentation of the need for their use may be required (213).

The possibility of postoperative alcohol withdrawal should be kept in mind, particularly if there is suspicion that the patient may have been a heavy drinker prior to surgery. Onset usually occurs 24 to 36 hour after the last ingestion of alcohol and is characterized by hypertension, tachycardia, hyperactivity, and agitation. This may progress to delirium tremens. Management includes the administration of benzodiazepines, thiamine administration, hypertension control, and general support (214).

Postoperative Cognitive Decline

The subject of cognitive decline following cardiac surgery has been one of considerable controversy. Clearly, adult patients who require cardiac surgery are, even before the surgery, frequently at risk for future cognitive deterioration due to age, vascular disease, and other associated problems. Likewise, the overall stress of any large surgical procedure or critical illness and life event may contribute to worsening of ongoing cognitive decline (215). Thus, it is difficult to quantitate and to directly assign causation of long-term cognitive changes directly to a preceding heart surgery procedure (216–218). Potential contributors to postoperative cognitive deterioration following heart surgery include cerebral microembolization, hypoperfusion, inflammation, hyperthermia, and edema in addition to individual patient susceptibility to such injurious factors (219). Performance of CABG procedures "off-pump" does not appear to be associated with a reduced incidence of subsequent cognitive dysfunction (220,221).

PERIPHERAL NERVE INJURY

Peripheral nerve injuries may occur during open-heart surgery. The most common injuries are to the upper extremity nerve supply, particularly the brachial plexus, although the risk of prolonged symptoms from this complication is well less than 1%. The mechanism of injury to the brachial plexus is not certain but is probably due to traction on the sternal halves with stretching of the lower nerve roots (C8–T1) (222). The most common form of brachial plexopathy is that of ulnar neuropathy and this occurs more often in older patients, men, and patients who are suffering from diabetes (223). Efforts to prevent these injuries have included opening the sternum only as wide as necessary, positioning the retractor low in the split sternum, use of the hands-up position, and maintenance of neutral head position, although consistent relationships between positioning and the development of brachial plexus injury have not been demonstrated. The usual presentation of this complication is numbness, sometimes with tingling, of the fifth finger and the medial portion of the fourth finger of the involved hand. Nerve conduction studies and electromyelography may be performed, although there is no specific treatment available. Reassurance of the patient is indicated, and, for some patients, this is reinforced when it is heard also from a consulting neurologist. The overall prognosis is very good with resolution of the symptoms in most patients. More than 75% of affected patients become asymptomatic within 4 months.

Saphenous neuropathy is the result of injury to the saphenous nerve, usually in the distal leg that occurs in association with open harvesting of the saphenous vein (224). It is characterized by anesthesia, hyperesthesia, and pain along the medial side of the calf and foot. Common early after surgery, the symptoms may persist for more than 18 months in a small proportion of affected patients. Most often the problem is not serious, resolves without specific treatment, and requires only reassurance of the patient.

Patients who undergo radial artery harvesting for coronary bypass surgery may experience postoperative neurologic deficits involving the hand. In one study, 5% of patients reported decreased thumb strength and 18% described sensation abnormalities (225). In our experience, the incidence is considerably lower. The most common complaint is skin numbness at the base of the thumb. Significant associations between the self-reported neurologic complications and diabetes, peripheral vascular disease, elevated creatinine levels, and smoking were demonstrated. The majority of patients with hand neurologic abnormalities following radial artery removal recover within months after the operation.

Vocal cord paralysis is an unusual complication that may be devastating, particularly if bilateral. Most often, vocal cord paralysis is transient and is characterized by temporary hoarseness but severe cases may result in severe airway problems. This complication is more frequently associated with aortic procedures and prolonged ventilation (226,227).

Another interesting, but rare, peripheral nerve complication may be present after surgery in patients who have undergone cardiac surgery. *Meralgia paresthetica* is characterized by a focal region of numbness and paresthesia on the anterolateral aspect of the thigh. The syndrome results from an injury to the lateral femoral cutaneous nerve, likely secondary to positioning of the legs during the operation. The symptoms usually resolve over time, although in rare patients surgical division of the nerve may be required (228).

COMPLICATIONS OF SAPHENOUS VEIN HARVESTING

Although the use of one or both internal mammary arteries as conduit for myocardial revascularization provides superior long-term results, it is still often necessary to use segments of the greater saphenous vein for additional conduits in patients who undergo multivessel coronary artery bypass procedures. Leg wound complications, predominantly minor, occur in nearly one fourth of patients in whom the saphenous vein is harvested.

As discussed previously, endoscopic vein harvesting techniques are associated with reduced complication rates (229,230). For harvesting of the vein, meticulous surgical technique and a good understanding of the anatomy of the leg's venous drainage are important. Risk factors associated with an increased incidence of leg wound problems with the open technique include female gender, peripheral vascular disease, diabetes, and postoperative intra-aortic balloon pump use (231). Careful preoperative evaluation of the leg to denote the presence of arterial insufficiency, the use of small noncontiguous incisions, avoidance of hematomas, and careful attention to proper incision closure technique are important factors in reducing the incidence of vein harvest site problems. For difficult patients (such as those with previous vein stripping, thrombophlebitis, or obesity), preoperative duplex ultrasound scanning with marking of the skin overlying the identified vein can provide a "map" to guide the surgeon in the operating room (232).

The most common complications of saphenous vein removal are infection, separation of the wound, cellulitis, abscess formation, lymphangitis, lymphocele, or lymph drainage from the wound. Postoperatively, some degree of distal leg edema is common; this usually resolves over a few weeks. Thus, patients are advised to keep the donor leg elevated when not ambulating. If the wound becomes infected, antibiotics are administered and open packing of the wound, often with a wound vacuum device, is performed as necessary. Although problems with the leg wound may seem trivial compared with the surgery performed directly on the heart, serious leg wound complications can lead to significant morbidity, patient discomfort, and prolonged hospitalization. Rarely, very major surgical reconstruction or even amputation may be required.

COMPLICATIONS RELATED TO THE USE OF THE RADIAL ARTERY

Use of the radial artery as bypass graft conduit is increasing due to apparent improved mid-term patency results that are comparable to other arterial grafts (233). Preoperative evaluation generally involves the use of the Allen's test or various modifications to ensure adequate collateral perfusion of the hand via the ulnar artery (see Chapter 1). With proper selection, ischemic complications are very rare. In one large series of over 6,600 patients with radial artery grafts, only two patients experienced fingertip ischemia (234). As discussed previously, however, neurologic complaints (usually numbness at the base of the thumb) are not rare but these usually resolve with time. Other potential complications include forearm hematoma, compartment syndrome, stitch abscesses, skin dehiscence, and infection. Overall, the incidence of nonneurologic complications, mostly minor, is <5% (235).

COMPLICATIONS RELATED TO INTERNAL MAMMARY ARTERY MOBILIZATION

One or both of the internal mammary (thoracic) arteries are utilized in over 95% of the coronary revascularization procedures performed at our institutions because of the proven long-term benefits of this conduit as compared with saphenous vein aortocoronary bypass grafts. It is remarkable that only rarely does the mobilization and distal division of this artery (which is the major blood supply to the sternum) contribute to wound or other postoperative complications.

As discussed previously, the use of bilateral internal mammary arteries in diabetic and other high-risk patients has been associated with an increased risk of sternal wound infections. Thus, the decision to use of both mammary arteries must be made with consideration of the associated risks and benefits.

Postoperative respiratory insufficiency may be worsened by the effects of mammary artery mobilization, likely as the result of injury to the phrenic nerve. Careful dissection and avoidance of thermal injury to the nerve during mobilization of the artery is important. If phrenic nerve paralysis persists more than 6 months, and if the patient is symptomatic, diaphragmatic plication is indicated and can be performed laparoscopically.

DEEP VENOUS THROMBOSIS AND PULMONARY EMBOLISM

The incidences of clinically apparent DVT and PE following cardiac surgery are not certain but appear to be lower than those for other major surgical procedures. The use of heparin during the operation and administration of antiplatelet drugs before and after surgery may help to reduce the incidence of clot formation. The only reported information in this regard pertains to CABG patients. The incidence of asymptomatic DVT following CABG surgery ranges from 16% to 48% (as determined by Doppler ultrasonography) while the incidence of PE ranges from 0.2% to 3.9% (236). The incidence of fatal PE following cardiac surgery has been reported to be as high as 0.5% (237). It is not clear, however, that routine thromboprophylaxis is indicated in the cardiac surgical population. Early postoperative administration of heparin (unfractionated or low molecular weight) does appear to be associated with an increased incidence of bleeding complications and tamponade (50). In our practices, we currently do not routinely administered prophylactic postoperative anticoagulation because of the low incidence of thromboembolic complications and the risk of anticoagulation in these patients. If however, the patient has a prolonged course or is bedridden for more than 48 hours, prophylaxis is considered (238).

Some patients are at increased risk for thromboembolic complications, including PE. These include those who are immobile (e.g., ventilator-dependent), have prolonged preoperative hospitalization, are obese, have prothrombotic conditions (including HIT), or other complicating factors. For such patients, anticoagulation with the appropriate agent at the appropriate dose is instituted. LMWH (subcutaneous) is preferred over unfractionated heparin, although it is more of a problem if bleeding occurs due to the longer duration of action when discontinued. If heparin is administered, the patient's platelet count should be serially checked due to the increased incidence of HIT in cardiac surgery patients. Nondrug measures such as properly fitted graduated compression stockings or intermittent pneumatic compression devices are also recommended (239).

It is important to remember that upper extremity DVT, involving the axillary and/or subclavian veins, may also occur and is frequently secondary to an indwelling catheter. These patients usually present with arm swelling and the diagnosis may be confirmed by ultrasound examination. Treatment involves anticoagulation, limb elevation, and the placement of a graduated compression arm sleeve. In some cases, catheter-directed thrombolysis or catheter suction thrombectomy may be performed (240).

PE is a common cause of death in hospitalized patients, but many cases also occur in postoperative patients following discharge from the hospital. The presentation may be that of catastrophic hemodynamic collapse due to a large embolus or the gradual development of dyspnea and chest pain due to smaller emboli. Sometimes the presentation can be subtle with reduced oxygen saturation as the only manifestation. Typically, the patient suffers respiratory insufficiency with unexplained hypoxemia. Leg swelling and warmth may also be present. A positive D-dimer test indicates that venous thrombosis and PE are possible diagnoses but this test is nonspecific and may occur with infection, cancer, trauma, and other inflammatory states (241). Although multiple different imaging techniques may be used to diagnose pulmonary emboli, the multichannel contrast-enhanced CT scan is a quick and reliable method of diagnosing or ruling out the presence of clot in the pulmonary veins (242). For patients with contrast allergy or significantly abnormal kidney function, a ventilation–perfusion lung scan is an alternative diagnostic technique.

Treatment of DVT with or without PE is initiated by treatment with subcutaneous LMWH, subcutaneous fondaparinux, or intravenous unfractionated heparin for at least 5 with transition to warfarin anticoagulation achieving prolongation of the INR to $\geqq 2.0$ for more than 24 hours (243). The warfarin is then continued for at least 3 months. Low molecular weight may be used instead of unfractionated heparin. For very desperately ill patients, an emergency embolectomy may be lifesaving (244). There is no role for systemic thrombolytic therapy for DVT or PE in patients who have recently undergone cardiac surgery due to the high risk of serious bleeding problems. Patients with contraindications to anticoagulation or patients who experience recurrence of pulmonary emboli despite anticoagulation are candidates for placement of an inferior vena caval filter.

References

1. Karthik S, Grayson AD, McCarron EE, et al. Reexploration for bleeding after coronary artery bypass surgery: risk factors, outcomes, and the effect of time delay. *Ann Thorac Surg* 2004;78:527–534.

2. Ranucci M, Bozzetti G, Ditta A, et al. Surgical reexploration after cardiac operations: why a worse outcome? *Ann Thorac Surg* 2008;86:1557–1562.
3. Moulton MJ, Creswell LL, Mackey ME, et al. Reexploration for bleeding is a risk factor to adverse outcomes after cardiac operations. *J Thorac Cardiovasc Surg* 1996;111:1037–1046.
4. Choong CK, Gerrard C, Goldsmith KA, et al. Delayed re-exploration for bleeding after coronary artery bypass surgery results in adverse outcomes. *Eur J Cardiothorac Surg* 2007;834–838.
5. Magovern JA, Sakert T, Benckart DH, et al. A model for predicting transfusion after coronary artery bypass grafting. *Ann Thorac Surg* 1996;61:27–32.
6. Despotis GJ, Filos KS, Zoys TN, et al. Factors associated with excessive postoperative blood loss and hemostatic transfusion requirements: a multivariate analysis in cardiac surgical patients. *Anesth Analg* 1996;82:13–21.
7. Alghamdi AA, Davis A, Brister S, et al. Development and validation of transfusion risk understanding scoring tool (TRUST) to stratify cardiac surgery patients according to their blood transfusion needs. *Transfusion* 2006;46: 1120–1129.
8. Moskowitz DM, Klein JJ, Shander A, et al. Predictors of transfusion requirements for cardiac surgical procedures at a blood conservation center. *Ann Thorac Surg* 2004;77:626–634.
9. Arora RC, Legare JF, Buth KJ, et al. Identifying patients at risk of intraoperative and postoperative transfusion in isolated CAZBG: toward selective conservation strategies. *Ann Thorac Surg* 2004;78:1547–1554.
10. Dietrich W, Dilthey G, Spannagl M, et al. Warfarin pretreatment does not lead to increased bleeding tendency during cardiac surgery. *J Cardiothorac Vasc Anesth* 1995;9:250–254.
11. Morris CD, Vega JD, Levy JH, et al. Warfarin therapy does not increase bleeding in patients undergoing heart transplantation. *Ann Thorac Surg* 2001;72: 714–718.
12. Davies LK. Cardiopulmonary bypass in infants and children: how is it different? *J Cardiothorac Vasc Anesth* 1999;13:330–345.
13. Wilkes MM, Navickis RJ, Sibbald WJ. Albumin versus hydroxyethyl starch in cardiopulmonary bypass surgery: a meta-analysis of postoperative bleeding. *Ann Thorac Surg* 2001;72:527–534.
14. Despotis G, Eby CV, Lublin DM. A review of transfusion risks and optimal management of perioperative bleeding with cardiac surgery. *Transfusion* (suppl) 2008;48:2S–30S.
15. Ascione R, Williams S, Lloyd CT, et al. Reduced postoperative blood loss and transfusion requirement after beating-heart coronary operations: a prospective randomized trial. *J Thorac Cardiovasc Surg* 2001;121:689–696.
16. Sellke FW, DiMaio JM, Caplan LR, et al. Comparing on-pump and off-pump coronary artery bypass grafting—numerous studies but few conclusions. *Circulation* 2005;111:2858–2864.
17. Meadows TA, Bhatt DL. Clinical aspects of platelet inhibitors and thrombus formation. *Circ Res* 2007;100:1261–1275.
18. Patrono C, Bachman F, Baigent C, et al. Expert consensus document on the use of antiplatelet agents. The task force on the use of antiplatelet agents in patients with atherosclerotic cardiovascular disease of the European society of cardiology. *Eur Heart J 2004*;25:166–181.
19. Anderson JL, Adams CD, Antman EM, et al. ACC/AHA 2007 guidelines for the management of patients with unstable angina/non-ST-elevation myocardial infarction—executive summary. *J Amer Coll Cardiol* 2007;50:652–726.

20. Ferraris VA, Ferraris SP, Moliterno DJ, et al. The Society of Thoracic Surgeons Practice Guideline Series: aspirin and other antiplatelet agents during operative coronary revascularization (executive summary). *Ann Thorac Surg* 2005;79:1454–1461.

21. Sun JCJ, Whitlock R, Cheng J, et al. The effect of preoperative aspirin on bleeding, transfusion, myocardial infarction, and mortality in coronary artery bypass surgery: a systematic review of randomized and observational studies. *Eur Heart J* 2008;1057–1071.

22. Ferraris VA, Ferraris SP, Saha SP, et al. Perioperative blood transfusion and blood conservation in cardiac surgery: the Society of Thoracic Surgeons and The Society of Cardiovascular Anesthesiologists clinical practice guideline. *Ann Thorac Surg* 2007;83:27–86.

23. Ferraris VA, Ferraris SP, Oji J, et al. Aspirin and postoperative bleeding after coronary artery bypass grafting. *Ann Surg* 2002;235:820–827.

24. Dacey LJ, Munoz JJ, Johnson ER, et al. Effect of preoperative aspirin use on mortality in coronary artery bypass grafting patients. *Ann Thorac Surg* 2000;1986–1990.

25. Bybee KA, Powell BD, Valeti U, et al. Preoperative aspirin therapy is associated with improved postoperative outcomes in patients undergoing coronary artery bypass grafting. *Circulation* 2005;112(suppl I):I-286–I-292.

26. Goldman S, Copeland J, Moritz T, et al. Starting aspirin therapy after operation: effects on early graft patency. *Circulation* 1991;84:520–526.

27. Mangano DT and the Multicenter Study of Perioperative Ischemia Research Group. Aspirin and mortality from coronary bypass surgery. *New Engl J Med* 2002;347:1309–1317.

28. Chua D, Ignaszewski A. Clopidogrel in acute coronary syndromes. *BMJ* 2009; 338:1180.

29. Thebault JJ, Kieffer G, Cariou R. Single-dose pharmacodynamics of clopidogrel. *Semin Thromb Hemostasis* 1999;25(suppl 2):3–8.

30. Berger JS, Frye CB, Harshaw Q, et al. Impact of clopidogrel in patients with acute coronary syndromes requiring coronary artery bypass surgery—a multicenter analysis. *J Am Coll Cardiol* 2008;52:1693–1701.

31. Purkayastha S, Athanasiou T, Malinovski V, et al. Does clopidogrel affect outcome after coronary artery bypass grafting? A meta-analysis. *Heart* 2006;92:531–532.

32. Filsoufi F, Rahmanian PB, Castillo JG, et al. Clopidogrel treatment before coronary artery bypass graft surgery increases postoperative morbidity and blood product requirements. *J Cardiothorac Vasc Anesth* 2008;22: 60–66.

33. Pickard AS, Becker RC, Schumock GT, et al. Clopidogrel-associated bleeding and related complications in patients undergoing coronary artery bypass grafting. *Pharmacotherapy* 2008;28:376–392.

34. Cannon CP, Mehta SR, Aranki SF. Balancing the benefit and risk of oral antiplatelet agents in coronary artery bypass surgery. *Ann Thorac Surg* 2005;80:768–779.

35. Mehta RH, Roe MT, Mulgund J, et al. Acute clopidogrel use and outcomes in patients with non-ST-segment elevation acute coronary syndromes undergoing coronary artery bypass surgery. *J Am Coll Cardiol* 2006;48:281–286.

36. Reichert MG, Robinson AH, Travis JA, et al. Effects of a waiting period after clopidogrel treatment before performing coronary artery bypass grafting. *Pharmacotherapy* 2008;28:151–155.

37. Lemmer JH Jr, Metzdorff MT, Krause AH Jr, et al. Emergency coronary artery bypass graft surgery in abciximab-treated patients. *Ann Thorac Surg* 2000;69: 90–95.
38. Singh M, Nuttall GA, Ballman KV, et al. Effect of abciximab on the outcome of emergency coronary artery bypass grafting after failed percutaneous coronary intervention. *Mayo Clin Proc* 2001;76:784–788.
39. De Carlo M, Maselli D, Cortese B, et al. Emergency coronary artery bypass grafting in patients with acute myocardial infarction treated with glycoprotein IIb/IIIa receptor inhibitors. *Int J Cardiol* 2008;123:229–233.
40. Lemmer JH Jr. Clinical experience in coronary bypass surgery for abciximab-treated patients. *Ann Thorac Surg* 2000;70:S33–S37.
41. Dyke CM, Bhatia D, Lorenz TJ, et al. Immediate coronary artery bypass surgery after platelet inhibition with eptifibatide: results from PURSUIT. *Ann Thorac Surg* 2000;70: 866–872.
42. Genoni M, Zeller D, Bertel O, et al. Tirofiban therapy does not increase the risk of hemorrhage after emergency coronary surgery. *J Thorac Cardiovasc Surg* 2001;122: 630–632.
43. Bizzarri F, Scolletta S, Tucci E, et al. Perioperative use of tirofiban hydrochloride (Aggrastat) does not increase surgical bleeding after emergency or urgent coronary artery bypass grafting. *J Thorac Cardiovasc Surg* 2001;122: 1181–1185.
44. Despotis GJ, Skubas NJ, Goodnough LT. Optimal management of bleeding and transfusion in patients undergoing cardiac surgery. *Semin Thorac Cardiovasc Surg* 1999;11:84–104.
45. Hirsh J, Bauer KA, Donati MB, et al. Parenteral anticoagulants. *Chest* 2008;133: 141S–159S.
46. Lemmer JH Jr, Despotis GJ. Antithrombin III concentrate to treat heparin resistance in patients undergoing cardiac surgery. *J Thorac Cardiovasc Surg* 2002;123:213–217.
47. Clark SC, Vitale N, Zacharias J, et al. Effect of low molecular weight heparin (Fragmin) on bleeding after cardiac surgery. *Ann Thorac Surg* 2000;69: 762–765.
48. McDonald SB, Renna M, Spitznagel EL, et al. Preoperative use of enoxaparin increases the risk of postoperative bleeding and re-exploration in cardiac surgery patients. *J Cardiovasc Vasc Anesth* 2005;19:4–10.
49. Henry TD, Satran D, Knox LL, et al. Are activated clotting times helpful in the management of anticoagulation with subcutaneous low-molecular-eight heparin? *Am Heart J* 2001;142:590–593.
50. Jones HU, Muhlestein JB, Jones KW, et al. Early postoperative use of unfractionated heparin or enoxaparin is associated with increased surgical re-exploration for bleeding. *Ann Thorac Surg* 2005;80:518–522.
51. Toh CH, Dennis M. Disseminated intravascular coagulation: old disease, new hope. *BMJ* 2003;327:974–977.
52. Fiser SM, Tribble CG, Kern JA, et al. Cardiac reoperation in the intensive care unit. *Ann Thorac Surg* 2001;71:1888–1893.
53. Rannuci M, Bozzetti G, Ditta A, et al. Surgical reexploration after cardiac operations: why a worse outcome? *Ann Thorac Surg* 2008;86:1557–1562.
54. Choong CK, Gerrard C, Goldsmith KA, et al. Delayed re-exploration for bleeding after coronary artery bypass surgery results in adverse outcomes. *Eur J Cardiothorac Surg* 2007;31:834–838.
55. McGrath T, Koch CG, Xu M, et al. Platelet transfusion in cardiac surgery does not confer increased risk for adverse morbid outcomes. *Ann Thorac Surg* 2008;543–553.

56. Price S, Prout J, Jaggar SI, et al. 'Tamponade' following cardiac surgery: terminology and echocardiography may both mislead. *Eur J Cardiothorac Surg* 2004;26:1156–1160.

57. Russo AM, O'Connor WH, Waxman HL. Atypical presentations and echocardiographic findings in patients with cardiac tamponade occurring early and late after cardiac surgery. *Chest* 1993;104:71–78.

58. Cheitlin MD, Armstrong WF, Aurigemma GP, et al. ACC/AHA/ASE 2003 guideline update for the clinical application of echocardiography: Summary article: a report of the American College of Cardiology/American Heart Association Task Force on Practice Guidelines. *Circulation* 2003;108:1146–1162.

59. Spodick DW. Acute cardiac tamponade. *N Engl J Med* 2003;684–690.

60. Charalambous CP, Ziptis CS, Keenan DJ. Chest reexploration in the intensive care unit after cardiac surgery: a safe alternative to returning to the operating theater. *Ann Thorac Surg* 2006;81:191–194.

61. Kuvin JT, Harati NA, Pandian NG, et al. Postoperative cardiac tamponade in the modern surgical era. *Ann Thorac Surg* 2002;74:1148–1153.

62. Mangi AA, Palacios IF, Torchiana DF. Catheter pericardiocentesis for delayed tamponade after cardiac valve operation. *Ann Thorac Surg* 2002;73: 1479–1483.

63. Tsang TSM, Barnes ME, Hayes SN, et al. Clinical and echocardiographic characteristics of significant pericardial effusions following cardiothoracic surgery and outcomes of echo-guided pericardiocentesis for management: Mayo Clinic experience 1979–1988. *Chest* 1999;116:322–331.

64. Gill R, Herbertson M, Vuylsteke A, et al. Safety and efficacy of recombinant activated factor VII: a randomized placebo-controlled trial in the setting of bleeding after cardiac surgery. *Circulation* 2009;120:21–27.

65. Karkouti K, Beattie WS, Arellano R, et al. Comprehensive Canadian review of the off-label use of recombinant activated factor VII in cardiac surgery. *Circulation* 2008;118:331–338.

66. Warren O, Mandal K, Hadjianastassiou V, et al. Recombinant activated factor Vii in cardiac surgery: a systematic review. *Ann Thorac Surg* 2007;83:707–714.

67. Dunkley S, Phillips L, McCall P, et al. Recombinant activated factor VII in cardiac surgery: experience from the Australian and New Zealand Haemostasis Registry. *Ann Thorac Surg* 2008;85:836–844.

68. Hardy J-F, Belisle S, Van der Linden P. Efficacy and safety of recombinant activated factor VIIU to control bleeding in nonhemophiliac patients: a review of 17 randomized controlled trials. *Ann Thorac Surg* 2008;86:1038–1048.

69. Johnson SJ, Ross MB, Moores KG. Dosing factor VIIa (recombinant) in nonhemophiliac patients with bleeding after cardiac surgery. *Am J Health-System Pharm* 2007;64: 1808–1812.

70. Rosner MH, Okusa MD. Acute kidney injury associated with cardiac surgery. *Clin J Am Soc Nephrol* 2006;1:19–32.

71. Ryckwaert F, Boccara G, Frappier J-M, Colson PH. Incidence, risk factors, and prognosis of a moderate increase in plasma creatinine early after cardiac surgery. *Crit Care Med* 2002;30:1495–1498.

72. Swaminathan M, Shaw AD, Phillips-Bute BG, et al. Trends in acute renal failure associated with coronary bypass surgery in the United States. *Crit Care Med* 2007;35: 2286–2291.

73. Cooper WA, O'Brien SM, Thourani VH, et al. Impact of renal dysfunction on outcomes of coronary artery bypass surgery: results from the Society of Thoracic Surgeons National Adult Cardiac Database. *Circulation* 2006;113: 1063–1070.

74. Gibson PH, Croal BL, Cuthbertson BH, et al. The relationship between renal function and outcome from heart valve surgery. *Am Heart J* 2008;156: 893–899.

75. Antunes PE, Prieto D, de Oliveira JF, et al. Renal dysfunction after myocardial revascularization. *Eur J Cardiothorac Surg* 2004;25:597–604.

76. Zakeri R, Freemantle N, Barnett V, et al. Relation between mild renal dysfunction and outcomes after coronary artery bypass grafting. *Circulation* 2005;112(9 suppl):I270–I275.

77. Karkouti K, Beattie WS, Wijeysundera DN, et al. Hemodilution during cardiopulmonary bypass is an independent risk factor for acute renal failure in adult cardiac surgery. *J Thorac Cardiovasc Surg* 2005;129:391–400.

78. Habib RH, Zacharias A, Schwann TA, et al. Role of hemodilutional anemia and transfusion during cardiopulmonary bypass in renal injury after coronary revascularization: implications on operative outcome. *Crit Care Med* 2005;33:1749–1756.

79. Ascione R, Lloyd CT, Underwood MJ, et al. On-pump versus off-pump coronary revascularization: evaluation of renal function. *Ann Thorac Surg* 1999; 68:493–498.

80. Schwann NM, Horrow JC, Strong MD, et al. Does off-pump coronary artery bypass reduce the incidence of clinically evident renal dysfunction after multivessel coronary revascularization? *Anesth Analg* 2004;99: 959–964.

81. Di Mauro M, Gagliardi M, Iaco AL, et al. Does off-pump coronary surgery reduce the postoperative acute renal failure? The importance of preoperative renal function. *Ann Thorac Surg* 2007;84:1496–1503.

82. Thakar CV, Arrigan S, Worley S, et al. A clinical score to predict acute renal failure after cardiac surgery. *J Am Soc Nephrol* 2005;16:162–168.

83. Mehta RH, Grab JD, O'Brien SM, et al. Bedside tool for predicting the risk of postoperative dialysis in patients undergoing cardiac surgery. *Circulation* 2006;114:2208–2216.

84. Wijeysundera DN, Karkouti K, Dupuis J-Y, et al. Derivation and validation of a simplified predictive index for renal replacement therapy after cardiac surgery. *JAMA* 2007;297:1801–1809.

85. Gill N, Nally JV, Fatica RA. Renal failure secondary to acute tubular necrosis: epidemiology, diagnosis, and management. *Chest* 2005;128:2847–2863.

86. Ranucci M, Ballota A, Kunki A, et al. Influence of the timing of cardiac catheterization and the amount of contrast media on acute renal failure after cardiac surgery. *Am J Cardiol* 2008;101:1112–1118.

87. Del Ducca D, Iqbal S, Rahme E, et al. Renal failure after cardiac surgery: timing of cardiac catheterization and other perioperative risk factors. *Ann Thorac Surg* 2007;84: 1264–1271.

88. Rosner MH. Analytic reviews: cardiac surgery as a cause of acute kidney injury: pathogenesis and potential therapies. *J Intensive Care Med* 2008;23:3–18.

89. Zacharias M, Gilmore IC, Herbison GP, et al. Interventions to protecting renal function in the perioperative period. *Cochrane Database Syst Rev* 2005; 20(3):CD003590.

90. Naughton F, Wijeysundera D, Karkouti K, et al. N-acetylcysteine to reduce renal failure after cardiac surgery: a systematic review and meta-analysis. *Can J Anesth* 2008;55:827–835.

91. Nigwekar SU, Kandla P. N-acetylcysteine in cardiovascular-surgery-associated renal failure: a meta-analysis. *Ann Thorac Surg* 209;87:139–147.

92. Karkouti K, Wijeysundera DN, Yau TM, et al. Acute kidney injury after cardiac surgery: focus on modifiable risk factors. *Circulation* 2009;119:495–502.
93. Gulbis BE, Spencer AP. Efficacy and safety of a furosemide continuous infusion following cardiac surgery. *Ann Pharmacother* 2006;40:1797–1803.
94. Ho KM, Sheridan DJ. Meta-analysis of furosemide to prevent or treat acute renal failure. *BMJ* 2006;333:420–423.
95. Mahesh B, Yim B, Robson D, et al. Does furosemide prevent renal dysfunction in high-risk cardiac surgical patients? Results of a double-blind prospective randomized trial. *Eur J Cardiothorac Surg* 2008;33:370–376.
96. Abuelo JG. Normotensive ischemic acute renal failure. *N Engl J Med* 2007;357: 797–805.
97. Woo EBC, Tang ATM, Gamel AE, et al. Dopamine therapy for patients at risk of renal dysfunction following cardiac surgery: science or fiction? *Eur J Cardiothorac Surg* 2002;22:106–111.
98. Marik PE. Low-dose dopamine: a systematic review. *Intensive Care Med* 2002;28:877–893.
99. Gill N, Nally Jr JV, Fatica RA. Renal failure secondary to acute tubular necrosis: epidemiology, diagnosis, and management. *Chest* 2005;128:2847–2863.
100. Demirkiliç U, Kuralay E, Yenicesu M, et al. Timing of replacement therapy for acute renal failure after cardiac surgery. *J Card Surg* 2004;19:17–20.
101. Bapat V, Sabetai M, Roxburgh J, et al. Early and continuous veno-venous hemofiltration for acute renal failure after cardiac surgery. *Interactive Cardiovasc Thorac Surg* 2004;3: 426–430.
102. Dittrich S, Dahnert I, Vogel M, et al. Peritoneal dialysis after infant open heart surgery: observations in 27 patients. *Ann Thorac Surg* 1999;68:160–163.
103. Jander A, Tkaczyk M, Pagowska-Klimek I, et al. Continuous veno-venous hemodiafiltration in children after cardiac surgery. *Eur J Cardiothorac Surg* 2007;31:1022–1028.
104. Elahi MM, Lim MY Joseph RN, et al. Early hemofiltration improves survival in post-cardiotomy patients with acute renal failure. *Eur J Cardiothorac Surg* 2004;26:1027–1031.
105. Fowler VG, O'Brien SM, Muhlbaier LW, et al. Clinical predictors of major infections after cardiac surgery. *Circulation* 2005;112(suppl I) I-358-I-365.
106. Chelemer SB, Prato S, Cox Jr PM, et al. Association of bacterial infection and red blood cell transfusion after coronary artery bypass surgery. *Ann Thorac Surg* 2002;73:138–142.
107. Braxton JH, Marrin CAS, McGrath PD, et al. 10-year follow-up of patients with and without mediastinitis. *Semin Thoracic Cardiovasc Surg* 2004;16:70–76.
108. Losanoff JE, Richman BW, Jones JW. Disruption and infection of median sternotomy: a comprehensive review. *Eur J Cardiothorac Surg* 2002;21:831–839.
109. Edwards FH, Engelman RM, Houck P, et al. The Society of Thoracic Surgeons Practice Guideline Series: antibiotic prophylaxis in cardiac surgery, Part I: Duration. *Ann Thorac Surg* 2006;81:397–404
110. Braxton JH, Marrin CAS, McGrath PD, et al. Mediastinitis and long-term survival after coronary artery bypass graft surgery. *Ann Thorac Surg* 2000;70: 2004–2007.
111. Eklund AM, Lyytikainen O, Klemets P, et al. Mediastinitis after more than 10,000 cardiac surgical procedures. *Ann Thorac Surg* 2006;82:1784–1789.
112. Filsoufi F, Rahmanian PB, Castillo JG, et al. Incidence, treatment strategies and outcome of deep sternal wound infection after orthotopic heart transplantation. *J Heart Lung Transplant* 2007;26:1084–1090.

113. Abboud CS, Wey SB, Baltar VT. Risk factors for mediastinitis after cardiac surgery. *Ann Thorac Surg* 2004;77:676–683.
114. Borger MA, Rao V, Weisel RD, et al. Deep sternal wound infection: risk factors and outcomes. *Ann Thorac Surg* 1998;65:1050–1056.
115. Alserius T, Anderson RE, Hammar N, et al. Elevated glycosylated haemoglobin (HbA$_{1c}$) is a risk marker in coronary artery bypass surgery. *Scand Cardiovasc J* 2008;42:392–398.
116. Crabtree TD, Codd JE, Fraser VJ, et al. Multivariate analysis of risk factors for deep and superficial sternal wound infection after coronary artery bypass grafting at a tertiary care medical center. *Semin Thorac Cardiovasc Surg* 2004;16:53–61.
117. Savage EB, Grab JD, O'Brien SM, et al. Use of both internal mammary arteries in diabetic patients increases deep sternal wound infection. *Ann Thorac Surg* 2007;83:1002–1007.
118. Toumpoulis IK, Theakos N, Dunning J. Does bilateral internal thoracic artery harvest increase the risk of mediastinitis? *Interactive Cardiovasc Thorac Surg* 2007;6:787–792.
119. Paul M, Raz A, Leibovici L, et al. Sternal wound infection after coronary artery bypass graft surgery: validation of existing risk scores. *J Thorac Cardiovasc Surg* 2007;133: 397–403.
120. Rahmanian PB, Adams DH, Castillo JG, et al. Tracheostomy is not a risk factor for deep sternal wound infection after cardiac surgery. *Ann Thorac Surg* 2007;84:1984–1991.
121. Curtis JJ, Clark NC, McKenney CA, et al. Tracheostomy: a risk factor for mediastinitis after cardiac operation. *Ann Thorac Surg* 2001;72:731–734.
122. Ko W, Lazenby D, Zelano JA, et al. Effects for shaving methods and intraoperative irrigation on suppurative mediastinitis after bypass operations. *Ann Thorac Surg* 1992;53:301–305.
123. Engelman R, Shahian D, Shemin R, et al. The Society of Thoracic Surgeons Practice Guideline Series: antibiotic prophylaxis in cardiac surgery, Part II: Antibiotic choice. *Ann Thorac Surg* 2007;83:1569–1576.
124. Reddy SLC, Grayson AD, Smith G, et al. Methicillin resistant *Staphylococcus aureus* infection following cardiac surgery: incidence impact, and identifying adverse outcome traits. *Eur J Cardiothorac Surg* 2007;32:113–117.
125. Dodds Ashley ES, Carroll DN, Engemann JJ, et al. Risk factors for postoperative mediastinitis due to methicillin-resistant *Staphylococcus aureus*. *Clin Infect Dis* 2004;38:1555–1560.
126. Cimochowski GE, Harostock MD, Brown R, et al. Intranasal mupirocin reduces sternal wound infection after open heart surgery in diabetics and nondiabetics. *Ann Thorac Surg* 2001;71:1572–1578.
127. Ridderstolpe L, Gill H, Granfeldt H, et al. Superficial and deep sternal wound complications: incidence, risk factors and mortality. *Eur J Cardiothorac Surg* 2001;20:1168–1175.
128. Tegnell A, Aren C, Ohman L. Coagulase-negative staphylococci and sternal infections after cardiac operation. *Ann Thorac Surg* 2000;69:1104–1109.
129. Misawa Y, Fuse K, Hasegawa T. Infectious mediastinitis after cardiac operations: computed tomographic findings. *Ann Thorac Surg* 1998;65: 622–624.
130. Molina JE, Nelson EC, Smith RRA. Treatment of postoperative sternal dehiscence with mediastinitis: twenty-four-year use of a single method. *Ann Thorac Surg* 2006;132: 782–787.

131. Rand Cochran RP, Aziz S, Hofer BO, et al. Prospective trial of catheter irrigation and muscle flaps for sternal wound infection. *Ann Thorac Surg* 1998;65:1046–1049.

132. Cicilioni OJ Jr, Stieg FH III, Papanicolaou G. Sternal wound reconstruction with transverse plate fixation. *Plast Reconstr Surg* 2005;115:1297–1303.

133. Sjogren J, Malmsjo M, Gustafsson R, et al. Poststernotomy mediastinitis: a review of conventional surgical treatments, vacuum-assisted closure therapy and presentation of the Lund university Hospital mediastinitis algorithm. *Eur J Cardiothorac Surg* 2006;898–905.

134. Song DH, WU LC, Lohman R, et al. Vacuum assisted closure for the treatment of sternal wounds: the bridge between debridement and definitive closure. *Plast Reconstr Surg* 2003;111:92–96.

135. Erez E, Katz M, Sharoni E, et al. Pectoralis major muscle flap for deep sternal wound infection in neonates. *Ann Thorac Surg* 2000;69:572–577.

136. Paletta CE, Huang DB, Fiore AC, et al. Major leg wound complications after saphenous vein harvest for coronary revascularization. *Ann Thorac Surg* 2000;70;492–497.

137. Athanasiou T, Aziz O, Al-Ruzzeh, et al. Are wound healing disturbances and length of hospital stay reduced with minimally invasive vein harvest? A meta-analysis. *Eur J Cardiothorac Surg* 2004;26:1015–1026.

138. Aziz O, Athanasiou T, Darzi A. Minimally invasive conduit harvesting: a systematic review. *Eur J Cardiothorac Surg* 2006;29:324–333.

139. Yun KL, Wu Y, Aharonian V, et al. Randomized trial of endoscopic versus open vein harvest for coronary artery bypass grafting: six-month patency rates. *J Thorac Cardiovasc Surg* 2005;129:496–503.

140. Lopes RD, Hafley GE, Allen KB, et al. Endoscopic versus open vein-graft harvesting in coronary-artery bypass surgery. *N Engl J Med* 2009;361:235–244.

141. Bouza E, Hortal J, Munoz P, et al. Infections following major heart surgery in European intensive care units: there is room for improvement. *J Hosp Infect* 2006;63:399–405.

142. Mizock BA. Risk of aspiration in patients on enteral nutrition: frequency, relevance, relation to pneumonia, risk factors, and strategies for risk reduction. *Curr Gastroenterol Reports* 2007;9:338–344.

143. Rello J. Bench-to-bedside review: therapeutic options and issuers in the management of ventilator-associated bacterial pneumonia. *Critical Care* 2005;259–265.

144. Leal-Noval SR, Marquez-Vacaro JA, Garcia-Curiel A, et al. Nosocomial pneumonia in patients undergoing heart surgery. *Crit Care Med* 2000;28:935–940.

145. Coffin Se, Klompas M, Classen D, et al. Strategies to prevent ventilator–associated pneumonia. *Infect Control Hosp* 2008;29:S31–S40.

146. American Thoracic Society. Guidelines for the management of adults with hospital-acquired, ventilator-associated and healthcare-associated pneumonia. *Am J Respir Crit Care* 2005;171:388–416.

147. Kac G, Durain E, Amrein C, et al. Colonization and infection of pulmonary artery catheter in cardiac surgery patients: epidemiology and multivariate analysis of risk factors. *Crit Care Med* 2001;29:971–975.

148. Merrer J, De Jonghe B, Golliot F, et al. Complications of femoral and subclavian venous catheterization in critically ill patients. *JAMA* 2001;286:700–707.

149. Taylor RW, Palagiri AV. Central venous catheterization. *Crit Care* Med 2007;1390–1396.

150. Khan JH, Lambert AM, Habib JH, et al. Abdominal complications after heart surgery. *Ann Thorac Surg* 2006;82:1796–1801.
151. Rodriguez F, Nguyen TC, Galanko JA. Gastrointestinal complications after coronary artery bypass grafting: a national study of morbidity and mortality predictors. *J Am Coll Surg* 2007;205:741–747.
152. Mangi AA, Christison-Lagay ER, Torchiana DF, et al. Gastrointestinal complications in patients undergoing heart operation. *Ann Surg* 2005;241:895–904.
153. Booth CM, Heyland DK, Paterson WG. Gastrointestinal promotility drugs in the critical care setting: a systematic review of the evidence. *Crit Care Med* 2002;30:1429–1435.
154. Gannon RH. Current strategies for preventing or ameliorating postoperative ileus: a multimodal approach. *Am J Health Syst Pharm* 2007;64(20 suppl 13): S8–12A.
155. Leier H. Does gum chewing help prevent impaired gastric motility in the postoperative period? *J Am Acad Nurs Pract* 2007;19:133–136.
156. Spirt M, Stanley S. Update on stress ulcer prophylaxis in critically ill patients. *Crit Care Nurse* 2007;26: 18–28.
157. Sibbing D, Morath T, Stegherr J, et al Impact of proton pump inhibitors on the antiplatelet effects of clopidogrel. *Throb Haemost* 2009 101(4):714–719.
158. Ho PM, Maddox TM, Wang L, et al. Risk of adverse outcomes associated with concomitant use of clopidogrel and proton pump inhibitors following acute coronary syndrome. *JAMA* 2009;301(9):937–944.
159. Gralnek IM, Barkun AN, Bardou M. Management of acute bleeding from a peptic ulcer. *N Engl J Med* 2008;359:928–937.
160. Klotz S, Vestring T, Rötker J, et al. Diagnosis and treatment of nonocclusive mesenteric ischemia after open heart surgery. *Ann Thorac Surg* 2001;72: 1593–1596.
161. Hasan S, Ratnatunga C, Lewis CT, et al. Gut ischemia following cardiac surgery. *Interact Cardiovasc Thorac Surg* 2004;3:475–478.
162. Chaudhuri N, James J, Sheikh A, et al. Intestinal ischemia following cardiac surgery: a multivariate risk model. *Eur J Cardiothorac Surg* 2006;29: 971–977.
163. Rady MY, Kodavatiganti R, Ryan T. Perioperative predictors of acute cholecystitis after cardiovascular surgery. *Chest* 1998;114:76–84.
164. Passage J, Joshi P, Mullany DV. Acute cholecystitis complicating cardiac surgery: case series involving more than 16,000 patients. *Ann Thorac Surg* 2007;83:1096–1101.
165. Perez A, Ito H, Farivar RS, et al. Risk factors and outcomes of pancreatitis after open heart surgery. *Am J Surg* 2005;190:401–405.
166. Gan TJ. Postoperative nausea and vomiting: can it be eliminated? *JAMA* 2002;1233–1236.
167. Ferraris VA, Ferraris SP, Moritz DM, et al. Oropharyngeal dysphagia after cardiac operations. *Ann Thorac Surg* 2001;71:1792–1796.
168. Barker J, Martino R, Reichardt B, et al. Incidence and impact of dysphagia in patients receiving prolonged endotracheal intubation after cardiac surgery. *Can J Surg* 2009;52:119–124.
169. Gundry SR, Borkon AM, McIntosh CL, et al. Candida esophagitis following cardiac operation and short-term antibiotic prophylaxis. *J Thorac Cardiovasc Surg* 1980;80:661–668.
170. Leffler DA, Lamont JT. Treatment of clositrium-associated disease. *Gastroenterology* 2009;136:1899–1912.

171. Thompson DF, Landry JP. Drug-induced hiccups. *Ann Pharmacother* 1997;31: 367–369.

172. Friedman NL. Hiccups: a treatment review. *Pharmacotherapy* 1996;16: 986–995.

173. Hansen BJ, Rosenberg J. Persistent postoperative hiccups: a review. *Acta Anaesth Scand* 1993;37:643–646.

174. McKhann GM, Grega MA, Borowicz LM, et al. Stroke and encephalopathy after cardiac surgery: an update. *Stroke* 2006;37:562–571.

175. Gottesman RF, McKhann GM, Hogue CW. Neurological complications of cardiac surgery. *Semin Neurol* 2008;28:703–715.

176. Katznelson R, Djaiani GN, Borger MA, et al. Preoperative use of statins is associated with reduced early delirium rates after cardiac surgery. *Anesthesiology* 2009;110:67–73.

177. Newman MF, Mathew JP, Grocott HP, et al. Central nervous system injury associated with cardiac surgery. *Lancet* 2006;368:694–703.

178. Brucerius J, Gummert JF, Borger MA, et al. Stroke after cardiac surgery: a risk factor analysis of 16,184 consecutive adult patients. *Ann Thorac Surg* 2003: 75:472–478.

179. Van der Linden J, Bergman P, Hadjinikolaou L. The topography of aortic atherosclerosis enhances its precision as a predictor of stroke. *Ann Thorac Surg* 2007;83:2087–2092.

180. Halkos ME, Poskas JD, Lattouf OM, et al. Impact of preoperative neurologic events on outcomes after coronary artery bypass grafting. *Ann Thorac Surg* 2008;86;504–510.

181. John R, Choudhri AF, Weinberg AD, et al. Multicenter review of preoperative risk factors for stroke after coronary artery bypass grafting. *Ann Thorac Surg* 2000;69:30–36.

182. Liddicoat JR, Redmond JM, Vassileva CM, et al. Hypothermic circulatory arrest in octogenarians: risk of stroke and mortality. *Ann Thorac Surg* 2000;69: 1048–1052.

183. Barbut D, Lo Y-W, Gold JP, et al. Impact of embolization during coronary artery bypass grafting on outcome and length of stay. *Ann Thorac Surg* 1997;63: 998–1002.

184. Salazar JD, Wityk RJ, Grega MA, et al. Stroke after cardiac surgery: short- and long-term outcomes. *Ann Thorac Surg* 2001;72:1195–1202.

185. Charlesworth DC, Likosky DS, Marrin DAS, et al. Development and validation of a prediction model for strokes after coronary artery bypass grafting. *Ann Thorac Surg* 2003;76:436–443.

186. Eagle KA, Guyton RA, Davidoff R, et al. ACC/AHA 2004 guideline update for coronary artery bypass graft surgery: summary article: a report of the American College of Cardiology/American Heart Association Task Force on Practice Guidelines (Committee to Update the 1999 Guidelines for Coronary Artery Bypass Graft Surgery). *J Am Coll Cardiol* 2004;44: 1146–1154.

187. Iglesia I, Murkin JM. Beating heart surgery or conventional CABG: are neurologic outcomes different? *Semin Thorac Cardiovasc Surg* 2001;13:158–169.

188. Sellke FW, DiMaio JM, Caplan LR, et al. Comparing on-pump and off-pump coronary artery bypass grafting: numerous studies but few conclusions: a scientific statement from the American Heart Association council on cardiovascular surgery and anesthesia in collaboration with the interdisciplinary working group on quality of care and outcomes research. *Circulation* 2005;111: 2858–2864.

189. Whitley WS. An argument for routine ultrasound screening of the thoracic aorta in the cardiac surgery population. *Semin Cardiothorac Vasc Anesth* 2008;12:290–297.

190. Zingone B, Rauber E, Gatti G, et al. The impact of epiaortic ultrasonographic scanning on the risk of perioperative stroke. *Eur J Cardiothorac Surg* 2006;29: 720–728.

191. Zingone B, Rauber E, Gatti G, et al. Diagnosis and management of severe atherosclerosis of the ascending aorta and aortic arch during cardiac surgery: focus on aortic replacement. *Eur J Cardiothorac Surg* 2007;31: 990–997.

192. Rosenberger P, Shernan SK, Löffler M, et al. The influence of epiaortic ultrasonography on intraoperative surgical management in 6051 cardiac surgical patients. *Ann Thorac Surg* 2008;85:548–553.

193. Kincaid EH, Jones TJ, Stump DA, et al. Processing scavenged blood with a cell saver reduces cerebral lipid microembolization. *Ann Thorac Surg* 2000; 1296–1300.

194. Grigore Am, Grocott HP, Mathew JP, et al. The rewarming rate and increased peak temperature alter neurocognitive outcome after cardiac surgery. *Anesth Analg* 2002;94:4–10.

195. Cook DJ. Cerebral hyperthermia and cardiac surgery: consequences and prevention. *Semin Thorac Cardiovasc Surg* 2001;13:176–183.

196. Svenarud P, Persson M., van der Linden J. Effect of CO2 insufflation on the number and behavior of air microemboli in open-heart surgery: a randomized clinical trial. *Circulation* 2004;109:1127–1132.

197. Martens S, Neuman K, Sodemann C, et al. Carbon dioxide field flooding reduces neurologic impairment after open heart surgery. *Ann Thorac Surg* 2008;85:543–547.

198. Mills NL, Ochsner JL. Massive air embolism during cardiopulmonary bypass. *J Thorac Cardiovasc Surg* 1980;80:708–717.

199. Ziser A, Adir Y, Lavon H, et al. Hyperbaric oxygen therapy for massive arterial air embolism during cardiac operations. *J Thorac Cardiovasc Surg* 1999;117: 818–821.

200. Shahian DM, Speert PK. Symptomatic visual deficits after open heart operations. *Ann Thorac Surg* 1989;48:275–279.

201. Shapira OM, Kimmel WA, Lindsey PS, et al. Anterior ischemic optic neuropathy after open heart operations. *Ann Thorac Surg* 1996;61:660–666.

202. Furster V, Ryden LE, Asinger RW, et al. ACC/AHA/ESC guidelines for the management of patients with atrial fibrillation. *J Amer Coll Cardiol* 2001;38: 1231–1265.

203. Lahtinen J, Biancari F, Salmela E, et al. Postoperative atrial fibrillation is a major cause of stroke after on-pump coronary artery bypass surgery. *Ann Thorac Surg* 2004;77:1241–1244.

204. Koster S, Hensens AG, van der Palen J. The long-term cognitive and functional outcomes of postoperative delirium after cardiac surgery. *Ann Thorac Surg* 2009;87:1469–1474.

205. Koster S, Oosterveld FJ, Hensens AG, et al. Delirium after cardiac surgery and predictive validity of a risk checklist. *Ann Thorac Surg* 2008;86: 1883–1887.

206. Norkiene I, Ringaitiene D, Misiuriene I, et al. Incidence and precipitating factors of delirium after coronary artery bypass grafting. *Scand Cardiovasc J* 2007;41:180–185.

207. Rudolph JL, Jones RN, Levkoff SE, et al. Derivation and validation of a preoperative prediction rule for delirium after cardiac surgery. *Circulation* 2009; 119:229–236.

208. Brucerius J, Gummert JF, Borger MA, et al. Predictors of delirium after cardiac surgery delirium: effect of beating-heart (off-pump) surgery. *J Thorac Cardiovasc Surg* 2004;127:57–64.

209. Katznels R, Djaiani GN, Morger MA, et al. Preoperative use of statins is associated with reduced early delirium rates after cardiac surgery. *Anesthesiology* 2009;110:67–73.

210. Odeh M, Oliven A. Central nervous system reactions associated with famotidine: report of five cases. *J Clin Gastroenterol* 1998;27:253–254.

211. Pandharipande P, Shintani A, Peterson J, et al. Lorezapam is an independent risk factor for transitioning to delirium in intensive care unit patients. *Anesthesiology* 2006;104:21–26.

212. Alagiakrishnan K, Wiens A. An approach to drug induced delirium in the elderly. *Postgrad Med J* 2004;80:388–393.

213. Chevrolet J-G, Jolliet P. Clinical review: agitation and delirium in the critically ill—significance and management. *Critical Care* 2007;11:214–218.

214. McKinley MG. Alcohol withdrawal syndrome: overlooked and mismanaged? *Crit Care Nurse* 2005;25:40–48.

215. Stevens RD, Nyquist PA. Coma, delirium, and cognitive dysfunction in critical illness. *Critical Care Clin* 2006;22:787–804.

216. Dupuis G, Kennedy E, Lindquist R, et al. Coronary artery bypass graft surgery and cognitive performance. *Am J Crit Care* 2006;15:471–479.

217. Rosengart TK, Sweet JJ, Finnin E, et al. Stable cognition after coronary artery bypass grafting: comparisons with percutaneous intervention and normal controls. *Ann Thorac Surg* 2006;82:597–607.

218. Selnes OA, Grega MA, Bailey, MM, et al. Neurocognitive outcomes 3 years after coronary artery bypass surgery: a controlled study. *Ann Thorac Surg* 2007; 84:1885–1896.

219. Grocott HP. Cognitive decline after cardiac surgery: revisiting etiology. *Semin Cardiothorac Vasc Anesth* 2005;9:123–129.

220. Hernandez F Jr, Brown JR, Likosky DS, et al. Neurocognitive outcomes of off-pump versus on-pump coronary artery bypass: a prospective randomized controlled trial. *Ann Thorac Surg* 2007;84:1897–1903.

221. Jensen BO, Hughes P, Rasmussen LS, et al. Cognitive outcomes in elderly high-risk patients after off-pump versus conventional coronary artery bypass grafting: a randomized trial. *Circulation* 2006;113:2790–2795.

222. Sharma AD, Parnley CL, Seeram G, et al. Peripheral nerve injuries during cardiac surgery: risk factors, diagnosis, prognosis, and prevention. *Anesth Analg* 2000;91:1358–1369.

223. Warner MA, Warner ME, Martin JT. Ulnar neuropathy: incidence, outcome, and risk factors in sedated or anesthetized patients. *Anesthesiology* 1994;81: 1332–1340.

224. Dayan V, Cura L, Cubas S, et al. Surgical anatomy of the saphenous nerve. *Ann Thorac Surg* 2008;85:896–900.

225. Denton TA, Trento L, Cohen M, et al. Radial artery harvesting for coronary bypass operations: neurologic complications and their potential mechanisms. *J Thorac Cardiovasc Surg* 2001;121:951–956.

226. Itagaki T, Kikura M, Sato S. Incidence and risk factors of postoperative vocal cord paralysis in 987 patients after cardiovascular surgery. *Ann Thorac Surg* 2007;83:2147–2152.

227. Joo D, Duarte VM, Ghadiali MT, et al. Recovery of vocal fold paralysis after cardiovascular surgery. *Laryngoscope* 2009;119:1435–1438.
228. Ivins GK. Meralgia paresthetica, the elusive diagnosis: clinical experience in 14 adult patients. *Ann Surg* 2000;232:281–286.
229. Athanasiou T, Aziz O, Al-Ruzzeh S, et al. Are wound healing disturbances and length of hospital stay reduced with minimally invasive vein harvest: a meta-analysis. *Eur J Cardiothorac Surg* 2004;26:1015–1026.
230. Bitondo JM, Daggett WM, Torchiana DF, et al. Endoscopic versus open saphenous vein harvest: a comparison of postoperative wound complications. *Ann Thorac Surg* 2002;73: 523–528.
231. Paletta CE, Huang DB, Fiore AC, et al. Major leg wound complications after saphenous vein harvest for coronary revascularization. *Ann Thorac Surg* 2000;70:492–497.
232. Lemmer JH Jr, Meng RL, Corson JD, et al. Preoperative saphenous vein mapping for coronary artery bypass. *J Card Surg* 1988;3:237–240.
233. Amano QA, Hirose H, Takahashi A, et al. Coronary artery bypass grafting using the radial artery: midterm results in a Japanese institute. *Ann Thorac Surg* 2001;72:120–125.
234. Tatoulis J, Royse AG, Buxton BF, et al. The radial artery in coronary surgery: a 5-year experience—clinical and angiographic results. *Ann Thorac Surg* 2002; 73:143–148.
235. Greene MA, Malias MA. Arm complications after radial artery procurement for coronary bypass operation. *Ann Thorac Surg* 2001;72:126–128.
236. Geerts WH, Bergqvist D, Pineo GF, et al. Prevention of venous thromboembolism. American College of Chest Physicians evidence-based clinical practice guidelines (8th edition). *Chest* 2008;133:381S–453S.
237. Shammas NW. Pulmonary embolus after coronary artery bypass surgery: a review of the literature. *Clin Cardiol* 2000;23:637–644.
238. Close V, Purohit M, Tanos, M, et al. Should patients post-cardiac surgery be given low molecular weight heparin for deep vein thrombosis prophylaxis? *Interact Cardiovasc Thorac Surg* 2006;5:624–629.
239. Goldhaber SZ, Schoepf UJ. Pulmonary embolism after coronary artery bypass. *Circulation* 2004;109:2712–2715.
240. Joffe HV, Goldhaber SZ. Upper-extremity deep vein thrombosis. *Circulation* 2002;106: 1874–1880.
241. Tapson VF. Acute pulmonary embolism. *N Engl J Med* 2008;358:1037–1052.
242. Konstantinides S. Acute pulmonary embolism. *N Engl J Med* 2008;359: 2804–2813.
243. Kearon C, Kahn SR, Agnelli G, et al. Antithrombotic therapy for venous thromboembolic disease. American College of Chest Physicians evidence-based clinical practice guidelines (8th edition). *Chest* 2008;133:454S–545S.
244. Putnam JB, Lemmer JH, Rocchini PA, et al. Embolectomy for acute pulmonary artery occlusion following Fontan procedure. *Ann Thorac Surg* 1988;45: 335–336.

6 Late Postoperative Management

CARDIAC REHABILITATION

For patients undergoing cardiac surgery the goal is to facilitate their return to as normal a lifestyle as possible, including employment when appropriate. Cardiac rehabilitation is a comprehensive, long-term program that involves medical evaluation, exercise, cardiac risk factor modification, education, and counseling designed to reduce the adverse physiological and psychological effects of, and the risk factors associated with, cardiac disease (1). Postoperative cardiac rehabilitation is carried out in three phases: inpatient (phase 1), early outpatient usually beginning within 1 to 2 months after surgery (phase 2), and long-term outpatient (phase 3). Properly conducted cardiac rehabilitation is safe, improves the patient's exercise capacity, should improve the ability of a patient to return to work, and improves the patient's general and cardiovascular disease long-term prognosis. Cardiac rehabilitation should be offered to all eligible patients and should include risk factor management where appropriate.

A well-organized program for cardiac rehabilitation addresses both the physical and the emotional needs of the cardiac surgery patient and begins with instruction in the preoperative period. An important element in cardiac rehabilitation is developing a positive patient attitude, starting with the assumption that rehabilitation to an active lifestyle and employment is the norm. Cardiac rehabilitation offers the patients graded exercise in a supervised environment up to the limit of their cardiac function. With continued conditioning, many of these patients, particularly those with heart failure that has been improved or corrected, should experience considerable improvement in exercise capacity over their preoperative status. This may, however, require a considerable effort over a period of time depending on the degree of preoperative disability. For most patients, postoperative cardiac rehabilitation begins in the hospital, a process that will continue when they are at home. Most initial rehabilitation programs for postoperative patients achieve only low-level exercise and low-level caloric expenditure during the inpatient portion of the program (2).

Ambulation is initiated as early as possible in the hospital after surgery. This is to decrease the amount of "deconditioning" and lack of mobility that develop with bed rest, to optimize pulmonary toilet and minimize atelectasis, and to decrease venous stasis in the lower extremities, consequently lowering the risk of thromboembolism. In addition, it has been demonstrated that patients achieve a better quality of life by 3 months following surgery if ambulation and rehabilitation are started early after surgery during the acute hospitalization (3). The program of ambulation varies from hospital to hospital, but, in general, it progresses to supervised stair climbing or exercise on a stationary bicycle before discharge. From both physical and emotional perspectives, the inpatient ambulation and phase 1 rehabilitation program introduces and prepares the patient for the outpatient program. As there is an emphasis on shortening the length of the hospital stay, generating a positive attitude toward rehabilitation and de-emphasizing cardiac illness may be important factors in reducing the number of postoperative in-hospital days. Providing the patient with information on what to expect after heart surgery is important and many resources are available including surgical society Web site links (4).

For patients who have undergone successful coronary artery bypass graft (CABG) procedures and who are asymptomatic, routine postoperative exercise stress testing is not indicated (5,6).

IMPROVING GRAFT PATENCY AFTER CABG

It is recognized that CABG is palliative and that atherosclerosis in the native coronary arteries often progresses. Up to 25% of saphenous vein bypass grafts will be occluded at the end of the first postoperative year; at 10 years, approximately 40% to 50% are closed (7). Graft occlusion is a complex subject, but factors that influence short-term graft patency include conduit used (arterial versus saphenous vein); the location, size, and quality of the recipient coronary artery; the technical quality of proximal and distal anastomoses; and the patient's atherosclerotic risk factors. Very early graft closure is often due to technical factors such as anastomotic stenosis or a very poor quality and/or small diameter coronary artery. Vein graft intimal hyperplasia can lead to subacute graft closure; this may be a response of the intima to the higher pressure present in the arterial circulation, while recurrent atherosclerosis leads to long-term graft closure (8). Arterial bypass grafts, in particular internal mammary and radial artery grafts, have patency rates that are clearly superior to those of vein grafts. In fact, more than 95% of left internal mammary artery grafts placed to the left anterior descending coronary artery remain functional 15 years after surgery (9). The degree of stenosis in the recipient coronary artery is a significant determinant of long-term patency. Grafts (arterial or venous) that are placed to an artery that is not significantly ($>$60%) blocked are much more likely to close early due to the presence of competitive flow in the native artery. In general, grafts to the left anterior descending coronary artery (arterial or venous) have higher long-term patency rates than do bypasses to the other major coronary arteries.

Postoperative efforts to improve graft patency have concentrated in two areas: platelet inhibitor drug treatment and atherosclerosis risk factor modification. Antiplatelet drugs can enhance graft patency; in particular, early postoperative administration of aspirin has been clearly demonstrated to improve vein graft patency rates. For this purpose, aspirin should be given within 6 hours of surgery (by rectal suppository) as long as the patient is not bleeding (10–12). When the patient is taking oral medications, enteric-coated aspirin is instituted. Because of aspirin's beneficial effect in the secondary prevention of subsequent clinical events in patients with coronary artery disease, the administration of aspirin is continued indefinitely (13). For selected patients, the addition of clopidogrel to aspirin may be considered. These include patients who presented with unstable angina pectoris and those who have indwelling drug-eluting coronary artery stents (14). We also consider adjunctive clopidogrel therapy for patients who have very severe diffuse coronary atherosclerosis and for those who required coronary endarterectomy at the time of operation. Likewise for patients with aspirin allergy, clopidogrel is indicated as an alternative antiplatelet agent (12).

Because recurrent atherosclerosis can occur both in the native circulation as well as in the bypass grafts, there is considerable emphasis on postoperative atherosclerosis risk factor modification. It is clear that secondary prevention efforts for patients with known coronary artery disease are of value and guidelines for patient management have been developed (15).

The risk factors known to accelerate atherosclerosis that can be controlled or modified include smoking, hypertension, dyslipidemia, physical inactivity, obesity, and diabetes. Younger patients with accelerated atherosclerosis and no other significant common risk factors should be screened either before surgery or 2 to 3 months after surgery for uncommon causes of premature atherosclerosis, such as coagulation system disorders or unusual risk factors such as elevated homocysteine, lipoprotein (a), C-reactive protein, and/or fibrinogen levels. Emphasizing the importance of eliminating controllable risk factors (such as smoking and atherogenic diet) and treating treatable risk factors (such as hypertension, diabetes, and dyslipidemia) are prominent parts of the cardiac rehabilitation process. The initial treatment of patients with dyslipidemia includes weight reduction, dietary modification with respect to fat and fiber intake, and aerobic exercise. Patients with an abnormal lipid profile should undergo further treatment. Patients with diabetes mellitus and coronary artery disease have an impaired long-term prognosis, and optimization of their risk factors and pharmacologic treatment regimen is very important (16).

With the availability of effective lipid-lowering medications such as the *statins* (hydroxymethylglutaryl–coenzyme A reductase inhibitors) and the *fibrates*, a greater degree of control over lipid metabolism is now possible. In fact, all patients undergoing CABG should receive statin therapy unless contraindications exist (14). In particular, low-density lipoprotein cholesterol should be kept below 70 mg/dL. When possible, CABG patients should undergo lipid profile evaluation prior to surgery. Statin administration prior to surgery is begun in patients with known coronary artery disease and then continued postoperatively. Although relatively safe, long-term treatment with lipid-lowering drugs does require careful follow-up. Statin therapy may cause increases in the patient's hepatic serum aminotransferase (i.e., aspartate aminotransferase and alanine aminotransferase) enzyme levels; this may occur in up to 3% of treated patients. Thus, liver function testing is required at 3 to 6 weeks after initiation of statin therapy (or increase in dosage) and should then be repeated every 3 to 6 months for at least the first year of therapy (17). Statins may potentiate the effect of warfarin (Coumadin) and should be used with care in patients with known liver disease. Another side effect of statin is uncomplicated myalgia; much more rare is severe rhabdomyolysis with renal failure. Other medications to treat dyslipidemias include the *fibrates* (often used for hypertriglyceridemia) and *niacin.*

Further long-term goals for patients with known coronary artery disease include regular exercise (30 minutes, 7 days per week), weight loss (body mass index < 25 kg/m^2), blood pressure control ($<140/90$ mm Hg), diabetes management (HbA$_{1c}$ < 6%), and complete cessation of smoking. Other recommended adjunctive medications for this patient group include beta-blockers, angiotensin-converting enzyme inhibitors, and annual influenza vaccination (16).

Clinical depression is common in patients with coronary artery disease, both before and after CABG. Preoperative anxiety and depression predict the occurrence of postoperative symptoms, which occur in 19% to 61% of patients (18). Preoperative antidepressant drug therapy (with selective serotonin reuptake inhibitors such as citalopram) is generally not recommended as these drugs may interact with other medications and may require several weeks before benefits occur. Postoperative management of significant depression may include a combination of antidepressant drug therapy, psychotherapy, and institution of a stress management program (19). Participation in cardiac rehabilitation is also of benefit for such patients.

COMPLICATIONS OF PROSTHETIC VALVES

Infection

Bacterial endocarditis is a potential risk in any patient who has undergone cardiac surgery, even after isolated mitral valve repair (17). The mechanism of endocarditis involves the deposition of fibrin and platelets at the site of endothelial damage or at the location of suture and/or a prosthetic valve cloth-sewing ring. Subsequent bacteremia can lead to bacterial adhesion to these lesions and proliferation of the bacterial colony resulting in prosthetic valve endocarditis (PVE). The cumulative risk of a patient developing PVE may be as high as 5% at 10 years following valve implantation (20). The diagnosis is based on positive blood cultures and, frequently, demonstration of abnormal valve function, periprosthetic abscess formation, and/or vegetations. The physical examination may reveal evidence of heart failure, new paravalvular leaks (regurgitant murmur), and/or evidence of metastatic infection. Any patient with a prosthetic valve who is febrile without an easily identifiable source must be considered as possibly having PVE. These patients should undergo multiple blood cultures, ideally during the onset of a fever spike. Echocardiography, most often transesophageal, is an important feature of making the diagnosis as this can demonstrate leakage around the valve and the presence of vegetations.

Treatment most often requires repeat replacement of the valve in addition to intensive and prolonged antibiotic therapy. Historically, PVE has been a highly lethal disease with reported mortality rates as high as 30%. However, with contemporary antibiotics and an aggressive surgical approach, the current potential for cure has become greater.

In an effort to reduce the incidence of PVE, patients with indwelling prosthetic valves have, in the past, been recommended to receive antibiotic therapy for situations in which they might become bacteremic. Theses recommendations have, however, been revised (21). Of note, the recommendation for prophylactic antibiotic treatment for patients with prosthetic valves undergoing dental procedures has been downgraded from Class I (treatment should be administered) to Class IIa (it is reasonable to administer treatment). Prophylactic antibiotic treatment is not recommended for patients with prosthetic valves undergoing nondental procedures such as endoscopic procedures, in the absence of active infection. Patients at risk who sustain open injuries require meticulous wound care and be monitored carefully for potential infection; the threshold to treat suspected early cellulitis should be lower for patients with indwelling prosthetic valves.

The treatment plan for PVE depends on the features of the presentation. Patients with fever and positive blood cultures but no hemodynamic deterioration are initially treated with appropriate antibiotic therapy. The drug is selected on the basis of culture data and optimized according to blood levels and quantitative bactericidal studies. If treatment results in complete fever resolution and if there is no evidence of prosthetic valve dysfunction, metastatic infection, or emboli, the antibiotics are continued for 6 weeks. Following this, the antibiotics are discontinued, and patients are observed and cultures are taken if a fever occurs.

Because of the presence of foreign material (the sewing ring of the prosthesis), PVE is less likely to be cured by antibiotics alone than is native valve endocarditis, particularly in cases that involve virulent organisms such as *Staphylococcus* sp. or fungi. Uncomplicated first-time PVE involving an antibiotic-sensitive organism does not require replacement (22). PVE due to *Streptococcus* species may be treatable with antibiotics alone unless the patient's fever fails to subside quickly and completely at which time surgery is likely indicated. Antimicrobial treatment of fungal PVE endocarditis fails in nearly all cases and surgery is required. In PVE due to the more virulent organisms, erosion of the cardiac tissues is more common, resulting in paravalvular leaks, abscess formation, and detachment of the valve or a recently placed intracardiac patch. Conduction system abnormalities (e.g., heart block) or a fistula from the aorta to the right atrium may develop in patients with aortic valve PVE, especially if caused by *Staphylococcus*. Thus, early operation is usually indicated for patients with PVE caused by organisms that are unlikely to be successfully treated with antimicrobial drugs. The occurrence of emboli despite antibiotic therapy is another indication for surgery. The presence of cerebral emboli may increase the surgical risk because of the possibility of intracranial hemorrhage at the site of necrotic brain tissue when the patient is anticoagulated for cardiopulmonary bypass.

Echocardiography, in particular transesophageal echocardiography, can delineate the status of valve function and the presence of vegetations and provide the detail needed for surgery. If the patient with PVE is being considered for surgery and has risk factors for coronary artery disease, coronary angiography may be needed. If, however, aortic valve vegetations are present, there is a risk of creating emboli; therefore, care must be taken in engaging the coronary ostia. High-resolution computed tomography angiography may provide details of the coronary anatomy in a less invasive manner for selected patients.

In general, when surgery is needed for PVE, the infection often extends beyond the prosthesis, and surgery must be aggressive to extirpate all infected tissue. The infected valve may be successfully replaced with a mechanical valve or a tissue valve, depending on the patient's age and other factors affecting life expectancy (such as coronary artery disease, ventricular function, renal failure). There has been considerable success using cryopreserved homografts for the treatment of aortic valve PVE, even under emergency conditions, particularly in patients in whom considerable tissue destruction has occurred (23,24).

Deterioration of Tissue Prosthetic Valves

Bioprosthetic heterograft valves, usually composed of porcine or bovine material mounted on a sewing ring, offer patients the advantage of a low (<1% annual) thromboembolic rate without the need for lifelong systemic anticoagulation. Although primary failure of tissue valves can occur early, the rate of failure generally begins to increase about 5 years after implantation. Younger patients, particularly those younger than 40 years, suffer deterioration of bioprosthetic valves more rapidly, with approximately half requiring replacement within 10 years of implantation (23). Bovine pericardial bioprostheses appear to have greater durability than porcine aortic bioprostheses. As a general rule, bioprosthetic valves are offered to patients aged between 60 and 65 years who do not have other reasons to require warfarin therapy. Younger patients may, however, after full discussion with the surgeon, request a bioprosthetic valve for lifestyle considerations (avoiding warfarin). Likewise, some older patients (particularly those younger than 70 years who do not have coronary artery disease) may, after full discussion with the surgeon, request implantation of a mechanical valve to improve their chances of avoiding a second valve replacement due to bioprosthetic valve failure. In the mitral position, porcine bioprosthetic valves may deteriorate prematurely in patients over a wide range of ages, including in the elderly. Thus, we more often use mechanical valves in the mitral position, even in older patients, unless the patient has a predictably limited expected lifespan. If the patient requires warfarin for other reasons (such as atrial fibrillation), a mechanical valve is usually recommended. Some patients on long-term warfarin therapy may, however, choose a tissue valve so that they can have a lower level of anticoagulation [international normalized ratio (INR) 2.0 to 3.0] and the drug can be discontinued for short periods of time with relative safety as compared to if a mechanical valve was in place. If there is a contraindication to long-term warfarin anticoagulation, it is necessary to use bioprosthetic aortic and mitral prostheses. The longevity of patients who have both valvular and coronary artery disease is significantly influenced by the natural history of the coronary atherosclerosis. Thus, in patients undergoing combined valve replacement and CABG, bioprosthetic valves are often used. This is because their long-term survival is more likely limited by the coronary artery disease (especially when extensive) than by future valve deterioration.

Tissue prostheses are subject to leaflet calcification or fracture, resulting in valve regurgitation or, less commonly, stenosis. This process usually develops gradually with progressive symptoms that lead the patient to seek medical attention. Most commonly, the presentation is that of congestive heart failure. Echocardiography is the initial diagnostic study when bioprosthetic valve failure is suspected to be present. Catastrophic sudden bioprosthetic valve failure is unusual.

Malfunction of Mechanical Valves

Low-profile mechanical valves incorporating pyrolytic carbon components are the most commonly used mechanical valve prostheses in the United States. The present generation of valves offers patients relatively low thromboembolic rates—less than those observed in prior decades with earlier mechanical prostheses (23); contemporary valves also have excellent flow characteristics, even in smaller sizes.

If the patient is inadequately anticoagulated for a significant period of time, mechanical prostheses are prone to thrombosis. This life-threatening complication may present as stroke, peripheral emboli, and/or prosthetic valve obstruction. It is more common with prosthetic valves in the mitral position as compared with those in the aortic position. Thrombolytic therapy (i.e., streptokinase or tissue plasminogen activator) can be used to treat prosthetic valve thrombosis, especially in very ill patients who are at high risk for surgery. There is, however, a significant risk of clot embolization (about 15% to 20%) and rethrombosis (25,26). Patients with large clots identified by echocardiography are less likely to have a successful result of thrombolytic therapy. Lytic therapy of thrombosed prosthetic tricuspid or pulmonary valves is more frequently successful than lytic therapy of clotted valves in the left side of the heart. This topic is also discussed in Chapter 1.

Pannus ingrowth leading to mechanical valve obstruction is a rare cause of late mechanical valve failure that may lead to the need for replacement of the prosthesis (27).

Paravalvular Leaks

A clinically significant leak around an implanted cardiac valve prosthesis is rare. The use of intraoperative transesophageal echocardiography (after weaning the patient from bypass but before closing the chest) provides for detection of paravalvular leaks in the operating room that may be a result of technical factors, which can be corrected at the time of primary implantation.

Occasionally, paravalvular leaks, particularly around mitral prostheses, may be silent. Trauma to the red blood cells can result in hemolytic anemia, and this may be the only clue that a paravalvular leak is present. Patients with persistent anemia after valve replacement should be evaluated by echocardiography for paravalvular leaks. Laboratory evaluation will often demonstrate fragmented erythrocytes, elevated lactate dehydrogenase level, and hemosiderin in the urine. Significant anemia, particularly if there is a transfusion requirement or hemodynamic compromise, mandates reoperation. Although it is tempting to close paravalvular leaks by primary suture, their boundaries are often rigid, consisting of the prosthetic sewing ring and a fibrotic or calcified annulus. Unless primary suture closes the defect with little tension, consideration must be given to closing a paravalvular leak with a patch or by re-replacement, often with a larger size prosthesis. Percutaneous transcatheter closure of a paraprosthetic leak may also be possible in some patients (28). Subclinical hemolysis may also occur because of a prosthetic valve, even in the absence of a paravalvular leak. This is more common with mechanical prostheses with a lower incidence in stented tissue valves. The presence of subclinical hemolysis is evidenced by elevated lactic dehydrogenase levels, although in the absence of a paravalvular leak, anemia does not usually occur (29).

Thromboembolism and Anticoagulation

Patients with prosthetic valves are at risk for thrombotic complications, and the risk is greater for valves in the mitral position than those in the aortic position. Although the risk is <1% per year for patients with biological (tissue) valves, mechanical valves are at higher risk and, thus, require lifelong warfarin anticoagulation. For patients with mechanical valves, good long-term anticoagulation control (minimizing variability in the degree of anticoagulation) is associated with improved long-term survival (30). Even with "adequate" warfarin treatment, the incidence of thromboemboli in patients with mechanical valves is 1% to 2% per year (31).

Long-term anticoagulation is achieved by the administration of the vitamin K antagonist warfarin. This drug is rapidly absorbed via the gastrointestinal tract, and its antithrombotic effect is due to reduction of endogenous prothrombin (Factor II) activity. Because prothrombin has a long half-life (approximately 3 days), the full antithrombotic effect of administered warfarin is not achieved quickly. In fact, since warfarin also inhibits other liver-derived factors that are anticoagulant in action but have shorter half-lives, a prothrombotic state may be induced early after warfarin administration, especially if a large dose is given (32). Therefore, a large loading dose (e.g., >10 mg) is not recommended and if rapid anticoagulation is needed, the patient should be bridged for a few days with intravenous unfractionated or subcutaneous low-molecular-weight heparin (LMWH) administration (33). Early administration of heparin to heart surgery patients is, however, associated with an increased incidence of the need for surgical re-exploration for postoperative bleeding (34). Therefore, in these situations the patient should be closely monitored. Unfractionated heparin may be preferred because of its shorter duration of action and easier reversibility should bleeding problems arise.

Previously, the prothrombin time was used to express the degree of anticoagulation. However, this laboratory test uses thromboplastin, and variability in thromboplastin responsiveness to warfarin-induced reductions in vitamin K-dependent clotting factors causes variability in prothrombin time determinations. To compensate for this variability in thromboplastin activity, the INR was developed (35). The optimum INR range for prosthetic valves has been the subject of numerous studies, reviews, and consensus committees (23,36). Currently recommended guidelines are shown in Table 6.1. These recommendations take into account the type of valve (mechanical versus tissue) and the presence or absence of additional risk factors such as prior thromboembolism, atrial fibrillation, left ventricular dysfunction, and the presence of a hypercoagulable condition. All patients with prosthetic heart valves should receive aspirin unless a contraindication is present (23). Patients who received a bioprosthetic valve and have no other indications for warfarin are treated with aspirin only. Patients with mechanical valves receive both warfarin and aspirin. This combined therapy reduces the rate of thromboembolism and total mortality but may increase the rate of bleeding complications somewhat (37). Low-dose aspirin (80 to 100 mg daily) may have a lower bleeding rate than does conventional dose. If aspirin cannot be administered because of allergy, clopidogrel should be considered.

Generally, patients who receive aortic valve bioprostheses do not routinely receive postoperative anticoagulation, other than aspirin treatment (38). Patients who receive tissue prosthetic valves in the mitral position may be at increased risk for thrombus formation and thus, unless contraindications exist, anticoagulation for 3 months is generally recommended, although this opinion is not universal (23,37). After 3 months has passed, as long as other risk factors (such as atrial fibrillation) are not present, the warfarin is discontinued and aspirin therapy is continued.

Anticoagulation treatment for patients with prosthetic valves begins when the patients are able to take medications orally. We generally start with a dose of 2.5 to 5.0 mg per day and follow the INR daily during the early postoperative period. The lower initial dose is used in patients who have had elevated right-sided filling pressures, any evidence of hepatic dysfunction, or long-standing cardiac cachexia. The dose is then increased by 1.0 to 2.5 mg every day or every other day until the INR begins to rise. At many hospitals, the pharmacists will determine the recommended daily dosage change on the basis of the daily INR and the individual patient's target value. Because of the lag time between the beginning of warfarin treatment and the achievement of a therapeutic INR level, some institutions begin treatment with LMWH during the early postoperative period for patients who have received

TABLE 6.1 Antithrombotic Therapy—Prosthetic Heart Valves[a]

	Mechanical Prosthetic Valves			Biological Prosthetic Valves		
	Warfarin, INR 2.0–3.0	Warfarin, INR 2.5–3.5	Aspirin, 50–100 mg	Warfarin, INR 2.0–3.0	Warfarin, INR 2.5–3.5	Aspirin, 75–100 mg
First 3 mo after valve replacement	+	++	+	++	+	+
After first 3 mo:						
Aortic valve	+		+			+
Aortic valve + risk factor[b]		+	+	+		
Mitral valve		+	+			+
Mitral valve + risk factor		+	+	+		+

INR, international normalized ratio; +, class I recommendation ("treatment should be administered"); ++, class IIa recommendation ("it is reasonable to administer treatment").

[a]Depending on the clinical status of patient, antithrombotic therapy must be individualized.

[b]Risk factors: atrial fibrillation, previous thromboembolus, left ventricular dysfunction, hypercoagulable state.

Adapted from Bonow RO, Carabello BA, Chatterjee K, et al. 2008 focused update incorporated into the ACC/AHA 2006 guidelines for the management of patients with valvular heart disease: a report of the American College of Cardiology/American Heart Association Task Force on Practice guidelines. *J Am Coll Cardiol* 2008;52:e1–e142. http://content.onlinejacc.org/cgi/content/full/52/13/e1.

mechanical valves. This is continued for a few days while the warfarin therapy is taking effect (39). For patients with aortic prostheses, we generally do not do this unless the INR remains suboptimal on the third or fourth postoperative day at which time, assuming no contraindications exist, we begin LMWH (typically enoxaparin at 1 mg/kg subcutaneous twice daily). For patients with mitral prostheses, LMWH is often begun on the second or third postoperative day. After discharge, the INR is checked regularly (initially two to three times per week, then weekly) until a stable level is demonstrated, at which time the interval between determinations may be lengthened. With continued patient recovery and, in particular, improvement in postoperative nutrition, the dose may need to be increased gradually above the amount needed during the early postoperative period. Some able and motivated patients may successfully self-manage their own INR levels with a home device using a predetermined warfarin dosing protocol (40,41).

A rare but serious potential side effect of warfarin therapy is skin necrosis (42,43). This typically begins a few days after the initiation of treatment and results in the development of hemorrhagic blisters or necrotic scars, particularly in areas with large quantities of adipose tissue (breast, hips, buttocks).

Many drugs may interfere with warfarin anticoagulation (and alter the INR) either by depressing or accelerating hepatic metabolism or by enhancing or interfering with warfarin–protein binding; prescribing physicians and patients should be aware of these (Table 6.2). Patients should also be aware that dietary intake of vitamin K may affect the INR; they should be urged to be relatively consistent in their dietary habits. Foods containing relatively large amounts of vitamin K include broccoli, parsley, cabbage, collard greens, mustard greens, peas, spinach, green tea, and pickles (44).

LONG-TERM ISSUES IN PATIENTS RECEIVING WARFARIN

Patients taking warfarin are at risk for hemorrhage, either related to excessive anticoagulation or secondary to other medical conditions. Management of the excessively prolonged INR anticoagulation takes into account magnitude of the INR and whether or not there is bleeding present (34). If the INR is >5.0 but <9.0 and there is no bleeding present, a dose or two of warfarin is omitted, the INR is followed closely, and warfarin is resumed at an adjusted dose when therapeutic. If the INR exceeds 5.0 without bleeding but the patient is at risk for bleeding or if urgent surgery is required, a small oral dose of vitamin K (phytonadione; 1 to 2.5 mg) may be given. It will take about 24 hours for the INR to be reduced. If the INR exceeds 9.0 without bleeding, warfarin should be held, a larger dose of oral vitamin K (3 to 5 mg) may be given,

TABLE 6.2	Drug Interactions with Warfarin
Drug	**Effect on Anticoagulation**
Acetaminophen	Increase
Allopurinol	Increase
Amiodarone	Increase
Barbiturate	Decrease
Carbamazepine	Decrease
Cholestyramine	Decrease
Cimetidine	Increase
Ciprofloxacin	Increase
Clofibrate	Increase
Dicloxacillin	Decrease
Gemfibrozil	Increase
Griseofulvin	Decrease
Lovastatin	Increase
Metronidazole	Increase
Nafcillin	Decrease
Neomycin	Increase
Omeprazole	Increase
Phenytoin	Decrease
Propafenone	Increase
Propoxyphene	Increase
Sucralfate	Decrease
Vitamin E	Increase
Vitamin K	Decrease
Zafirlukast	Increase

Note: This list includes many of the drugs that might be administered to heart surgery patients but does not include all drugs that are known to affect warfarin's action.

and when the INR is within therapeutic range, warfarin may be restarted at a lower dose with more frequent INR monitoring. In general, if serious bleeding is not present, oral vitamin K is preferred to the intravenous route although low-dose intravenous vitamin K does appear to be safe (45). If the INR is very elevated and serious bleeding is present, intravenous vitamin K, 10 mg, is given by slow infusion and is supplemented with fresh frozen plasma or prothrombin complex concentrate, as dictated by the clinical circumstance. Vitamin K is avoided, if at all possible, in patients who have mechanical prosthetic valves in place as rapid normalization of the INR may precipitate valve thrombosis. Following correction of the INR (and management of bleeding), reinstitution of anticoagulation may be begun with heparin infusion; this may require additional time to overcome resistance to warfarin caused by the previously administered vitamin K.

Pregnancy presents a special problem in patients who require warfarin anticoagulation for prosthetic heart valves (46). Warfarin crosses the placenta and may cause fetal wastage, bleeding, and teratogenicity (47,48). Therefore, for women with mechanical heart valves who become pregnant it is suggested that they receive adjusted twice daily dose of LMWH or unfractionated heparin throughout pregnancy. Alternatively, after 12 weeks, warfarin may be restarted (the risk of teratogenicity is reduced) and then replaced again by heparin when the patient is close to delivery. During the times of heparin treatment, anticoagulation can be achieved by using an aggressive adjusted-dose unfractionated subcutaneous heparin protocol (monitoring the activated prothrombin time or the anti-Xa heparin level) or by using a weight-adjusted subcutaneous LMWH protocol (monitoring anti-Xa levels to adjust the dose). Neither form of heparin appears to cross the placenta. With use of this regimen, warfarin treatment is used beginning week 13 and up to the middle of the last trimester. Alternative regimens include the use of subcutaneous unfractionated heparin or LMWH throughout the entire pregnancy. Of note, low-dose aspirin (75 to 100 mg daily) is also recommended for pregnant women with mechanical prosthetic valves (49).

PERICARDITIS AND DELAYED PERICARDIAL TAMPONADE

Postoperative pericardial effusions can occur in any patient who has undergone cardiac surgery, whether the pericardium was left open or closed, even if the pleural spaces were entered during sternotomy. The boundaries of the pericardial space will seal in the first 1 to 2 weeks after surgery; thus, despite what appears to be adequate drainage at the time of operation, the pericardial space can once again become "closed." Serous or serosanguineous effusions can occur from pericarditis. Sometimes, the presence of evolving postoperative pericarditis may be suggested while the patients are still in the hospital by the presence of pain, a pericardial rub, and/or fever. Such patients are treated with a nonsteroidal antiinflammatory agent such as indomethacin. Indomethacin has the potential for renal toxicity, and therefore, the patient's creatinine level should be followed, especially if heart failure is present.

Pericarditis and pericardial effusions may also develop in the weeks after surgery. The presence of a significant pericardial effusion 3 to 4 weeks after surgery is not unusual and late tamponade may occur (49–51). Pericardial effusion also occurs commonly in children following cardiac surgery (52). When seeing the patient postoperatively, the surgeon must be alert to nonspecific complaints such as malaise, slow progress, lack of energy, or sometimes nausea and anorexia. Heart sounds may be muffled on examination. The neck veins may be distended, and paradox may be present when the blood pressure is determined. The QRS voltage of the electrocardiogram may be diminished. Fluid retention and weight gain may occur despite use of diuretics, and the serum creatinine and blood urea nitrogen levels may be elevated. The problem of delayed tamponade appears to be more common in patients who have had valve surgery and who are taking warfarin. The development of an inordinately elevated INR level is a clue to the presence of tamponade. This may occur because of elevated venous pressure and hepatic congestion with resultant increased sensitivity to warfarin. If subacute cardiac tamponade is at all suspected, an urgent echocardiogram is indicated. While echocardiography can readily detect pericardial effusion, the echocardiographic signs of tamponade (such as right ventricular diastolic collapse) do not need to be present in order to have a physiologically significant pericardial effusion.

Management of symptomatic postoperative effusions or tamponade may be either by percutaneous echocardiographically guided catheter drainage or by surgery (53–55). Surgical management usually involves placement of a tube via the subxiphoid approach, the so-called pericardial window or subxiphoid pericardiostomy. For many postoperative patients, this approach may be preferable to catheter drainage due to the presence of adhesions and fluid loculations in the pericardial space that may inhibit successful catheter drainage. Furthermore, the presence of bypass grafts may make the needle approach more dangerous. In the case of recurrent effusions refractory to medical therapy and repeated percutaneous drainage, creation of a true pericardial "window" that drains into the pleural space may be indicated (56). This surgically created pericardial defect allows for drainage of the pericardial fluid into the pleural space where there is more room and surface area for absorption. In very unusual cases, delayed pericardial tamponade may be the result of chylous effusions (57,58). Initial management is conservative with pericardiocentesis, institution of a low-fat or no-fat diet, or, if needed, intravenous hyperalimentation. In refractory cases, surgery, including thoracic duct ligation and pleuropericardial window creation, may be necessary. Once discharged from the hospital after treatment of delayed pericardial effusions, the patient should undergo a follow-up echocardiogram to ensure that the effusion has not recurred.

A late complication of postoperative pericarditis is pericardial constriction (59). In this condition, the heart becomes encased by the thickened, noncompliant pericardium with resultant impaired diastolic filling of the ventricles and venous congestion. The patient presents with fatigue, dyspnea, weight gain, ascites, liver enlargement, and edema. Echocardiography (to demonstrate abnormal ventricular filling), computed tomography (to evaluate pericardial thickness), and cardiac catheterization are used to make the diagnosis (60). Treatment of constrictive pericarditis usually involves partial pericardiectomy, a procedure with significant morbidity and mortality, but long-term relief from symptoms is achieved in most patients (61–63).

References

1. Leon AS, Franklin BA, Costa F, et al. Cardiac rehabilitation and secondary prevention of coronary heart disease: an American Heart Association scientific statement from the Council on Clinical Cardiology (Subcommittee on Exercise, Cardiac Rehabilitation, and Prevention) and the Council on Nutrition, Physical Activity, and Metabolism (Subcommittee on Physical Activity), in collaboration with the American Association of Cardiovascular and Pulmonary Rehabilitation. *Circulation* 2005;111:369–376.

2. Savage PD, Brochu M, Scott P, et al. Low caloric expenditure in cardiac rehabilitation. *Am Heart J* 2000;140:527–533.

3. Myles PS, Hunt JO, Fletcher H, et al. Relation between quality of recovery in hospital and quality of life at 3 months after cardiac surgery. *Anesthesiology* 2001;95:862–867.

4. The Society of Thoracic Surgeons. Patient information: what to expect after heart surgery. http://www.sts.org/sections/patientinformation/adultcardiacsurgery/heartsurgery/.

5. Gibbons RJ, Balady GJ, Bricker JT, et al. ACC/AHA 2002 guideline update for exercise testing: summary article. A report of the American College of Cardiology/American Heart Association Task Force on Practice Guidelines (Committee to Update the 1997 Exercise Testing Guidelines). *J Am Coll Cardiol* 2002;40: 1531–1540. American College of Cardiology Website.

6. Krone RJ, Harrison RM, Chaitman BR, et al. Risk stratification after successful coronary revascularization: the lack of a role for routine exercise testing. *J Am Coll Cardiol* 2001;38:136–142.

7. Barner HB. Operative treatment of coronary atherosclerosis. *Ann Thorac Surg* 2008;85:1473–1482.

8. Parang P, Arora R. Coronary vein graft disease: pathogenesis and prevention. *Can J Cardiol* 2009;25:e57–e62.

9. Tatoulis J, Buxton BF, Fuller JA. Patencies of 2,127 arterial to coronary conduits over 15 years. *Ann Thorac Surg* 2004;77:93–101.

10. Goldman S, Copeland J, Moritz, et al. Starting aspirin therapy after operation: effects on early graft patency. *Circulation* 1991;84:520–526.

11. Dunning J, Versteegh M, Fabbri A, et al. Guideline on antiplatelet and anticoagulation management in cardiac surgery. *Eur J Cardiothorac Surg* 2008;34: 73–92.

12. Ferraris VA, Ferraris SP, Moliterno DJ, et al. The Society of Thoracic Surgeons practice guideline series: aspirin and other antiplatelet agents during operative coronary revascularization (executive summary). *Ann Thorac Surg* 2005;79: 1454–1461.

13. Eagle KA, Guyton RA, Davidoff R, et al. ACC/AHA 2004 guideline update for coronary artery bypass surgery: a report of the American College of Cardiology/American Heart Association Task Force on Practice Guidelines (Committee to Update the 1999 Guidelines for Coronary Artery Bypass Graft Surgery). *Circulation* 2004;110:e340–e437.

14. Becker RG, Meade TW, Berger PB, et al. The primary and secondary prevention of coronary artery disease. American College of Chest Physicians Evidence-Based Clinical Practice Guidelines (8th edition). *Chest* 2008;133:776S–814S.

15. Smith SC, Allen J, Blair SN, et al. AHA/ACC guidelines for secondary prevention for patients with coronary and other atherosclerotic disease: 2006 update. *Circulation* 2006;113:2363–2372.

16. Marso SP. Optimizing the diabetic formulary: beyond aspirin and insulin. *J Am Coll Cardiol* 2002;40:652–661.

17. Gillinov MA, Faber NC, Sabik JF, et al. Endocarditis after mitral valve repair. *Ann Thorac Surg* 2002;73:1813–1816.

18. Pignay-Demaria V, Lesperance F, Demaria RG, et al. Depression and anxiety and outcomes of coronary artery bypass surgery. *Ann Thorac Surg* 2003;75: 314–322.

19. Freedland KE, Skala JA, Carney RM, et al. Treatment of depression after coronary artery bypass surgery: a randomized controlled trial. *Arch Gen Psychiatry* 2009;66:387–396.

20. Mahesh B, Angelini G, Caputo M, et al. Prosthetic valve endocarditis. *Ann Thorac Surg* 2005;80:1151–1158.

21. Wilson W, Taubert KA, Gewitz M, et al. Prevention of infective endocarditis: guidelines from The American Heart Association Rheumatic Fever, Endocarditis, and Kawasaki Disease Committee, Council on Cardiovascular Disease in the Young, and the Council on Clinical Cardiology, Council on Cardiovascular Surgery and Anesthesia, and Quality of Care and Outcomes Research Interdisciplinary Working Group. *Circulation* 2007;116:1736–1754. http://circ.ahajournals. org/cgi/reprint/116/15/1736.

22. Bonow RO, Carabello BA, Chatterjee K, et al. 2008 focused update incorporated into the ACC/AHA 2006 guidelines for the management of patients with valvular heart disease: a report of the American College of Cardiology/American Heart Association Task Force on Practice guidelines. *J Am Coll Cardiol* 2008;52: e1–e142. http://content.onlinejacc.org/cgi/content/full/52/13/e1.

23. Lupinetti FM, Lemmer JH Jr. Emergency aortic valve replacement for endocarditis: comparison of allografts and prosthetic valves. *Am J Cardiol* 1991; 68:637–641.

24. Sabik JF, Lytle BW, Blackstone EH, et al. Aortic root replacement with cryopreserved allograft for prosthetic valve endocarditis. *Ann Thorac Surg* 2002;74: 650–659.

25. Butchart EG, Gohlke-Barwolf C, Antunes MJ, et al. Recommendations for the management of patients after heart valve surgery. *Eur Heart J* 2005;26:2463–2471.

26. Tong AT, Roudaut R, Ozkan M, et al. Transesophageal echocardiography improves risk assessment of thrombolysis of prosthetic valve thrombosis: results of the PRO-TEE registry. *J Am Coll Cardiol* 2004;43:77–84.

27. Rizzoli G, Guglielmi C, Toscano G, et al. Reoperations for acute prosthetic thrombosis and pannus: an assessment of rates, relationship, and risk. *Eur J Cardiothorac Surg* 1999;16:74–80.

28. Latson LA. Transcatheter closure of paraprosthetic valve leaks after surgical mitral and aortic valve replacements. *Expert Rev Cardiovasc Ther* 2009;7:507–514.

29. Mecozzi G, Milano AD, De Carlo M, et al. Intravascular hemolysis in patients with new-generation prosthetic heart valves: a prospective study. *J Thorac Cardiovasc Surg* 2002;123:550–556.

30. Butchart EG, Payne N, Li H-H, et al. Better anticoagulation control improves survival after valve replacement. *Ann Thorac Surg* 2002;123:715–723.

31. McAnulty JH, Rahimtoola SH. Antithrombotic therapy for valvular heart disease. In: O'Rourke RA, Fuster V, Alexander RW, et al., eds. *Hurst's the heart manual of cardiology*. New York: McGraw-Hill, 2001:483–492.

32. Harrison L, Johnston M, Massicotte MP, et al. Comparison of 5-mg and 10-mg loading doses in initiation of warfarin therapy. *Ann Intern Med* 1997;126: 133–136.

33. Ansell J, Hirsh J, Hylek E, et al. Pharmacology and management of the vitamin K antagonists. American College of Chest Physicians Evidence-Based Clinical Practice Guidelines (8th edition). *Chest* 2008;133:160S–198S.

34. Jones HU, Muhlestein JB, Jones KW, et al. Early postoperative use of unfractionated heparin or enoxaparin is associated with increased surgical re-exploration for bleeding. *Ann Thorac Surg* 2005;80:518–522.

35. Hirsh J, Fuster V. Guide to anticoagulant therapy. Part 2. Oral anticoagulants. *Circulation* 1994;89:1469–1480.

36. Salem DN, O'Gara PT, Madias C, et al. Valvular and structural heart disease. American College of Chest Physicians Evidence-Based Clinical Practice Guidelines (8th edition). *Chest* 2008;133:593S–629S.

37. Massel D, Little SH. Risks and benefits of adding anti-platelet therapy to warfarin among patients with prosthetic heart valves: a meta-analysis. *J Am Coll Cardiol* 2001;37: 569–578.

38. Jamieson WRE, Moffatt-Bruce SD, Skarsgard P, et al. Early thrombotic therapy for aortic valve bioprostheses: is there an indication for routine use? *Ann Thorac Surg* 2007;83:549–557.

39. Kulik A, Rubens FD, Wells PS, et al. Early postoperative anticoagulation after mechanical valve replacement: a systematic review. *Ann Thorac Surg* 2006;81: 770–781.

40. Hamad MAS, van Eekelen E, van Agt T, et al. Self-management program improves anticoagulation control and quality of life: a prospective randomized study. *Eur J Cardiothorac Surg* 2009;35:265–269.

41. Eitz T, Schenk S, Fritzsche D, et al. International normalized ratio self-management lowers the risk of thromboembolic events after prosthetic heart valve replacement. *Ann Thorac Surg* 2008;85:949–955.

42. Chan YC, Valenti D, Mansfield AO, et al. Warfarin-induced skin necrosis. *Br J Surg* 2000;87:266–272.

43. Roujeau JC, Stern RS. Severe adverse cutaneous reactions to drugs. *N Engl J Med* 1994;331:1272–1285.

44. Booth SL, Sadowski JA, Pennington JAT. Phylloquinone (vitamin K) content of food in the US Food and Drug Administrations Total Diet Study. *J Agric Food Chem* 1995;43: 1574–1579.

45. Yiu KH, Siu CW, Jim MH, et al. Comparison of the efficacy and safety profiles of intravenous vitamin K and fresh frozen plasma as treatment of warfarin-related over anticoagulation in patients with mechanical heart valves. *Am J Cardiol* 2006;97:409–411.

46. Lee CN, Wu CC, Lin PY, et al. Pregnancy following cardiac prosthetic valve replacement. *Obstet Gynecol* 1994;83:353–356.

47. Vitale N, DeFeo M, DeSanto LS, et al. Dose-dependent fetal complications of warfarin in pregnant women with mechanical heart valves. *J Am Coll Cardiol* 1999;33:1637–1641.

48. Bates SM, Greer IA, Pabinger I, et al. Venous thromboembolism, thrombophilia, antithrombotic therapy and pregnancy. American College of Chest Physicians Evidence-Based Clinical Practice Guidelines (8th edition). *Chest* 2008;133: 844S–886S.

49. Meurin P, Weber H, Renaud N, et al. Evolution of the postoperative pericardial effusion after day 15: the problem of the late tamponade. *Chest* 2004;125: 2282–2287.

50. Kuvin JT, Harati NA, Pandian NG, et al. Postoperative cardiac tamponade in the modern surgical era. *Ann Thorac Surg* 2002;74:1148–1153.

51. Pepi M, Muratori M, Barbier P, et al. Pericardial effusion after cardiac surgery: incidence, site, size and hemodynamic consequences. *Br Heart J* 1994;72: 327–331.
52. Cheung EWY, So SA, Tang KKY, et al. Pericardial effusion after open heart surgery for congenital heart disease. *Heart* 2003;89:780–783.
53. Buchanan CL, Sullivan VV, Lampman R, et al. Pericardiocentesis with extended catheter drainage: an effective therapy. *Ann Thorac Surg* 2003;76: 817–820.
54. Mangi AA, Palacios IF, Torchiana DF. Catheter pericardiocentesis for delayed tamponade after cardiac valve operation. *Ann Thorac Surg* 2002;73:1479–1483.
55. Allen KB, Faber LP, Warren WH, et al. Pericardial effusion: subxiphoid pericardiostomy versus percutaneous catheter drainage. *Ann Thorac Surg* 1999;67: 437–440.
56. O'Brien PKH, Kucharczuk JC, Marshall B, et al. Comparative study of subxiphoid versus video-thoracoscopic pericardial "window." *Ann Thorac Surg* 2005;80:2013–2019.
57. Thomas CS Jr, McGoon DC. Isolated massive chylopericardium following cardiopulmonary bypass. *J Thorac Cardiovasc Surg* 1971;61:945–948.
58. Dib C, Tajik J, Park S, et al. Chylopericardium in adults: a literature review over the past decade (1996–2006). *J Thorac Cardiovasc Surg* 2008;136:650–656.
59. Killian DM, Furiasse JG, Scanlon PJ, et al. Constrictive pericarditis after cardiac surgery. *Am Heart J* 1989;118:563–568.
60. Myers RB, Spodick DH. Constrictive pericarditis: clinical and pathophysiologic characteristics. *Am Heart J* 1999;138:219–232.
61. Maisch B, Seferovic PM, Ristic AD, et al. Guidelines on the diagnosis and management of pericardial diseases: executive summary. The Task Force on the Diagnosis and Management of Pericardial Diseases of the European Society of Cardiology. *Eur Heart J* 2004;25:587–610.
62. Ling LH, Oh JK, Schaff HV, et al. Constrictive pericarditis in the modern era: evolving clinical spectrum and impact on outcome after pericardiectomy. *Circulation* 1999;100:1380–1386.
63. Chowdhury UK, Subramaniam GK, Kumar AS, et al. Pericardiectomy for constrictive pericarditis: a clinical, echocardiographic, and hemodynamic evaluation of two surgical techniques. *Ann Thorac Surg* 2006;81:522–530.

7

Management of Infants and Children

Jeff L. Myers

OVERVIEW

A prompt and accurate anatomic diagnosis is essential for proper surgical management of the patient with congenital heart disease. Clinical presentation, physical examination, and even the chest x-ray and electrocardiogram are informative, but rarely diagnostic. For most patients, echocardiography can elucidate the anatomic basis for proper patient management. When the diagnosis remains unclear, magnetic resonance imaging (MRI), computed tomography (CT), or angiography may be required.

Cardiac catheterization and angiography were once the diagnostic gold standard for congenital lesions. Although very effective for defining anatomy, measuring gradients, and quantifying shunts, cardiac catheterization is associated with increased morbidity when compared with echocardiography. Although it may not define the anatomy of some malformations as well as catheterization, echocardiography is superior to others, and it permits frequent reassessments, including early intra- and postoperative evaluation, and for many lesions, high-quality echocardiography eliminates the need for catheterization (1). Advances in CT and MRI have significantly increased the ability to noninvasively identify even subtle anatomic features such as coronary artery patterns.

Brief Review of Common Lesions

Septal Defects

The most common congenital heart anomaly requiring operative correction is the ventricular septal defect (VSD). Preoperative evaluation is usually accomplished by echocardiography, which can assess the number and location of defects and estimate right ventricular (RV) pressure. Surgery for restrictive lesions may be delayed if there is evidence of a progressive decrease in size. Defects with unrestricted blood flow may produce pulmonary hypertension and should therefore be closed by 3 to 4 months of age. In patients who present late (older than 6 months), cardiac catheterization may be needed to assess the pulmonary vascular resistance (PVR). This is especially true if echocardiographic evidence of increased pulmonary artery pressure exists. While a more complicated postoperative course would be anticipated, patients with pulmonary hypertension are considered operable if the PVR falls in response to vasodilators such as oxygen or inhaled nitric oxide.

Atrial septal defects (ASDs) may be closed by either percutaneous devices or surgical correction. Symptomatic secundum ASDs and patent foramen ovales are now frequently closed by devices. Contraindications to device closure include inadequate margins to seat the device, large defects, and infants who are too small to accommodate the device and delivery system. Ostium primum defects, sinus venosus defects, and unroofed coronary sinus defects are also not appropriate for device closure. Sinus venosus defects can be closed by multiple techniques including a single patch, double patch, or a Warden procedure. The Warden procedure incorporates translocation of the superior vena cava (SVC) to the right atrial (RA) appendage to avoid an incision across the SVC–RA junctions and potential damage to the arterial supply to the sinoatrial node.

Atrioventricular Canal

Echocardiography accurately defines complete atrioventricular (AV) canal defects and gives critical information about AV valve anatomy and function. The size of the two ventricles must be assessed to ascertain that they are "balanced" to permit a biventricular repair. As in the case of VSDs, preoperative catheterization may be useful in evaluating the degree of the patient's PVR, particularly when repair is delayed beyond 4 or 5 months of age. The onset of pulmonary hypertension is particularly early in patients with trisomy 21. In these patients, we sometimes perform cardiac catheterization to define pulmonary hemodynamics, particularly in those older than 6 to 9 months. Postoperative care can be challenging if there is AV valve regurgitation or significant pulmonary hypertension in the postoperative period. These patients are especially prone to having spells of pulmonary vascular hypertensive crises postoperatively. This aspect of postoperative management may be aided by a pulmonary artery catheter placed at the time of surgery, not only for the postoperative measurement of pulmonary artery pressure but also to permit blood sampling to measure pulmonary artery saturation and hence detect any residual shunts. The catheter is placed through the RV infundibulum, through the pulmonary valve, and into the pulmonary artery. Because AV valve function is sometimes an issue after correction, proper postoperative monitoring of left atrial and RA pressures is useful for assessing the mitral and tricuspid valves, respectively.

Partial AV canals are characterized by an ostium primum defect and a cleft anterior mitral leaflet without a VSD component. Physiologically these lesions behave more like ASDs with very little risk of pulmonary hypertension. Repair early in life is still preferred since chronic mitral regurgitation is associated with a less pliable anterior leaflet and the potential for a suboptimal repair.

Tetralogy of Fallot

Patients with tetralogy of Fallot (TOF) may require angiography, particularly to define the anatomy of the pulmonary arteries and coronary arteries. Although much of this information can be ascertained by a high-quality echocardiogram, if there is any doubt as to the size of the branch pulmonary arteries, angiography may be needed. It may also be used to define anomalous coronary arteries crossing the right ventricular outflow tract (RVOT). For most patients with TOF, primary complete repair is performed. In neonates with small pulmonary arteries, a systemic-to-pulmonary shunt may be constructed to the central pulmonary arteries or an RVOT reconstruction may be utilized, leaving the VSD open initially. In this situation, we employ a polytetrafluoroethylene monocusp to provide protection to the right ventricle in the initial postoperative period. Continuity of the RVOT is beneficial because it allows for rehabilitation of hypoplastic branch pulmonary arteries in the catheterization laboratory.

When a complete repair is performed, particular attention is paid to the function of the right ventricle in the postoperative period. Since the repair frequently requires transannular reconstruction of the outflow tract with a ventriculotomy, these patients are at risk for low cardiac output and must be ventilated, carefully monitored, and supported with inotropic agents. Particularly when corrections have been carried out early in the first few months of life, RV dysfunction may be managed by leaving open a patent foramen ovale or fenestrating the VSD patch. Thus, if right heart failure occurs after surgery, elevated right-sided pressure produces a right-to-left shunt that will help maintain cardiac output but with some systemic desaturation. As RV function recovers during the first 3 to 5 days after surgery, this shunt diminishes as RV pressure falls.

Pulmonary Atresia with Ventricular Septal Defect

Pulmonary atresia with VSD may be considered a very severe form of TOF. It is distinct from TOF in that the pulmonary arteries are often abnormal in size with abnormal arborization. The source of pulmonary blood flow is used to classify the defect. Type A is defined having the pulmonary blood flow supplied by the native pulmonary arteries; type B is supplied by a combination of pulmonary arteries and major aortopulmonary collaterals (MAPCAs); and type C is supplied only by MAPCAs. Cardiac catheterization is useful in defining the ventricular anatomy and the size and location of the pulmonary arteries. Prostaglandin E_1 (PGE_1) infusion can be employed in the neonatal period to open the ductus arteriosus. Operation early in life may consist of complete repair or palliation with a shunt and complete correction delayed until the child is larger. Complete repair is usually reserved for patients with central pulmonary arteries with a central area > 50% of normal for the patients' age, the pulmonary arteries must supply at least ten segments (roughly the equivalent of one lung), and if a single pulmonary artery is present, it must be of normal size and reach all segments of that lung. If palliation is required, for patients with atresia limited to the pulmonary valve, the valve may be perforated and dilated in the catheterization laboratory. Patients with more significant atresia may require surgical valvotomy, an outflow tract patch, or a right ventricle-to-pulmonary artery conduit. RV outflow into the central pulmonary arteries can promote arterial growth and allows access to the branch pulmonary arteries for rehabilitation in the catheterization laboratory. In patients with type C anatomy, single or multiple stage unifocalization of the MAPCAs is required as part of the complete repair.

Pulmonary Atresia with Intact Ventricular Septum

Pulmonary atresia with intact ventricular septum (IVS) differs from pulmonary atresia with VSD in that the tricuspid valve is rarely normal and RV development is heterogeneous with some degree of hypoplasia in almost all patients. Ventriculocoronary connections are present in approximately 45% of patients. Almost 10% will have coronary artery stenosis and therefore have an "RV-dependent" coronary circulation. Major aortopulmonary collaterals are rare. PGE_1 is useful in the newborn to stabilize the patient by increasing pulmonary blood flow. If the anatomy is suitable, pulmonary valvotomy is performed both to improve pulmonary perfusion and, it is hoped, to stimulate RV growth. A systemic-to-pulmonary shunt procedure is frequently required as well. Many patients will have severe underdevelopment of the right ventricle and require a univentricular repair via the Fontan pathway.

Transposition of the Great Arteries

Transposition of the great arteries is the commonest cause of cyanosis present in the neonatal period. As soon as the diagnosis is suspected, PGE_1 is begun to improve mixing across the ductus. If mixing remains inadequate, an atrial septostomy (either in the catheterization laboratory or with echocardiography guidance) can be performed. Echocardiography is always performed to confirm the diagnosis and define anatomic detail, including the presence of concomitant lesions and left ventricular outflow tract (LVOT) obstruction, and to define the coronary artery anatomy. In patients with an IVS, the left ventricle rapidly becomes unable to tolerate systemic pressures postoperatively, and an arterial switch operation should therefore be carried out within the first 2 weeks of life. In patients with a VSD, this can be delayed if necessary since the left ventricle remains exposed to systemic pressures throughout the preoperative period and remains "trained" to handle postoperative hemodynamics. The presence of pulmonary stenosis complicates the surgical management since an arterial switch would result in outflow obstruction of the neo-LVOT. The Rastelli operation creates an intracardiac tunnel to produce an initially unobstructed LVOT. However, there is progressive LVOT obstruction and significant long-term mortality. More recently, the Nikaidoh operation (and variants) has been used in an attempt to decrease the incidence of delayed LVOT obstruction and improve long-term survival. This operation consists of translocation of the aortic root posteriorly, creating near normal geometry of the LVOT. Reconstruction of the RVOT is then performed anteriorly, again creating an essentially normal (and unobstructed) arrangement between the right ventricle and pulmonary arteries.

Coarctation of the Aorta and Interrupted Aortic Arch

Coarctation of the aorta varies in its presentation from profound congestive failure and peripheral hypoperfusion in neonates to asymptomatic hypertension in older children. In the critically ill newborn, PGE_1 may palliate severe coarctation until operation is performed, as it opens the ductus and restores distal aortic perfusion from the pulmonary artery. Echocardiography is usually adequate in the neonate to detect the presence of the coarctation and any associated intracardiac defects. Surgical correction may be postponed for a few days in newborns if the PGE_1 is effective in restoring peripheral perfusion. This allows a semielective operation to be done on a stable patient. In older children, operation is done electively, usually to treat hypertension. While no strict guidelines for asymptomatic infants exist, a loss of luminal diameter of 50% should be repaired. Echocardiography-derived gradients are more difficult to use as hard guideline in infants, but a gradient >20 to 30 mm Hg in the absence of peripheral pulses will usually require elective repair. Delay of elective operations may be preferable until 2 to 3 months of age to allow for maturation of the ductal tissue. While preparing in the operating room (OR), we allow topical cooling to a temperature of 35°C for a degree of spinal cord protection. Repair by a simple end-to-end anastomosis is adequate for a discrete coarctation with a relatively normal-sized arch. An extended end-to-end repair with the anastomosis carried onto the underside of the arch to the level of the left common carotid artery is preferred for patients with arch hypoplasia. Despite the method chosen and the adequacy of the repair, recoarctation rates remain between 5% and 10%. These can almost always be successfully treated with balloon dilatation in the cardiac catheterization laboratory. Treatment goals are a gradient <10 mm Hg and no requirement for hypertensive medications.

Interrupted aortic arch results in antegrade perfusion through the aortic valve of structures proximal to the interruption and perfusion through the ductus arteriosus of structures distal to the interruption. The type is defined by the location of the interruption with type A occurring distal to the left subclavian artery, type B between the left subclavian and left carotid arteries, and type C between the left carotid and innominate arteries. Preoperative management is similar to infants with severe coarctation, and circulatory collapse is common in these patients. Operative correction is usually made on bypass through a sternotomy, although type A interruptions can be repaired through a left thoracotomy.

Patent Ductus Arteriosus

Patent ductus arteriosus (PDA) is encountered commonly in premature infants with respiratory distress syndrome. Echocardiography establishes the diagnosis and excludes other significant intracardiac conditions. In the newborn, indomethacin or ibuprofen may be used to attempt closure of the ductus without surgery, but is contraindicated in the presence of renal failure or intracranial bleeding. Operation is also usually performed for severe congestive heart failure requiring inotropic support in which some urgency is present. The operation is usually performed in the neonatal intensive care unit (NICU) with clipping of the PDA to avoid the bleeding risks involved with circumferential dissection and suture ligation. Division is not necessary. In children, operation should be performed electively because of the long-term risk of endocarditis, as well as the risk of developing pulmonary vascular obstructive disease with a large patent ductus. Surgical management should include ligation and division. Alternatively, older children may be treated by percutaneous closure. Controversy exists regarding "silent PDAs" that are picked up incidentally and are both asymptomatic and not associated with a murmur. It is appropriate to monitor these lesions without elective closure.

Aortopulmonary Window

Aortopulmonary window (AP window) is a defect between the aorta and pulmonary artery associated with essentially normal aortic and pulmonary valves (in distinction to truncus arteriosus). The large left-to-right shunt continues to worsen as the PVR falls in the neonatal period and has a presentation similar to a large unrestricted VSD. More than half of AP window patients have associated cardiac anomalies and commonly have associated distal arch obstruction or interrupted aortic arch, which will worsen the left-to-right shunt. Presentation after infancy has a high association with pulmonary hypertension, and Eisenmenger syndrome may develop within the first years of life. Closure of the defect can be performed through the aorta, pulmonary artery, or the AP window itself. Some defects, especially in older patients, may be closed with a percutaneous device. These patients are at risk for pulmonary hypertension postoperatively and should be treated appropriately.

Truncus Arteriosus

Truncus arteriosus is an uncommon defect present in the neonatal period with congestive failure caused by excessive pulmonary blood flow. In place of the aortic and pulmonary valves, a single truncal valve is present. Total correction is generally performed in neonates and certainly by 2 or 3 months of age. The repair is constructed such that the truncal valve is used for left ventricular (LV) outflow. If operation is delayed, pulmonary vascular obstructive disease is likely to develop rapidly, and in this setting, postoperative management may be challenging because of pulmonary hypertension. Truncus with interrupted aortic arch is a particularly difficult lesion with an extremely high morbidity and mortality.

Total Anomalous Pulmonary Venous Connection

The presentation of total anomalous pulmonary venous connection (TAPVC) is dependent on the anatomy and degree of obstruction to venous return. All subtypes (infracardiac, supracardiac, cardiac, and mixed) may present with obstruction and present as a surgical emergency. The severity of the patient's symptoms is directly related to the degree of pulmonary venous obstruction, with severely obstructed pulmonary veins resulting in patient presentation in the newborn period. Operation is performed urgently in all cases of obstructed TAPVC, as there are few temporizing measures. PGE_1 is avoided, as restoration of ductal patency can worsen pulmonary congestion in the presence of obstructed pulmonary veins. Cardiac catheterization is also avoided because of the adverse effects of the hyperosmolar load on the obstructed pulmonary circulation. The most critical element of postoperative care is management of the lungs because of the effects of pulmonary venous obstruction and resulting pulmonary hypertension and lung injury. Invariably, several days of ventilation are required after surgery. Patients with unobstructed TAPVC may be operated upon electively and will behave similar to patients with ASD, with their symptoms determined by the degree of right-to-left shunting.

Aortic Stenosis

Aortic stenosis, depending on its severity, may cause symptoms at any age. Severe stenosis in infancy produces profound congestive failure and acidosis and requires emergency intervention. This extreme form is best managed with prompt echocardiographic diagnosis, followed by a brief period of medical stabilization with ventilation and vasopressor support before percutaneous or operative valvotomy. Milder forms of stenosis may be followed until symptoms occur or until the patient develops a sufficiently severe gradient that makes sudden death a risk. In general lesions with a mean gradient by echocardiography >50 mm Hg, a decrement in LV function, or significant LV dilatation should undergo elective surgical management. Attempts are made at a repair, and an acceptable result may include a degree of residual stenosis or insufficiency as a preferred alternative to placement of an artificial valve. The use of a pulmonary autograft (Ross operation) has unique benefits in this patient population since it will not fail by early calcification and has the potential for significant growth in many patients.

Univentricular Heart

The term univentricular heart encompasses a wide variety of anatomic configurations that share the common feature of having a single functional ventricular chamber. The associated defects and resultant physiology determine the clinical effects, degree of cyanosis, and approach to patient management. Usually, an initial palliative operation is required to increase or decrease pulmonary blood flow, with the aim of eventually carrying out a Fontan type of procedure to put the pulmonary and systemic circulations in series.

Tricuspid Atresia

Tricuspid atresia is a type of univentricular cardiac lesion characterized by the absence of the tricuspid valve and thus absence of the normal connection between the right atrium and right ventricle. The right ventricle is invariably hypoplastic. Associated defects determine the physiologic consequences of tricuspid atresia. Pulmonary blood flow may be increased, decreased, or normal depending on associated anatomic features, and the degree of cyanosis is similarly variable. Most patients have diminished pulmonary blood flow and require treatment with PGE_1 and systemic-to-pulmonary artery shunting in the neonatal period. Eventually, a Fontan operation is performed.

Hypoplastic Left Heart Syndrome

Hypoplastic left heart syndrome (HLHS) results in univentricular physiology based on an anatomic right ventricle associated with unimpeded pulmonary blood flow and systemic blood flow that is ductus dependent. Consequently, upon ductal closure, these infants can present with profound circulatory collapse and severe systemic acidosis. Initial management consists of intubation, PGE_1 to open the ductus arteriosus, inotropic support, bicarbonate administration to correct acidosis, and ventilatory management to limit pulmonary blood flow. With appropriate management, these very ill neonates can be stabilized to permit surgery under controlled and optimized conditions. They are usually treated by the Norwood procedure to produce balanced parallel circulations, followed by staged conversion to a Fontan procedure. The Norwood procedure was first described with a modified Blalock–Taussig (BT) shunt to establish pulmonary blood flow in conjunction with an aortic arch reconstruction that incorporates the pulmonary valve to function as a neoaortic valve. Recently, many centers have replaced the BT shunt with a Sano shunt from the right ventricle to the pulmonary artery, resulting in a decreased perioperative mortality for many surgeons. A new hybrid procedure has been proposed and may allow for palliation of high-risk neonates. This procedure uses a stent in the ductus arteriosus to maintain systemic blood flow and bilateral pulmonary artery bands to regulate pulmonary blood flow. The indications for this procedure continue to evolve. Alternatively, patients with HLHS may receive transplants as their preferred treatment.

PREOPERATIVE PREPARATION

Although patient weight has gradually become less of a predictor, the patient's preoperative condition remains highly associated with outcomes in neonatal corrections. The need for truly emergent operation has become rare because of improvements in diagnosis and management, especially the contributions of PGE_1 and effective resuscitation, which allows for stabilization of most of the anomalies that cause severe circulatory collapse. Laboratory studies usually include blood gases, electrolytes, glucose, calcium, and hematocrit. A specimen for blood crossmatching is obtained as well. Typically, a chest x-ray, electrocardiogram, and echocardiogram are performed as part of the initial diagnostic investigation. Cardiac catheterization is required infrequently but should remain an option in patients in whom the diagnosis or physiologic details remain unclear.

Critically ill neonates are likely to develop profound metabolic acidosis as an early indicator of poor cardiac output. This should be corrected with bicarbonate infusion as the ductus is being opened with PGE_1. Respiratory acidosis should be treated with mechanical ventilation to lower the patient's Pco_2. Intubation may also be necessary if apnea develops as a side effect of PGE_1 and should be routinely performed when transferring patients between hospitals while on PGE_1.

	Lesions Palliated by PGE₁ Infusion

Lesions with inadequate pulmonary blood flow
    Tetralogy of Fallot
    Pulmonary atresia
    Tricuspid atresia

Lesions with inadequate systemic blood flow
    Coarctation
    Interrupted aortic arch
    Critical aortic stenosis
    Hypoplastic left heart syndrome

Lesions with inadequate mixing
    Transposition of the great arteries

PGE_1, prostaglandin E_1.

All babies, particularly premature infants, have difficulty with thermal autoregulation; thus, they are at risk for hypothermia. This can further aggravate hypoperfusion. Radiant warming devices with temperature control servomechanisms permit maintenance of normal body temperature without impeding access to the patient.

Catecholamine and milrinone support may be required in patients with significant myocardial dysfunction during the resuscitation period. In these patients, normalization of pH is of even greater importance since adrenergic inotropic support is not effective in an acidic environment.

Ductus-Dependent Lesions

A considerable number of congenital heart defects that previously required urgent operative treatment in the neonatal period are now palliated by opening the ductus arteriosus and maintaining its patency with PGE_1 (Table 7.1) (2). This may be useful in patients with inadequate pulmonary blood flow (such as those with pulmonary or tricuspid atresia or TOF); inadequate systemic blood flow (such as those with coarctation, critical aortic stenosis, or HLHS); or transposition of the great arteries as well as other less common conditions. PGE_1 is administered intravenously at 0.01 to 0.1 μg/kg per minute. The lowest effective dose is used to prevent side effects, which include hypotension, seizures, fever, and apnea.

OPERATIVE CONSIDERATIONS

Monitoring Lines

Adequate intravenous (IV) access must be ensured to permit safe initiation of the operation; additional transthoracic lines for postoperative use are placed easily during the procedure. Conventional percutaneous catheterization of peripheral lines is usually possible, but cutdowns may be required as well, particularly in neonates. Scalp vein catheters are precarious and should not be relied on for any critical medication or fluid infusion.

Peripheral arterial cannulation is generally accomplished by percutaneous insertion into the radial artery, although cutdown is sometimes required, particularly in the neonate. A right radial catheter is preferred for operations in which the left subclavian or femoral arteries will be occluded or distal to a clamp, resulting in loss of the arterial tracing. A 22-gauge catheter is adequate for small children and most infants, and this can be maintained for several days with proper nursing care. Although 24-gauge catheters may seem easier to insert, they are at higher risk for kinking and becoming nonfunctional; efforts should be made to insert at least a 22-gauge catheter. Percutaneous insertion may be facilitated by the use of a straight, flexible guidewire (0.015 in). Alternatively, if this produces a poor arterial pressure tracing or if blood withdrawal is difficult, a short 22-gauge catheter may be exchanged over a guidewire to a 2.5-Fr catheter inserted up to 2 to 3 cm into the radial artery. This will usually yield better blood withdrawal and improve the phasic arterial pressure tracing. Femoral artery and vein cannulation may be used as an alternative but is less desirable in patients expected to require cardiac catheterization in the future and in whom preservation of femoral access is critical.

Patients undergoing uneventful operation for relatively simple defects generally require no additional catheters beyond those inserted preoperatively. At the conclusion of the more complex operative procedures, we often use a variety of transthoracic lines that permit more accurate hemodynamic monitoring and provide additional access for administration of volume and drugs. An RA catheter can be inserted easily via a pursestring suture in the right atrium, and it is brought out to the surface by a separate stab wound. Similarly, a left atrial catheter may be placed through a pursestring suture in the right superior pulmonary vein (see Fig. 2.4). Meticulous line care is required to minimize the risk of air embolization from left atrial catheters, and their use should be limited to monitoring. All transthoracic lines of this type should be removed before withdrawal of the patient's mediastinal drainage tubes, lest excessive bleeding from the heart lead to tamponade. This should not be done unless blood is available for transfusion and coagulation values are adequate. The complication rate from these lines is far less than 1% (3) and justifies their use in appropriate patients.

Umbilical artery catheters are often helpful in the pre- and postoperative management of neonates (4). Often, the umbilical vessels can provide access for cardiac catheterization, and at the conclusion of catheterization, umbilical artery and vein catheters may be inserted for subsequent intra- and postoperative use (Fig. 7.1). Multiple-lumen

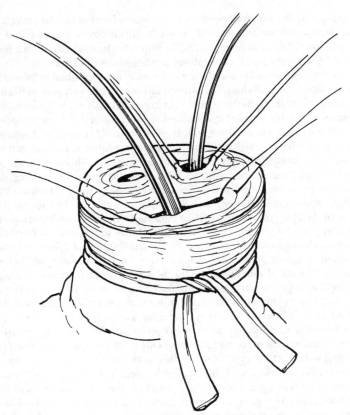

FIGURE 7.1 Insertion of umbilical artery and vein catheters for neonatal monitoring and fluid and drug infusion. After a sterile prep and draping, the umbilicus is amputated to within 5 to 8 mm of the skin line. Two umbilical arteries and an umbilical vein (larger vessel) can be identified in the cross section. Silk traction sutures (3-0 or 4-0) are placed through the edges of the cut vessels as shown, and gentle upward countertraction is exerted. An artery and the vein are then catheterized with a commercially available umbilical vessel catheter. The amount of each catheter one should insert to result in the catheter tip being at the level of the diaphragm can be estimated from the following formulas:

Artery: Inserted length (cm) = 8.5 + [1.6 × shoulder–umbilical length (cm)]
Vein: Inserted length (cm) = 5.0 + [0.6 × shoulder–umbilical length (cm)]

Shoulder–umbilical length is measured on a perpendicular line from the baby's shoulder to a transverse line drawn through the umbilicus. The traction sutures can be tied around each catheter to secure the insertion. To complete the procedure, umbilical tape is tied around the base of the umbilicus at the skin line to ensure a good seal around each catheter. (From Dunn P. Localization of the umbilical catheter by postmortem measurement. *Arch Dis Child* 1966;41:69. Adapted from *The Harriet Lane handbook*. Chicago, IL: Year Book Medical Publishers, 1984.)

catheters may also be used via umbilical access (5). Proper positioning of these lines, preferably below the level of the renal arteries, should be radiologically confirmed. It is desirable to remove umbilical artery lines as soon as possible, as they have been implicated in the development of necrotizing enterocolitis and arterial thrombosis (6), particularly in premature infants. We generally remove them after patients are extubated or other access has been established in the perioperative period. Usually, patients are not fed until they are removed, although this practice varies from institution to institution. Similarly, umbilical venous lines may lead to portal vein thrombosis and should be removed within a few days after insertion, as the risk of this complication increases after 5 or 6 days of use, particularly if the line is used for transfusion (7). These lines are removed by first discontinuing heparinized saline infusion. Beginning with the umbilical venous line, these lines are slowly withdrawn until a small amount of bleeding is noted around each catheter. The catheter is then advanced back in 1 to 2 mm. After approximately 15 minutes, they may be completely withdrawn, as the umbilical vessels will have clotted.

POSTOPERATIVE CARE

Assessment of Cardiovascular Status

The evaluation of the small child or infant after cardiac surgery is a demanding task requiring the utmost vigilance and attention to subtle changes. Unlike the adult patient, cardiac output is not directly measured and must be inferred from the clinical course and supported by laboratory results.

Physical Examination

One of the most important indicators of tissue perfusion in the infant is the distribution of skin temperature. Often, a distinct gradation in skin temperature from abdominal wall, to thigh, to calf, and to foot can be detected as the patient's cardiac output varies. The presence and volume of the peripheral pulses are a good index of cardiac output; inspection of the skin color and capillary refill of the nail beds is also valuable. Particularly in neonates, central fever with a cool periphery is a sign of low cardiac output that requires prompt attention.

Calculated ventilatory tidal volumes based on the patient's body weight may be misleading. Visual examination of the chest and auscultatory examination of the lung fields give important information regarding the adequacy of ventilation and can provide an early warning of impending difficulty. When the patient is mechanically ventilated, chest excursion should be smooth and symmetric, and the lung fields should sound clear. A chest x-ray in response to an abnormal examination may reveal an inappropriate position of the endotracheal tube, important pleural effusions, or significant atelectasis. After extubation, the infant's breathing pattern should remain smooth, and there should be no nasal flaring, intercostal retraction, or use of accessory muscles.

Hepatomegaly is a common sign of congestive failure. The liver edge is easily palpated in most children, and it will rise and fall in response to treatment. Peripheral edema is common after cardiopulmonary bypass and does not always signify failure; however, it is an important indicator of total body fluid and generally signifies a need for diuresis. Serial assessment of the tension of the cranial fontanelles, which are not fused in neonates, provides another method of assessing fluid status.

Auscultation of the heart in the young patient is difficult because of the rapid heart rate and respiratory rate. Nevertheless, it is important for surgeons caring for such patients to familiarize themselves with each patient's particular auscultatory findings to permit identification of changes in heart sounds that may indicate a physiologically important alteration. A new or changing murmur, presence or resolution of a gallop, and appearance of a friction rub should be noted and compared with previous examinations.

Mixed Venous Saturation

Mixed venous oxygen saturation (Svo_2) varies with the patient's oxygen consumption and extraction, hemoglobin concentration, arterial oxygen saturation, and cardiac output. If the first four factors are constant, changes in Svo_2 can be followed as an approximate indicator of cardiac output. In the setting of congenital heart surgery, this assumes that there are no new or residual left-to-right shunts that can falsely elevate Svo_2. We have found it most helpful to rely on fluctuations of Svo_2 over time rather than on an isolated value as the most valuable indicator of cardiac performance (8). Therefore, an Svo_2 should be drawn immediately upon arrival to the intensive care unit (ICU) to establish a baseline. We also have found the Svo_2 to be most helpful when used in conjunction with other parameters such as base deficit and serum lactate. In addition to its use to monitor fluctuations of Svo_2 over time, a sudden rise in saturation with diminution of peripheral perfusion can also signify opening of a left-to-right shunt, such as a residual VSD following VSD or tetralogy repair. In general, patients with good cardiac output and without residual shunts maintain an Svo_2 above 60%.

We have added near-infrared spectrometry (NIRS) to our postoperative assessment of cardiac output. This allows for continuous monitoring of cerebral oxygenation. The measured values are a combination of arterial and venous blood, and a fall in the cerebral NIRS may be altered by a change in hemoglobin, or oxygen delivery, consumption or extraction. If hemoglobin values and oxygen extraction and consumption remain constant, the fall in the cerebral NIRS value may be an early indicator of decreased oxygen delivery and therefore decreased cardiac output (9). A fall in NIRS values can then be confirmed by measurement of serum lactate, base deficit, and Svo_2 coupled with a changing clinical picture.

Treatment of Low Cardiac Output

Hypovolemia occurs commonly after operations for congenital heart defects; bleeding, blood sampling, vasodilation from rewarming, and diuresis all contribute to this. Appropriate infusions of blood, colloid, and crystalloid are administered to correct volume deficits and maintain appropriate oxygen-carrying capacity. Left atrial and/or pulmonary artery catheters are useful in assessing the need for and results of volume replacement. Excessive volume loading can produce deleterious effects, however, and this adverse response to excessive fluid administration is most likely in infants and in more complex cardiac defects (10). As a general rule, infants and young children do not respond favorably to high levels of preload as do adults, and we rarely push the central venous pressure above 10 mm Hg or the left atrial pressure above 15 mm Hg, relying more heavily on catecholamine administration to improve cardiac output.

The general use of pharmacologic agents in the treatment of low cardiac output is discussed in Chapter 3. Dopamine and dobutamine are useful in stimulating the myocardium without causing vasoconstriction at moderate doses. Epinephrine has traditionally been used as a second-line drug when the above agents produce unsatisfactory results. However, recent data has been shown that dopamine has a deleterious effect on the balance between oxygen consumption and delivery that is not seen with epinephrine in patients undergoing the Norwood procedure for HLHS (11). This has pushed epinephrine toward the frontline of adrenergic inotropes for single-ventricle patients and decreased the enthusiasm for dopamine as a first-line drug for the treatment of low cardiac output in many centers. Milrinone can be used in conjunction with adrenergic inotropes to provide a synergistic inotropic effect in addition to decreasing systemic vascular resistance. It is also especially useful in pediatric patients, as it reduces PVR. Occasionally, nitroglycerin, nitroprusside, or PGE_1 is added for systemic afterload reduction. The target systolic arterial blood pressure, of course, is age related, ranging from 50 to 60 mm Hg in the neonates to 80 to 100 mm Hg in the young children.

Tamponade Physiology

Cardiac tamponade represents a life-threatening complication in children as it does in adults. Fluid (usually blood in the immediate postoperative period) collects in the pericardial space preventing diastolic filling. This results in a decrease in stroke volume and cardiac output. The volume of fluid required to produce tamponade in children is, of course, much smaller; therefore, the surgeon must have a lower threshold for reopening the sternum when this occurs. The difficulty lies in making the diagnosis of tamponade, particularly in the absence of intracardiac pressure measurements, which often facilitate the diagnosis in adult patients. Tamponade must be suspected in any child who demonstrates diminished tissue perfusion and elevated venous pressure in the postoperative period without an identifiable cause. The index of suspicion must be particularly high when these findings occur in an otherwise stable child following removal of intracardiac monitoring lines. Tamponade may be heralded by mediastinal drainage tubes that suddenly stop draining or by temporary pacing wires that falter. Although sometimes difficult to accurately measure, new onset of pulsus paradoxus in spontaneously breathing patients should increase the index of suspicion. Echocardiography does not have the sensitivity to rule out tamponade secondary to small accumulations but will often demonstrate large collections that require drainage. Prompt sternal reopening, either in the OR or, if needed, in the ICU is the most effective treatment. Sometimes, exploration is necessary to rule out this diagnosis even when the clinical signs are very "soft" and echocardiography is nondiagnostic.

Infants are especially prone to develop tamponade physiology because of cardiac compression even in the absence of mediastinal blood. A small amount of cardiac edema, swelling of the mediastinal tissues, or elevation of the diaphragm from ascites can produce this syndrome. Leaving the sternum open after surgery may prove lifesaving (12) and does not appear to be associated with complications if closed before 5 to 6 days. Also, we sometimes place a peritoneal dialysis drain at the time of surgery (through the sternotomy incision) to drain ascites and help avoid elevation of the diaphragm. This drain can also be used for early peritoneal dialysis when renal function is impaired in the first few postoperative days. Some have advocated continuous fluid removal early after surgery in critically ill infants as a means of alleviating the consequences of edema. This may be achieved by continuous ultrafiltration or early dialysis (13,14). Late tamponade due to pericardial effusion can occur following operations for congenital heart disease and, in some patients, can be life threatening (15,16). Prior to hospital discharge and at the first postoperative office visit, the neck veins should be examined and the patient should be checked for pulsus paradox.

Aspirin (16) or steroids (17) may be useful for the treatment of postoperative pericardial effusions in this setting.

Residual Lesions

Residual lesions include those anatomic abnormalities that are not repaired at operation because of technical difficulty, unacceptable risk, or incomplete diagnosis and those that are deliberately left uncorrected for physiologic reasons. Typical examples include ASD or VSD that are incompletely closed owing to technical error, resulting in excessive pulmonary blood flow. Other residua include a persistent gradient across a coarctation repair or persistent valvular stenosis after aortic or pulmonary valvotomy. Knowledge of residual lesions obtained by postoperative monitoring or echocardiography can guide the timing of late postoperative restudy (18).

Treatment of these conditions must be individualized according to the patient's symptoms, physical findings, and results of invasive and noninvasive studies. Residual lesions must be considered after operation if the patient has a worse-than-expected clinical course. If a patient is not progressing after surgery as expected, the adequacy of repair and the presence of residual lesions must be determined. Echocardiography is an essential first step in this process. If necessary, cardiac catheterization may be required. If a poor clinical course leads to restudy, and a significant residual lesion is found, it can be corrected either in the catheterization laboratory or by reoperation.

As mentioned above, sometimes defects are deliberately left unrepaired or incompletely repaired. An example is the incomplete closure of an ASD or VSD to allow right-to-left shunting when RV function is impaired (19) or a fenestration in patients after a Fontan procedure (20). Leaving residual right-to-left shunts in such situations has decreased the morbidity and mortality for right-sided failure sometimes observed following these types of operations.

Pulmonary Management

Pulmonary care in the young patient usually begins in the OR with intubation. Although practices vary from institution to institution, if intubation is anticipated to be of short duration (intraoperative or early postoperative extubation), it may be done via the oral route, using an appropriately sized uncuffed tube (Table 7.2). The endotracheal tube is of the appropriate size if it maintains a good seal up to 25 to 30 cm H_2O airway pressure but "leaks" at higher airway pressures. Cuffed tubes are now available in pediatric sizes and are frequently used even in neonatal patients. The connections between the endotracheal tube and the

TABLE 7.2	Endotracheal Tube (ETT) Size and Intubation Guidelines

Age	Internal Diameter (mm)[a]
Premature infant[b]	2.5–3.0[c]
Term infant[b]	3.0–3.5
3 mo–1 yr	4.0
1–2 yr	4.5
2–15 yr	$\dfrac{16 + \text{age (years)}}{4}$

[a]If no leak is present at airway pressures >30 cm H_2O, change to the next smaller tube.
[b]The head should not be extended for placement of the ETT in newborns due to anatomic differences compared with older patients.
[c]Most premature neonates can accept a 3.0 ETT. 2.5 ETTs have increased airway resistance and are difficult to suction adequately.
Adapted from *The Harriet Lane Handbook*. Chicago, IL: Year Book Medical Publishers, 1984.

ventilator must be flexible enough to permit motion of the patient's head without moving the tube within the trachea. Failure to make provision for this may lead to unplanned tube removal or trauma to the airway. It is essential that patients requiring mechanical ventilation be provided with sufficient analgesia and sedation to prevent vigorous movements. Particularly in patients with postoperative pulmonary hypertension, high-dose sedation with narcotics such as fentanyl (at least 10 μg/kg per hour) or morphine (0.1 mg/kg per hour) combined with pharmacologic paralysis (vecuronium 0.1 mg/kg per hour) is usually necessary for the appropriate ventilatory control of the pulmonary circulation.

Maintenance of endotracheal tube patency is critical. In particular, small-caliber endotracheal tubes such as 3- or 3.5-mm tubes are prone to plugging at their distal tip with dried secretions. Particularly if surgery involved pulmonary artery branch mobilization, small amounts of blood may be present initially in the airway secretions and can contribute to plugging. Maintenance of tube patency requires routine irrigation and suctioning if blood is present. Irrigation with alkalinized saline may help mobilize secretions adherent to the endotracheal tube. Unexplained increases in P_{CO_2} in patients on pressure-cycled ventilators or unexplained increases in peak airway pressure in patients on volume-cycled ventilators should raise suspicion of partial endotracheal tube obstruction. Hand ventilation will sometimes help detect tube obstruction. If there is uncertainty, changing the endotracheal tube will resolve this important issue.

The postoperative care of children following cardiac surgery, particularly the care of the neonate, involves very close attention to respiratory care and ventilatory management (21,22). Atelectasis should be prevented by ensuring adequate tidal volume and providing appropriate chest physiotherapy. Endotracheal suctioning is important, but it must be used with great caution in the hemodynamically precarious patient. Vigorous airway suctioning can produce alveolar derecruitment or induce pulmonary hypertensive crises resulting in hypoxia, pulmonary vascular spasm, and cardiovascular collapse (23). To prevent pulmonary hypertensive crisis, premedication with additional narcotic plus manual hyperventilation with 100% oxygen may be needed before suctioning is performed. Even when appropriately performed, suctioning may not succeed in removing a mucous plug or clot that is acting as a "ball valve" on the tip of the tube.

Formerly, the only mechanical ventilators used for pediatric patients were of the pressure-cycled type. These ventilators deliver gas until a given pressure is reached, followed by an expiratory phase. In neonates after cardiopulmonary bypass, inspiratory pressures of 15 to 20 cm H_2O are commonly required. Positive end-expiratory pressure (PEEP) of 3 to 5 cm H_2O is used to prevent alveolar collapse and improve functional residual capacity. The ventilatory rate typically is 15 to 20 per minute. In uncomplicated patients, we generally employ the intermittent mandatory ventilation mode because this allows the patient to establish his or her own breathing pattern. The inspiratory/expiratory ratio (I/E) is usually 1:2.

Volume-cycled ventilators use a similar ventilatory rate, PEEP, and I/E ratio. The tidal volume is about 12 to 15 mL/kg. The inspiratory pressures must be monitored and limits set to guard against barotrauma. High-frequency jet ventilation, although not in common use in postoperative cardiac infants, may be of value in selected cases of severe pulmonary failure, acute respiratory distress syndrome, refractory pulmonary hypertension, or after a Fontan procedure (24). More recently, we have employed pressure-regulated volume control modes. The decelerating inspiratory flow pattern automatically adjusts the inspiratory pressure for changes in compliance and resistance resulting in a guaranteed tidal volume at the lowest possible pressure (22).

The fractional inspired oxygen (FIO_2) is reduced as rapidly as possible to prevent both complications specific to newborns (Table 7.3) and the acute lung injury associated with hyperoxic ventilation in all patients.

TABLE 7.3	Potential Complications of Ventilating Neonates with High Concentrations of Oxygen

Retrolental fibroplasias
Excessive pulmonary blood flow in patients with left-to-right shunts
Increased pulmonary congestion in the presence of obstructed total anomalous pulmonary venous drainage

Ideally, the FIO_2 is reduced below 0.40. It is more important to individualize this in pediatric patients than in adults because of the unique physiologic requirements imposed by some of their cardiac anomalies.

Pulmonary Hypertension

Pulmonary hypertension is typically encountered in patients with large left-to-right shunts and those with left-sided obstructive lesions such as mitral stenosis, cor triatriatum, and obstructed total anomalous pulmonary venous return. If left untreated for significant periods of time, PA pressure may rise to systemic levels or higher and become irreversible (Eisenmenger syndrome); these patients are inoperable. One of the tasks of preoperative catheterization is to separate those patients with fixed elevation of PVR from those in whom the PVR falls to operable levels in response to oxygen and/or inhaled nitric oxide. Some of these latter borderline-operable patients will, thus, be operated on, and they demand great attention postoperatively.

The most important component of the treatment of postoperative pulmonary hypertension is proper ventilatory management. Since oxygen is a powerful vasodilator, the FIO_2 is kept high, and hypercarbia and acidosis are avoided; a degree of respiratory alkalosis also helps to lower pulmonary artery pressure. The patient should receive adequate sedation and paralysis to prevent voluntary resistance to ventilation and precipitation of pulmonary hypertensive crisis. These measures are often sufficient to maintain maximum pulmonary vasodilatation. Vigorous hand ventilation of the patient with 100% oxygen can alleviate episodes of pulmonary vascular spasm that appear periodically and may be lifesaving. IV vasodilators such as nitroglycerin and nitroprusside or PGE_1 may also be used but are limited by systemic hypotension. Milrinone is another valuable agent for lowering pulmonary artery resistance, and its positive inotropic effect may provide additional benefits.

Inhaled nitric oxide has been used with good results to treat postoperative pulmonary hypertension as it appears to be a truly selective, potent pulmonary vasodilator (25). Since its approval for clinical use, nitric oxide has become a first-line treatment for significant pulmonary hypertension at many institutions. It is administered by a special ventilator apparatus in doses ranging from 1 to 80 ppm. Data suggest that most patients respond to doses in the range of 5 to 40 ppm, and keeping the dose under 40 ppm minimizes potential complications such as alveolar injury, nitrogen dioxide generation, and methemoglobin formation (26). Withdrawal of nitric oxide therapy must be done gradually and with monitoring of clinical status because of the potential for rebound pulmonary hypertension (27). Oral sildenafil is effective in transitioning patients with significant rebound from inhaled nitric oxide.

Parallel Circulations and Control of the Pulmonary Circulation

One of the most challenging problems for postoperative management in congenital heart surgery is the care of patients with parallel circulations. Parallel circulations are encountered after palliation of any single-ventricle lesion, such as after the Norwood operation for HLHS or after creation of a systemic-to-pulmonary shunt in complex lesions. In these patients, the systemic saturation achieved depends on the relative amounts of pulmonary and systemic blood flow, which is expressed as the ratio $\dot{Q}_p/\dot{Q}_s$. Figure 7.2 shows an example of the systemic saturation achieved as a function of $\dot{Q}_p/\dot{Q}_s$, assuming a completely mixed circulation such as that encountered in single-ventricle physiology and, for the purpose of illustration, assuming a systemic saturation of 50%. Note that 100% saturation is approached asymptotically so that very high ratios of $\dot{Q}_p/\dot{Q}_s$ are required to achieve high levels of systemic saturation. It is important to note that increasing systemic saturation is obtained not only by increasing pulmonary blood flow but also by decreasing systemic flow. This has particularly important implications in the management of the neonate. *In utero*, there is relatively little pulmonary blood flow. As a result, a fetus with single-ventricle physiology needs only to pump to the systemic circulation plus the blood flow to the placenta. The neonatal single ventricle has therefore not accommodated

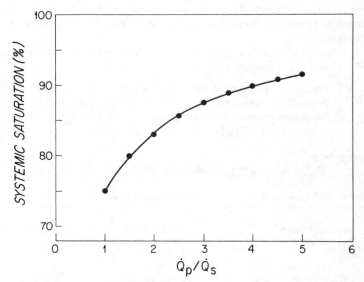

FIGURE 7.2 Illustration of systemic saturation achieved as a function of the pulmonary-to-systemic flow ratio ($\dot{Q}_p/\dot{Q}_s$). Note that 100% saturation is approached asymptotically.

to pumping large volume loads such as may be the case in parallel circulations. Furthermore, there is evidence to suggest that single ventricles with RV morphology may be less efficient than single ventricles with LV morphology, the former situation encountered in the HLHS. In these neonates, a higher systemic saturation may signify not only increasing $\dot{Q}_p$ but also decreasing $\dot{Q}_S$. Thus, neonates with single-ventricle physiology are capable of being well saturated but having a consequent low output state and acidosis. In essence, whatever blood flow goes through the lungs does not necessarily go through the systemic circulation and vice versa.

Central to managing these neonates is the control of pulmonary blood flow so as to maintain adequate systemic perfusion while having adequate saturation for oxygen transport. With time, the neonatal single ventricle adapts to increasing volume load and meets the demands of the systemic circulation while providing substantial amounts of pulmonary blood flow. However, early after such operations as the Norwood procedure, it may be particularly challenging to maintain adequate systemic perfusion. This issue is further complicated by the fact that early after creation of a surgically placed systemic-to-pulmonary shunt, it is desirable to maintain systemic output and pressure to help maintain shunt patency and coronary flow.

A key management strategy for "balancing" the systemic and pulmonary circulations in these neonates is through careful postoperative ventilatory management, usually aimed initially at restricting pulmonary blood flow.

There are three key ventilatory parameters that have important effects on the pulmonary circulation (see Table 7.4):

1. **F$_{IO_2}$**. Particularly in the neonate, the pulmonary circulation will respond to increasing concentrations of inspired oxygen by vasodilation; conversely, decreasing inspired oxygen concentrations down to room air will result in some pulmonary vasoconstriction.

TABLE 7.4	Control of Pulmonary Blood Flow
Factors That Increase $\dot{Q}_p$	**Factors That Decrease $\dot{Q}_p$**
↑ F$_{IO_2}$	↓ F$_{IO_2}$
Alkalosis; Hypocarbia	Acidosis; Normocarbia or mild hypercarbia
Mean airway pressure	Mean airway pressure
↓ PEEP	↑ PEEP
↓ I/E ratio	↑ I/E ratio
↓ Tidal volume	↑ Tidal volume

F$_{IO_2}$, fractional inspired oxygen; I/E ratio, inspiratory/expiratory ratio; PEEP, positive end-expiratory pressure; $\dot{Q}_p$, pulmonary blood flow.

In extreme circumstances, FIO_2 may be decreased to 0.17 to 0.18 by blending in nitrogen to achieve control of excessive pulmonary blood flow.

2. **pH and carbon dioxide.** Respiratory alkalosis and hypocarbia may produce pulmonary vasodilation (28), and conversely, normocarbia and normal pH may produce some increase in PVR.

3. **Airway pressure.** By direct mechanical effect, increasing airway pressure also opposes pulmonary blood flow. The airway pressure can be varied in two ways. PEEP can be added or removed to increase or decrease the mean airway pressure. Pulmonary blood flow may also be decreased by increasing the relative amount of time the ventilator spends in inspiration versus expiration (I/E ratio). A similar effect to increasing the mean airway pressure (and hence decrease pulmonary blood flow) can be achieved by using very large tidal volumes (20 to 25 mL/kg); however, inspired CO_2 (1% to 4%) must be added to normalize PCO_2 (29).

To illustrate, after the Norwood procedure for first-stage palliation of HLHS, it is sometimes necessary to limit pulmonary blood flow. The single ventricle with RV morphology requires time to accommodate pumping to parallel circulations, and in these neonates, excessive systemic saturation is common and is usually accompanied by poor systemic perfusion and acidosis. Thus, these infants are frequently ventilated immediately after surgery with room air. The ventilatory rate and total volume are adjusted, so that normocarbia results and hyperventilation is avoided. PEEP may be added up to 5 to 7 cm H_2O, and a relatively long inspiratory time is selected, so that the I/E ratio is 1:2 to 1:3. Cardiac performance is then maximized by ensuring optimal filling pressures and by the use of inotropic agents. In general, achieving precise control of ventilatory parameters early after surgery usually requires continuous narcotic sedation and pharmacologic paralysis. Oxygen-carrying capacity is optimized by raising the hematocrit level to about 40%. Finally, the systemic vascular resistance may be actively lowered by the use of α-adrenergic antagonists such as phenoxybenzamine. The use of α-antagonists is now routine in many programs after stage I palliation.

In contrast, patients who have undergone a Fontan procedure must have PVR minimized (30). These patients are ventilated after surgery with little or no PEEP and with short inspiratory times; atelectasis may be minimized by the use of intermittent ventilatory sighs or by intermittent hand ventilation. Hypoxia is assiduously avoided. In-series circulations after a Fontan procedure function best with spontaneous ventilation (31), and accordingly, efforts should be made to extubate these patients as early as possible after operation.

Extubation of the postoperative patient requires hemodynamic stability, freedom from severe edema, smooth respiratory motion of the chest wall with spontaneous breathing, and acceptable blood gases. Most patients are extubated after a short period of time. We do not think infants should have the additional stress of a continuous positive airway pressure trial, because this requires a great deal of effort as the baby attempts to overcome the combined resistance of continuous positive airway pressure and a small-caliber endotracheal tube. Airway edema and consequent obstruction may be more of a problem following prolonged intubation or in babies who have been very active prior to extubation and more likely to have tube-related airway trauma. The IV administration of dexamethasone (0.5 mg/kg) several hours before and after tube removal in infants assists in reducing airway edema and may help to prevent reintubation. Racemic epinephrine inhalation (2.25%, 1 mL in 5 mL of saline) also helps control postextubation stridor due to upper airway edema. In addition to airway edema, intraoperative phrenic nerve injury and the resulting diaphragmatic paralysis may also result in acute respiratory failure following extubation.

Tracheostomy may be required in the care of some infants who cannot be separated from the ventilator after several weeks. It often seems that tracheostomy, by providing a shorter airway pathway and permitting easier suctioning for removal of secretions, permits weaning from the ventilator in a short time. Meticulous surgical technique is required for this procedure. Injury to the cricoid cartilage must be avoided to prevent subglottic stenosis, the proper size tube should be inserted, and the device must be secured in place to avoid trauma to the skin and trachea. No one except the responsible surgical team should attempt removal or repositioning of the tube for the first 5 to 7 days; after that time, the tube can be removed easily for cleaning and reinserted. We have also performed a cricoid split for failure to extubate in a select group of patients; specifically patients with trisomy 21 with associated subglottic airway compromise (32).

Cardiac Rhythm Management

Arrhythmias can occur frequently following correction of congenital cardiac defects in children and include a wide range of brady- and tachyarrhythmias, with an overall incidence approaching 50% (33). Some arrhythmias may be related anatomically to surgery, such as heart block following VSD closure or tachyarrhythmias following procedures involving extensive suture lines in the atria, like Fontan procedures or atrial switch procedures for transposition.

As in the case of adult patients, bradyarrhythmias are managed by pacing. Pacing electrodes may be placed on the atria and ventricles, and smaller-caliber electrodes are available for use in pediatric patients.

Despite smaller cardiac dimensions, efforts should be made to avoid unipolar pacing because of higher thresholds and lower reliability. In particular, atrial pacing electrodes should be sufficiently far apart to yield an adequate signal for atrial sensing to permit DDD pacing. The RA free wall near the AV groove and the cephalic atrial wall between the atrial appendages produce optimum temporary pacing wire properties in pediatric patients (34). We have employed bipolar pacing leads (Model 6495, Medtronic, Inc., Minneapolis, MN) in smaller children with the intention of decreasing the number of sutures required to affix the leads to the atrium and ventricle and potentially the risk of bleeding with removal. All pacing leads should be tested for appropriate sensing and pacing prior to leaving the OR and confirmed upon arrival to the ICU.

Among the tachyarrhythmias occurring after pediatric cardiac surgery, junctional ectopic tachycardia (JET) can produce substantial morbidity because of its effect on overall cardiac performance. It should be aggressively treated. This tachyarrhythmia appears as a regular rhythm at a rate that can vary between 150 and 250 beats per minute. Although P-wave activity may be difficult to recognize during JET, this rhythm is characterized by AV dissociation (35). An atrial electrogram using the atrial pacing leads is particularly helpful in the diagnosis. JET is managed by first ensuring that sympathetic tone is minimized. Adequate sedation should be ensured, and doses of catecholamine inotropic agents should be minimized. Pancuronium exerts a vagolytic action, and if it is being used for muscle relaxation, it should be switched to another agent. Systemic cooling to approximately 34°C may be of value in small infants, and if topical cooling is used, adequate muscle relaxation should be used to block shivering. Cooling of the ventilator gases will help in cooling the patient.

Increasingly, amiodarone is being used to control JET, as well as other tachyarrhythmias that may be poorly tolerated. In the postoperative setting, if simple measures such as cooling and minimizing adrenergic drug infusions are ineffective in controlling JET, IV amiodarone loading and maintenance infusion should be instituted if the arrhythmia is poorly tolerated, as manifested by evidence of low cardiac output (36,37). We also will frequently give the loading dose in the OR if significant arrhythmias occur during separation from bypass. If hemodynamic instability is encountered, the patient can be briefly supported by reinstituting bypass.

Fluids, Electrolytes, and Nutrition

Routine Fluid and Electrolyte Management

Postoperatively, intelligent fluid administration requires careful consideration of the patient's cardiac output, systemic and pulmonary pressures, filling pressures, urine output, and blood loss. In the immediate postoperative period, our initial plan of volume replacement dictates infusion of red blood cells and/or plasma equal in volume to that lost via mediastinal drainage and blood sampling on an hour-by-hour basis. The volume expander chosen is dictated by the desired hematocrit level: normal in acyanotic patients and elevated in cyanotic patients.

Usual full maintenance fluid requirements in a child are 100 mL/kg per day for the first 10 kg of body weight, plus 50 mL/kg per day for the second 10 kg, plus 20 mL/kg per day for weight more than 20 kg. In patients after cardiopulmonary bypass, this calculated volume is reduced by half because of the tendency for these patients to retain large volumes of excess water. Dextrose, 5% in water ($\pm$0.2 N saline), with 20 mEq/L of potassium chloride added on day 2, is generally used for maintenance fluids.

Further alterations in volume and composition of intravenously administered fluids depend on the clinical situation and measurements of hematocrit, electrolytes, and blood gases. It must be recalled that hyponatremia is almost always dilutional and requires fluid restriction, although small infants may require some sodium administration. Fluid restriction may be difficult because of the large number of IV lines that are at risk of occlusion if flow rates are low. Syringe infusion pumps with digital control are the most reliable devices for precise administration of small volumes of fluid as well as critical medications. For most arterial and central venous lines, at least 1.5 to 2.0 mL per hour is required to maintain patency. Arterial lines should receive saline or 0.5 N saline without dextrose; other lines should receive 5% or 10% dextrose. Heparin is usually added (1 U/mL) but must be discontinued in any patient suspected of having heparin-induced thrombocytopenia.

Nutritional Management

The typical child who undergoes an uneventful open heart surgery should be able to begin clear liquids by mouth a short time (6 hours) after the endotracheal tube is removed. If liquids are well tolerated, a regular diet for age may be resumed later that day. Postoperative ileus is unusual in most pediatric cardiac patients, and there is no reason to withhold nourishment. One exception to this rule is the patient undergoing repair of coarctation (below). Most neonates may similarly begin sugar solution after extubation, with a rapid progression to breast milk or formula.

The more critically ill infant poses a more difficult problem in nutritional management, and a need for prolonged ventilation makes normal feeding impossible. Whenever possible, we prefer to use the patient's gastrointestinal tract as a route for alimentation. Feedings are started via an orogastric tube with 5% dextrose or balanced electrolyte solution (e.g., Pedialyte®) with frequent residuals measured to guard against gastric dilatation. Formula may then be initiated at increasing volumes and concentrations until the infant is receiving 120 to 140 kcal/kg per day. If additional volume must be administered to reach this nutritional intake, diuretics may be needed. Diarrhea or stools positive for reducing substances require discontinuation of the feedings, followed by resumption at a slightly lower rate or concentration. Intolerance to formula mandates formula changes. It is not necessary to hold enteral feeds in patients requiring adrenergic support, especially trophic feeds that may prevent gut translocation of bacteria (38).

IV hyperalimentation may be needed if the gastrointestinal tract is not usable. Central administration is preferable, as higher solute concentrations can be given with less volume. Lipids are added to increase the calorie intake.

Glucose

Glucose homeostasis is frequently deranged in infants with severe congenital heart defects. This derangement may be most severe when circulatory arrest is employed (39). Hyperglycemia is particularly common in the postoperative period, and this may lead to osmotic diuresis, dehydration, and increase in serum osmolarity, which may lead to cerebral hemorrhage. Plasma glucose values above 200 mg/dL may not need to be treated beyond reducing the rate or concentration of dextrose-containing IV solutions. Glucose levels above 250 mg/dL require the IV administration of regular insulin, 0.1 to 0.2 U/kg, every 6 to 12 hours until glucose levels stabilize. Standing orders for "sliding scale" insulin should never be used in infants because of the risk of dangerous hypoglycemia. Hypoglycemia must be prevented by frequent monitoring of glucose levels in patients receiving insulin, and dextrose infusions should be administered if the levels fall below 100 mg/dL. The small glycogen stores in neonates and limited capacity for gluconeogenesis make hypoglycemia the greater danger. Neonates may not manifest any clinical evidence of hypoglycemia until serum glucose levels fall below 30 mg/dL, at which point the patient is at risk for cerebral insult. This is completely preventable in most cases by using maintenance solutions containing 10% dextrose and by estimating blood glucose frequently using bedside monitoring. When plasma glucose levels fall below 50 mg/dL despite these precautions, the patient should receive small dextrose-containing fluid boluses through a secure central venous catheter, and the concentration of dextrose in the maintenance solutions should be increased to $\geq$10%.

Calcium

Hypocalcemia most commonly occurs in neonates and may cause irritability, seizures, and abnormalities of cardiac rhythm. The immature neonatal myocardium does not concentrate calcium efficiently and is dependent on higher levels of extracellular calcium. Therefore, measurement of ionized, not total, calcium is critical and is the best guide to calcium replacement. Replacement may be particularly necessary when blood products have been administered. Calcium supplementation can be provided as a 10% calcium gluconate infusion and should be infused slowly 1 to 2 mL/kg at a time preferably through a central venous line. Particularly in neonates, hypocalcemia may be recurrent, especially if the DiGeorge syndrome is present; in this circumstance, it can be added to the maintenance solutions (calcium gluconate, 2 g/L).

Hypomagnesemia may coexist very rarely with hypocalcemia, and it should be suspected when symptomatic hypocalcemia does not respond to calcium infusion alone (40). Although laboratory measurements of serum magnesium levels are, at best, an uncertain indicator of total body magnesium, levels below 1.4 mEq/L are abnormal and mandate parenteral replacement.

Potassium

Hypokalemia is most commonly due to urinary losses and administration of bicarbonate ion. Unlike adult cardiac patients, who are often very sensitive to hypokalemia, children rarely develop ventricular irritability because of moderately low serum potassium levels. Unless the potassium falls below 3.0 mEq/L, additional potassium supplementation is usually unnecessary. Enteral administration of potassium is preferred to IV administration if the gastrointestinal route is available and the deficit is modest. Intravenously administered potassium chloride requires a central venous catheter and should be given slowly at a dose of 0.1 to 0.2 mEq/kg over 20 to 30 minutes, followed by redetermination of the potassium level.

More dangerous is significant hyperkalemia, which most commonly occurs because of renal failure and metabolic acidosis. Elevated serum potassium levels lead to progressive electrical instability of the heart and eventually to cardiac arrest. Hyperkalemia may be palliated temporarily by the administration of calcium, bicarbonate, and/or glucose and insulin. These measures, however, only shift the potassium to the intracellular compartment. Removal of potassium is best accomplished with vigorous diuresis, if possible, or the use of ion exchange resins (Kayexalate) as enemas. Kayexalate is prepared as a slurry (1 g/mL of sorbitol solution), and it is administered through an indwelling rectal tube. Dialysis is not an efficient method of rapid potassium removal but may be used to stabilize the serum concentration while other measures take effect.

Special Problems

Coagulation Disorders and Transfusion

Younger patients are at greater risk than adults for capillary leak and excessive peripheral edema after cardiopulmonary bypass. As extreme anemia and dilution of serum oncotic pressure encourage edema formation, we usually use a blood prime in our bypass circuit in infants and small children. We also add steroids in an effort to minimize the inflammatory component of cardiopulmonary bypass.

Patients with congenital heart defects are more likely than most individuals to have abnormal preoperative coagulation tests (41). This is particularly evident in cyanotic patients. In most respects, replacement of blood products in the pediatric patient undergoing cardiac operation follows the same principles used for adults. Some cardiac surgeons believe that there is a beneficial effect of transfusing fresh whole blood in achieving hemostasis immediately after open heart surgeries and that this benefit surpasses that of component therapy. There is some objective evidence to support this belief (42), but it is often impractical in practice owing to the time required to perform screening serologic tests. It is useful to remove as much free water as possible by hemofiltration while on bypass to "make room" for fresh frozen plasma and platelet transfusions in these patients. Alternately, modified ultrafiltration can be employed after discontinuation of bypass either in addition to, or instead of, conventional hemofiltration.

Paradoxical Hypertension After Coarctation Repair

Despite technically adequate surgical correction of aortic coarctation, severe hypertension in the early postoperative period occurs in 37% to 63% of patients (43). Proposed mechanisms of this hypertension include elevated sympathetic activity (44,45) and elevated renin (46). It is interesting to note that paradoxical hypertension does not occur after balloon dilatation of the coarctation (47). Postoperative hypertension is less of a problem in neonatal coarctation repair.

Preoperative treatment with β-blockers effectively prevents this paradoxical hypertension (48). The patient begins atenolol (1 mg/kg per day) orally, starting 2 weeks before operation. When hypertension does occur after coarctation repair, we prefer to treat it as we would other forms of systemic hypertension, with nitroprusside infusion beginning at 0.5 μg/kg per minute and increasing as needed in addition to achieve IV β-blockade. Alternatively, if hypertension is not easily controlled, IV esmolol (49) or labetalol (50) can be used. We restart atenolol when oral intake has begun for additional pressure control and to assist in weaning nitroprusside. Particularly in older patients, persistent hypertension may be a significant problem. In these patients, high-dose β-blockade combined with potent antihypertensives such as angiotensin-converting enzyme inhibitors or calcium channel blocking agents may be needed.

Blood pressure control in these patients is important to prevent the complication of mesenteric arteritis, which commonly followed coarctation repair in past years. In these patients, who were generally older than the patients operated on now, hypertension occurred "paradoxically" after several days. Mesenteric arteritis may result in intestinal necrosis. For this reason, we do not permit oral intake after coarctation repair until the abdomen is soft and bowel sounds are vigorous.

Temperature Regulation

Neonates do not effectively regulate their body temperature because of their relatively large surface area, limited subcutaneous fat, and inability to generate heat by shivering. This is part of the rationale for ligation of PDAs in the NICU to prevent hypothermia during transport. Use of radiant warming devices prevents hypothermia in these patients while permitting access for necessary care. Automatic radiant heaters incorporate skin temperature probes to regulate warming by using skin temperature in a servomechanism feedback system. Either elevation or depression of body temperature may be a sign of infection.

Effects of Profound Hypothermia and Circulatory Arrest

Neurologic issues in pediatric cardiac surgery are the most devastating and most feared complications. Although the neurologic risk of surgery to correct relatively simple defects is very low, studies have shown that operations for very complex lesions, particularly single-ventricle lesions, and operations done using prolonged circulatory arrest are associated with greater decrements in neurocognitive function (51). In the extreme, operations for complex congenital cardiac defects, particularly those requiring prolonged hypothermic circulatory arrest, can produce devastating neurologic complications, including choreoathetosis (52). Choreoathetosis may be a result of cooling to 16°C and lower. Maintaining temperatures above this appears to significantly reduce the incidence of this complication.

Many situations exist where using profound hypothermia and circulatory arrest are of benefit. This technique has been applied in a wide variety of congenital heart defects and permits operating in a bloodless field without the obstruction that perfusion cannulas may create in the smaller patient. Some surgeons are concerned that this technique may lead to cerebral injury and developmental delay, perhaps to a very subtle degree (51). Therefore, other strategies such as low-flow perfusion and selective cerebral perfusion are being utilized to avoid this technique, even when complex aortic arch surgery is required.

Because neurologic complications can be devastating, this area has been the subject of considerable investigation. Some studies suggested that subtle changes in cognitive function occur with use of circulatory arrest and that this may be related to excessively short periods of core cooling on bypass before circulatory arrest is effected (53); more recent studies have suggested that use of circulatory arrest is associated primarily with long-term issues of motor coordination (54). Studies have shown that neurologic function may be improved early following hypothermic circulatory arrest if pH–stat blood gas management is used during cardiopulmonary bypass (55). Control of blood glucose levels and pH during reperfusion may also be of particular importance in avoiding cerebral injury (56). We also use NIRS cerebral oximetry as a guide to maintaining adequate oxygen delivery during circulatory arrest. Together, all of these measures have helped improve neurologic outcomes following surgery for congenital heart defects (57).

Seizure Activity

Infants are at high risk for seizures after cardiac operations because of electrolyte imbalance, osmotic shifts, anoxic cerebral insult, or air or thrombotic emboli through persistent shunts. These most commonly occur after the use of deep hypothermic arrest. Seizure activity in babies may vary from obvious tonic–clonic motions to subtle eye, tongue, or mouth movements. In the neonate or infant who is mechanically ventilated and with adjunct pharmacologic paralysis, seizures may be masked and may be manifested only by tachycardia, hypertension, mydriasis, or bronchorrhea; the sudden appearance of any of these signs should raise suspicion of seizure activity in the paralyzed patient. In all cases, vigorous treatment is indicated to prevent the cerebral consequences of unchecked seizures. Initial control may be obtained with intravenously administered diazepam (0.1 mg/kg). Phenobarbital, the preferred maintenance agent, should be given intravenously in two loading doses of 10 mg/kg each, followed by a maintenance dose of 5 mg/kg per day divided into b.i.d. doses. Phenytoin (20 mg/kg IV loading dose and 5 mg/kg per day divided b.i.d.) is an alternative maintenance agent (58).

CT scanning, MRI, or ultrasound of the brain in neonates may be needed to exclude the possibility of intraventricular hemorrhage. Sudden changes in serum osmolarity may predispose the infant to this problem. Therefore, no more than 5 to 6 mOsm/kg per hour should be given in any 1 hour to neonates. Hyperventilation and steroids are used for treatment of this condition.

Renal Failure

We generally strive to maintain a urine output of approximately 1 mL/kg per hour in children after cardiac operations. Oliguria combined with rising blood urea nitrogen and creatinine levels indicates renal failure. Renal failure in the neonatal period usually results from prerenal causes: low cardiac output, sepsis, and hypovolemia. Postrenal factors such as obstructive uropathy may need to be considered and excluded with ultrasound. Correction of the underlying cause will correct the renal dysfunction in most cases. Peritoneal dialysis is indicated for severe volume overload or persistent metabolic acidosis. Some surgeons advocate early aggressive dialysis in infants to prevent the edema formation and fluid and electrolyte problems common in these patients (13).

Sepsis

Bacterial sepsis is unfortunately common in the newborn period and may further complicate the care of the patient with congenital heart defects. *Streptococcus* sp. are probably the most common cause of neonatal sepsis, followed by the common hospital-acquired pathogens such as *Staphylococcus* and *Pseudomonas*. Rising or falling temperature, lethargy, pallor, mottling, decreasing platelet count, hemodynamic instability, and poor feeding are typical manifestations of sepsis. The nonspecificity of these signs and the frequency with which they occur in cardiac patients without sepsis are testimony to the difficulty in prompt diagnosis of sepsis. Laboratory studies may reveal elevated or decreased white blood cell count, thrombocytopenia, hyperglycemia, and acidosis (59).

The surgeon must maintain a high index of suspicion regarding the presence of infection, even during the first postoperative night and particularly in the postoperative patient with multiple indwelling lines and foreign material within the heart. Avoidance of septic complications is achieved by minimizing the number of invasive devices and the length of time they are used, meticulous nursing procedures, and prophylactic change of lines that must be in place for a prolonged time. When infection is suspected, vigorous attempts should be made to identify the source with blood, urine, and sputum cultures; chest radiographs; and possibly CT scans. Meningitis must also be considered, and cerebrospinal fluid cultures should be obtained.

After cultures have been obtained, the routine antibiotic regimen is changed, and broad-spectrum antibiotics may be instituted, usually vancomycin and an aminoglycoside. More specific coverage may be determined by the culture results. Doses of antibiotics used may require modification according to the patient's renal function. This may be abnormal because of the immaturity of the kidneys, as well as renal injury related to the underlying illness or operative complications.

Postoperative Investigations

Postoperative Echocardiography

Echocardiography, because of the detailed anatomic information it can provide and its noninvasive nature, is a nearly ideal technique for post-operative investigation of patients with congenital heart defects. We have found echocardiography to be most useful in assessing ventricular function and determining the presence of significant blood and fluid collections. Injections of saline-containing microbubbles provide an echocardiographic contrast medium to demonstrate the presence of intracardiac shunts. Color flow Doppler facilitates shunt detection and the estimation of valve regurgitation and stenosis. Alternatively, trans-esophageal echocardiography can be used, particularly if mediastinal drainage tubes obscure transthoracic echocardiography windows. Caution must be exercised, particularly in infants, to make sure that inadvertent endotracheal tube dislodgement does not occur during echocardiography probe manipulation. Transthoracic echocardiography, with or without transesophageal echocardiography, has made early postoperative cardiac catheterization of critically ill infants virtually unnecessary.

References

1. Pfammatter JP, Berdat P, Hammerli M, et al. Pediatric cardiac surgery after exclusively echocardiography-based work-up. *Int J Cardiol* 2000;74:185–190.
2. Freed MD, Heymann MA, Lewis AB, et al. Prostaglandin E$_1$ in infants with ductus arteriosus-dependent congenital heart disease. *Circulation* 1981;64:899–905.
3. Gold JP, Jonas RA, Lang P, et al. Transthoracic intracardiac monitoring lines in pediatric surgical patients: a ten-year experience. *Ann Thorac Surg* 1986;42: 185–191.
4. Butt WW, Whyte H. Blood pressure monitoring in neonates: comparison of umbilical and peripheral artery catheter measurements. *J Pediatr* 1984;105: 630–632.
5. Pinheiro JM, Fisher MA. Use of a triple-lumen catheter for umbilical venous access in the neonate. *J Pediatr* 1992;120:624–626.
6. Marsh JL, King W, Barrett C, et al. Serious complications after umbilical artery catheterization for neonatal monitoring. *Arch Surg* 1975;110:1203–1208.
7. Kim JH, Lee YS, Kim SH, et al. Does umbilical vein catheterization lead to portal venous thrombosis? Prospective US evaluation in 100 neonates. *Radiology* 2001;219:645–650.
8. Schranz D, Schmitt S, Oelert H, et al. Continuous monitoring of mixed venous oxygen saturation in infants after cardiac surgery. *Intensive Care Med* 1989;15: 228–232.
9. Bhutta AT, Ford JW, Parker JG, et al. Noninvasive cerebral oximeter as a surrogate for mixed venous saturation in children. *Pediatr Cardiol* 2007;28:34–41.
10. Burrows FA, Williams WG, Teoh KH, et al. Myocardial performance after repair of congenital cardiac defects in infants and children. Response to volume loading. *J Thorac Cardiovasc Surg* 1988;96:548–556.

11. Li J, Zhang G, Holtby H, et al. Adverse effects of dopamine on systemic hemodynamic status and oxygen transport in neonates after the Norwood procedure. *J Am Coll Cardiol* 2006;48:1859–1864.

12. Tabbutt S, Duncan BW, McLaughlin D, et al. Delayed sternal closure after cardiac operations in a pediatric population. *J Thorac Cardiovasc Surg* 1997;113: 886–893.

13. Zobel G, Stein JI, Kuttnig M, et al. Continuous extracorporeal fluid removal in children with low cardiac output after cardiac operations. *J Thorac Cardiovasc Surg* 1991;101: 593–597.

14. Thompson LD, McElhinney DB, Findlay P, et al. A prospective randomized study comparing volume-standardized modified and conventional ultrafiltration in pediatric cardiac surgery. *J Thorac Cardiovasc Surg* 2001;122: 220–228.

15. Kron IL, Rheuban K, Nolan SP. Late cardiac tamponade in children. A lethal complication. *Ann Surg* 1984;199:173–175.

16. Beland MJ, Paquet M, Gibbons JE, et al. Pericardial effusion after cardiac surgery in children and effects of aspirin for prevention. *Am J Cardiol* 1990;65: 1238–1241.

17. Wilson NJ, Webber SA, Patterson MW, et al. Double-blind placebo-controlled trial of corticosteroids in children with postpericardiotomy syndrome. *Pediatr Cardiol* 1994;15:62–65.

18. Lang P, Chipman CW, Siden H, et al. Early assessment of hemodynamic status after repair of tetralogy of Fallot: a comparison of 24 hour (intensive care unit) and 1 year postoperative data in 98 patients. *Am J Cardiol* 1982;50: 795–799.

19. DiDonato RM, Jonas RA, Lang P, et al. Neonatal repair of tetralogy of Fallot with and without pulmonary atresia. *J Thorac Cardiovasc Surg* 1991;101: 126–137.

20. Bridges ND, Mayer JE Jr, Lock JE, et al. Effect of baffle fenestration on outcome of the modified Fontan operation. *Circulation* 1992;86:1762–1769.

21. Meliones J, Kern F, Schulman S. Pathophysiologic approach to respiratory support for patients with congenital heart disease: pediatric cardiovascular intensive care. *Prog Pediatr Cardiol* 1995;4.

22. Kocis KC, Dekeon MK, Rosen HK, et al. Pressure-regulated volume control vs. volume control ventilation in infants after surgery for congenital heart disease. *Pediatr Cardiol* 2001;22:233–237.

23. Hopkins RA, Bull C, Haworth SG, et al. Pulmonary hypertensive crises following surgery for congenital heart defects in young children. *Eur J Cardiothorac Surg* 1991;5:628–634.

24. Kocis KC, Meliones JN, Dekeon MK, et al. High-frequency jet ventilation for respiratory failure after congenital heart surgery. *Circulation* 1992;86(suppl III): III27–III32.

25. Frostell C, Fratacci M-D, Wain JC, et al. Inhaled nitric oxide. A selective pulmonary vasodilator reversing hypoxic pulmonary vasoconstriction. *Circulation* 1991;83:2038–2047.

26. Atz AM, Wessel DL. Delivery and monitoring of inhaled nitric oxide. *Curr Opin Crit Care* 1997;3:243–249.

27. Atz AM, Adatia I, Wessel DL. Rebound pulmonary hypertension after inhalation of nitric oxide. *Ann Thorac Surg* 1996;62:1759–1764.

28. Morray JP, Lynn AM, Mansfield PB. Effect of pH and pCO_2 on pulmonary and systemic hemodynamics after surgery in children with congestive heart disease and pulmonary hypertension. *J Pediatr* 1988;113:474–479.

29. Jobes DR, Nicolson SC, Steven JM, et al. Carbon dioxide prevents pulmonary overcirculation in hypoplastic left heart syndrome. *Ann Thorac Surg* 1992;54:150–151.

30. O'Brien P, Elixson EM. The child following the Fontan procedure: nursing strategies. *AACN Clin Issues Crit Care Nurs* 1990;1:46–58.

31. Lofland GK. The enhancement of hemodynamic performance in Fontan circulation using pain free spontaneous ventilation. *Eur J Cardiothorac Surg* 2001;20:114–118.

32. Eze NN, Wyatt ME, Hartley BE. The role of the anterior cricoid split in facilitating extubation in infants. *Int J Pediatr Otorhinolaryngol* 2005;69:843–846.

33. Valsangiacomo E, Schmid ER, Schüpbach RW, et al. Early postoperative arrhythmias after cardiac operation in children. *Ann Thorac Surg* 2002;74:792–796.

34. Kashima I, Aeba R, Katogi T, et al. Optimal position to atrial epicardial leads for temporary pacing in infants after cardiac surgery. *Ann Thorac Surg* 2001;71:1945–1948.

35. Gillette PC. Diagnosis and management of postoperative junctional ectopic tachycardia. *Am Heart J* 1989;118:192–194.

36. Figa FH, Gow RM, Hamilton RM, et al. Clinical efficacy and safety of intravenous amiodarone in infants and children. *Am J Cardiol* 1994;74:573–577.

37. Perry J, Fenrich AL, Hulse JE, et al. Pediatric use of intravenous amiodarone: efficacy and safety in critically ill patients from a multicenter protocol. *J Am Coll Cardiol* 1996;27:1246–1250.

38. Sanchez C, Lopez-Herce J, Carillo A, et al. Transpyloric enteral feeding in the post-operative of cardiac surgery in children. *J Pediatr Surg* 2006;41:1096–102.

39. Benzing G III, Francis PD, Kaplan S, et al. Glucose and insulin changes in infants and children undergoing hypothermic open-heart surgery. *Am J Cardiol* 1983;52:133–136.

40. Satur C, Stubington S, Jennings A, et al. Magnesium flux during and after open heart operations in children. *Ann Thorac Surg* 1995;59:921–927.

41. Colon-Otero G, Gilchrist GS, Holcomb GR, et al. Preoperative evaluation of hemostasis in patients with congenital heart disease. *Mayo Clin Proc* 1987;62:379–385.

42. Mohr R, Martinowitz U, Lavee J, et al. The hemostatic effect of transfusing fresh whole blood versus platelet concentrates after cardiac operations. *J Thorac Cardiovasc Surg* 1988;96:530–534.

43. Fox S, Pierce WS, Waldhausen JA. Pathogenesis of paradoxical hypertension after coarctation repair. *Ann Thorac Surg* 1980;29:135–141.

44. Benedict CR, Grahame-Smith DG, Fisher A. Changes in plasma catecholamines and dopamine beta-hydroxylase after corrective surgery for coarctation of the aorta. *Circulation* 1978;57:598–602.

45. Sealy WC. Paradoxical hypertension after repair of coarctation of the aorta: a review of its causes. *Ann Thorac Surg* 1990;50:323–329.

46. Rocchini AP, Rosenthal A, Barger AC, et al. Pathogenesis of paradoxical hypertension after coarctation resection. *Circulation* 1976;54:382–387.

47. Choy M, Rocchini AP, Beekman RH, et al. Paradoxical hypertension after repair of coarctation of the aorta in children: balloon angioplasty versus surgical repair. *Circulation* 1987;75:1186–1191.

48. Gidding SS, Rocchini AP, Beekman R, et al. Therapeutic effect of propranolol on paradoxical hypertension after repair of coarctation of the aorta. *N Engl J Med* 1985;312:1224–1228.

49. Smerling A, Gerson WM. Esmolol for severe hypertension following repair of aortic coarctation. *Crit Care Med* 1990;18:1288–1290.

50. Bojar RM, Weiner B, Cleveland RJ. Intravenous labetalol for control of hypertension following repair of coarctation of the aorta. *Clin Cardiol* 1988;11: 639–641.

51. Forbess JM, Visconti KJ, Hancock-Friesen C, et al. Neurodevelopmental outcome after congenital heart surgery: results from an institutional registry. *Circulation* 2002;106(suppl I):I95–I102.

52. DeLeon G, Ilbawi M, Arcilla R, et al. Choreoathetosis after deep hypothermia without circulatory arrest. *Ann Thorac Surg* 1990;50:714–719.

53. Bellinger DC, Wernovsky G, Rappaport LA, et al. Cognitive development of children following early repair of transposition of the great arteries using deep hypothermic circulatory arrest. *Pediatrics* 1991;87:701–707.

54. Bellinger DC, Wypij D, Kuban KC, et al. Developmental and neurologic status of children 4 years of age after heart surgery with hypothermic circulatory arrest or low-flow cardiopulmonary bypass. *Circulation* 1999;100:526–532.

55. duPlessis AJ, Jonas RA, Wypij D, et al. Perioperative effects of alpha-stat versus pH-stat strategies for deep hypothermic cardiopulmonary bypass infants. *J Thorac Cardiovasc Surg* 1997;114:991–1001.

56. Ekroth R, Thompson RJ, Lincoln C, et al. Elective deep hypothermia with total circulatory arrest: changes in plasma creatine kinase BB, blood glucose, and clinical variables. *J Thorac Cardiovasc Surg* 1989;97:30–35.

57. Menache CC, duPlessis AJ, Wessel DL, et al. Current incidence of acute neurologic complications after open-heart operations in children. *Ann Thorac Surg* 2002;73:1752–1758.

58. Painter MJ, Bergman I, Crumrine P. Neonatal seizures. *Pediatr Clin North Am* 1986;33:91–109.

59. Donovan EF. Perioperative care of the surgical neonate. *Surg Clin North Am* 1985;65: 1061–1081.

Mechanical Cardiac Support and Transplantation

Marco E. Larobina and Bruce R. Rosengard

In patients with heart failure, there is a subgroup of patients who fail maximal medical therapy. For these patients, mechanical devices to support the failing heart may be lifesaving. Mechanical circulatory support (MCS) may permit recovery of the failing myocardium or may function as a bridge to transplantation. Short-term support is most commonly instituted in the setting of postcardiotomy cardiogenic shock, acute myocardial infarction, myocarditis, and primarily graft failure after transplantation. In contrast, long-term mechanical support is most commonly used in patients with chronic heart failure or in those patients in whom acute heart failure does not sufficiently recover after short-term support.

The indications, management, and outcomes of all of these categories differ and must be treated as separate entities. All patients requiring MCS are characterized by left, right, or biventricular heart failure, which results in elevated filling pressures, poor cardiac output, and the consequent compromise of end organ perfusion (Table 8.1). The ensuing multiorgan failure, in the inadequately supported patient, inevitably leads to death.

Irrespective of the etiology of the patient's cardiac failure, initial therapy involves optimization of cardiac output by adjustment of preload, afterload, and contractility using volume resuscitation, diuretics, dialysis, inotropic agents, vasodilators, pacing, chronotropes, and antiarrythmic medications. In the chronic heart failure setting, further interventions such as biventricular pacing can be used in some patient subsets to improve myocardial performance.

Failure of the aforementioned measures necessitates MCS and/or consideration of cardiac transplantation. The choice among the use of intra-aortic balloon counterpulsation, extracorporeal membrane oxygenation (ECMO), a ventricular assist device (VAD), or transplantation is dependent on the length of time support is contemplated, patient comorbidity, and the setting in which support is to be deployed.

INTRA-AORTIC BALLOON COUNTERPULSATION

The most commonly used method of MCS is intra-aortic balloon counterpulsation, commonly called the *intra-aortic balloon pump* (IABP). Appropriately timed inflation and deflation of the balloon in the proximal

TABLE 8.1	Definition of Ventricular Failure						
	CVP	**PAP**	**PCWP**	**MAP**	**CI**	**End-Organ Perfusion**	**Additional Features**
LV failure	<10	>25	>15–20	<70	<1.8	Poor	Pulmonary edema
RV failure	>15	<25	<15	<70	<1.8	Poor	Ascites, peripheral edema
Biventricular failure	>15		>15–20	<70	<1.8	Poor	Pulmonary edema, ascites, peripheral edema

CI, cardiac index (liters/min/m^2); CVP, central venous (right atrial) pressure; PAP, mean pulmonary artery pressure; PCWP, pulmonary capillary wedge pressure; MAP, mean arterial pressure.

descending aorta leads to a reduction in systemic afterload and myocardial oxygen consumption as well as improved coronary perfusion. Therefore, the IABP is useful in the setting of unstable angina and low cardiac output of any etiology. Balloon pump support is particularly advantageous in patients with severe mitral valve regurgitation or postinfarction ventricular septal defect, as it improves the forward ejection of left ventricular blood into a lowered resistance circuit, thus reducing the severity of the regurgitation or left-to-right shunting. International IABP registry data reports that the duration of assistance varied from 1 to 89 days with a mean of 53 hours (1). IABP support in children has been reported but is generally not the support method of choice because of size issues. In children, other methods such as ECMO are usually preferred (2,3).

Insertion of Intra-Aortic Balloon Pump

In most patients, the IABP is inserted percutaneously via the femoral artery (Fig. 8.1) using the Seldinger technique. The insertion can be either imaging guided (fluoroscopy or TEE) or performed blindly. Insertion without a sheath reduces the diameter of the artery occupied by the device and reduces the risk of ischemic complications. Either a 34 or 40 mL IABP is advanced into the thoracic aorta, with the tip placed just distal to the takeoff of the left subclavian artery. Balloon inflation and deflation are timed to the cardiac cycle using either the electrocardiogram or the arterial pressure waveform. Deflation of the balloon during early systole provides afterload reduction (decreased impedance to ventricular emptying), with a resultant increase in cardiac output of up

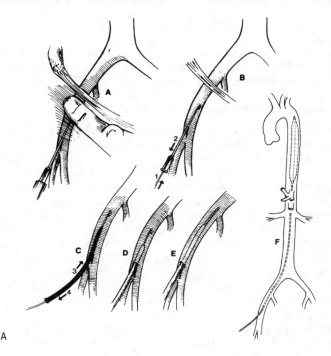

A

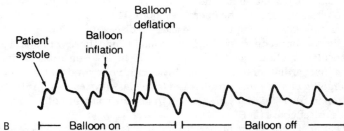

B |⊢——— Balloon on ———|⊢|⊢——— Balloon off ———|

FIGURE 8.1 Percutaneous insertion of an intra-aortic balloon pump via the femoral artery. **(A):** Insertion technique. If a femoral arterial line is not already present, the femoral artery is localized with a needle and syringe. Ideally, the artery should be entered immediately below the inguinal ligament (A). A guidewire is introduced via the needle (or femoral arterial line, if present) and into the iliofemoral tree (B). The needle is withdrawn over the guidewire, using gentle pressure to prevent bleeding around the insertion site, and dilators are serially introduced over the guidewire to dilate the femoral puncture site (C). An intra-aortic balloon pump insertion sheath is then inserted over the final dilator (D, E). The dilator is removed, and the balloon is inserted into the sheath. The balloon is then directed into the descending aorta (F). Passage of the balloon can be facilitated if a long guidewire is used (150 cm) to help negotiate the balloon through the iliofemoral arterial system. **(B):** Proper balloon timing is shown in this tracing of arterial blood pressure. Balloon inflation occurs during patient diastole, and balloon deflation occurs as the patient's heart ejects so as to produce mechanical afterload reduction.

to approximately 20%. Inflation of the balloon is timed to occur at the dicrotic notch of the arterial waveform and results in increased coronary artery perfusion pressure and flow.

Indications for Use of the Intra-Aortic Balloon Pump

IABP counterpulsation can be beneficial for all etiologies of cardiogenic shock. In acute myocardial infarction or perioperative infarction, the use of the IABP is clearly preferable to inotropes due to the reduction in myocardial oxygen consumption that it produces. In the postcardiotomy situation, an IABP is typically inserted when the patient's cardiac index is <1.8 to 2.0 L per minute per square meter despite moderate doses of inotropic drugs and in the absence of hypovolemia or reversible conditions such as tamponade. Aortic valve insufficiency, aortic dissection, and thoracic aortic aneurysm are contraindications for IABP insertion. Severe atherosclerosis of the descending aorta (which can be visualized by transesophageal echocardiography) and an abdominal aortic aneurysm may also be relative contraindications due to the risk of peripheral embolization of dislodged plaque or cholesterol emboli.

Preoperative placement of an IABP may be initiated in high-risk patients for whom there is a significant likelihood of postoperative IABP requirement. In this situation, the IABP is often inserted in the cardiac catheterization laboratory using fluoroscopy to guide placement, often en route to the operating room. This is particularly useful for patients with iliofemoral atherosclerotic disease or tortuous vessels. Candidates for preoperative IABP insertion include those with poor left ventricular function (ejection fraction <25% to 30%), unstable angina, acute myocardial infarction, and those with poor surgical targets or undergoing challenging repeat coronary bypass procedures. IABP utilization in such situations has proven to improve patient outcome and to be cost-effective (4–6).

Patients undergoing higher-risk surgical procedures such as repeat operation with patent but diseased vein grafts or with moderately impaired left ventricular function do not necessarily require a preoperative IABP but are at an increased risk for needing support to wean from cardiopulmonary bypass (CPB). In these patients, placement of a femoral arterial catheter after the induction of anesthesia facilitates subsequent placement of an IABP should it be required. For patients with severe aortoiliac occlusive disease or other conditions preventing femoral artery insertion, it is possible to place an IABP retrograde through the ascending aorta (Fig. 8.2) (3,7).

Complications of Intra-Aortic Balloon Pump

Major complications such as limb ischemia, hemorrhage, balloon gas leak, and death related to the balloon insertion or manipulation occur

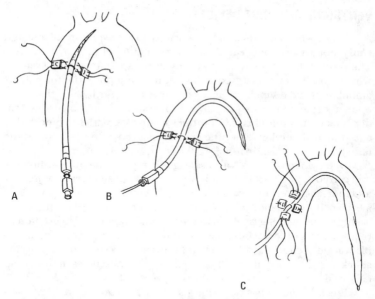

FIGURE 8.2 Technique for transthoracic intra-aortic balloon placement. With use of two concentric purse string sutures, a guidewire and dilators are introduced into the ascending aorta and passed around the aortic arch into the descending aorta. An insertion sheath is placed over the guidewire and dilators and directed beyond the brachiocephalic vessels **(A)**. The intra-aortic balloon pump catheter and balloon are then introduced over the guidewire, via the sheath, into the descending aorta **(B)**. The position must be estimated visually by the surgeon so that the proximal extent of the balloon is beyond the left subclavian artery **(C)**. The sheath is then withdrawn from the aorta, and the purse string sutures are tightened using short tourniquets. The balloon may be subsequently removed by withdrawing the balloon catheter out the aortotomy, achieving digital control of the aortotomy site, and tightening and tying down the purse string sutures.

in approximately 3% of patients (see Benchmark Registry data). The most common complication is leg ischemia (3,8), particularly in patients with peripheral vascular occlusive disease and poor preoperative left ventricular function. Conditions such as hypertension, diabetes, and female gender are potential contributors. For the ischemic limb, surgical intervention is usually required. Early IABP removal with thromboendarterectomy and femoral artery repair is usually required. If the leg is ischemic but the patient is IABP dependent, revascularization may be accomplished by construction of a femoral artery-to-femoral artery crossover graft. An alternative is to sew a vascular graft as a "chimney" off of the larger iliac artery and to remove the IABP from the femoral artery.

VENTRICULAR ASSIST DEVICES

A patient, who remains in a low-output state despite inotropic and IABP support may be a candidate for escalation of therapy to a VAD. The term VAD encompasses a variety of pump and cannula systems which vary in complexity, cost, ease of use, and potential for patient ambulation and rehabilitation. Recent developments include the development of percutaneously deployed VAD systems. The choice of system depends on the anticipated duration of support, patient comorbidity and prognosis, and whether the device will serve as a bridge or be the last step (i.e., the "destination") in the treatment algorithm.

Deployment of a VAD as a salvage therapy in the postcardiotomy and cardiogenic shock settings is associated with significant morbidity and mortality rates in excess of 50% (9). In contrast, the use of VADs as a bridge to transplant can be performed either in the cardiogenic shock scenario or semielectively in patients with recurrent heart failure requiring multiple hospital readmissions. Success in achieving transplantation occurs in 70+% of patients (10). The presence of cardiogenic shock or right ventricular failure predicts worse outcomes in this group (11), as does the necessity for BiVAD support (12).

Elective VAD insertion can also be performed to achieve pulmonary vascular remodeling in patients with chronically elevated pulmonary vascular resistance in whom orthotopic heart transplant presents an unacceptable risk of post-transplant right ventricular failure (13). The use of VADs in these scenarios allows for much more refined patient selection and preparation for subsequent transplantation, significantly reducing morbidity and mortality.

Ventricular Assist Device Classes and Systems

A myriad of device technologies are either available or in advanced development and are broadly divided into short-term versus long-term support devices and pulsatile versus nonpulsatile devices (Table 8.2). More recent development has centered on the percutaneously/peripherally inserted VAD, which obviates the need for sternotomy and CPB. In this book, we have focused primarily on devices for which we have clinical experience.

Devices for Short-Term Support

The short-term devices are cheaper and simpler both to insert and manage postoperatively, but are extracorporeal in location and therefore severely restrict patient management beyond the immediate intensive care setting. Short-term devices are available either as pulsatile or as continuous flow systems. On-site perfusion support is often required,

TABLE 8.2	Ventricular Assist Devices				
		Cost	Location	Ambulation	Anticoagulation
Short-term continuous flow					
Biomedicus		+	Extracorporeal	No	Heparin
Levitronix CentriMag		++	Extracorporeal	No	Heparin
Short/intermediate-term pulsatile					
Abiomed BVS 5000		+	Extracorporeal	No	Heparin
Abiomed AB5000		++	Paracorporeal	Yes	Heparin
Long-term pulsatile					
Thoratec PVAD		+++	Paracorporeal	Yes	Aspirin, warfarin
Thoratec IVAD		+++	Intracorporeal	Yes	Aspirin, warfarin
HeartMate I XVE		+++	Intracorporeal	Yes	Aspirin
Long-term continuous flow					
HeartMate II		+++	Intracorporeal	Yes	Aspirin, warfarin
Percutaneous VADs					
Impella		++	Intracorporeal	No	Heparin
TandemHeart		++	Extracorporeal	No	Heparin

although highly trained nursing staff can obviate the need for this in experienced centers. Cannulation to support the left, right, or both ventricles can be performed depending on the clinical situation.

Early short-term left-sided VAD support was in the form of a centrifugal pump with atrioaortic or ventriculoaortic cannulation (14,15). The cannulae can exit either directly through the sternotomy or through separate incisions to facilitate chest closure. Left-sided inflow cannula placement can be either from the left atrium or from the LV apex, and the outflow cannula is placed into the aorta. This VAD system requires continuous anticoagulation with intravenous heparin. Right-sided support is similarly accomplished with right atrial or ventricular inflow cannulation with outflow into the pulmonary artery.

The Levitronix Centrimag™ is a centrifugal blood pump with a magnetically levitated rotor designed to be frictionless and reduce device related blood trauma. The flow characteristics are intended to produce minimal areas of stasis within the pump to reduce the thromboembolic risk. Multiple reports have documented both adequate hemodynamic performance and clinical success in multiple settings (16–18).

Pulsatile short-term support can be provided using the the Abiomed BVS 5000 Biventricular Support System (Abiomed, Danvers, MA). This extracorporeal device is connected by transcutaneous cannulae to the patient, with the blood pump and drive console being located at the patient's bedside (see Table 8.2) (19,20). The pump has a dual chamber configuration ("atrium" and "ventricle") and integral polymer trileaflet valves. It uses a pneumatic drive; these extracorporeal pumps are inexpensive.

The device has been primarily utilized in the postcardiotomy cardiogenic shock scenario as a bridge to recovery, a bridge to more definitive long-term support, or as a bridge to transplant (21). Use as a bridge to recovery in myocarditis and as a primary bridge to transplant in the non–postcardiotomy setting has also yielded clinical success (20).

The Abiomed AB5000 is a pulsatile paracorporeal device consisting of a blood pump sac and integral trileaflet polymer valves, similar to the BVS 5000. It provides intermediate term support and can be operated from the same drive console as the BVS 5000.

Percutaneous Ventricular Assist Devices

Recent developments include the advent of the percutaneously deployed assist devices, which include the TandemHeart™ (CardiacAssist, Inc. Pittsburgh, PA) and the Impella™ System (Abiomed). The TandemHeart system requires percutaneous placement of an inflow cannula transseptally into left atrium, with a return cannula to the descending aorta. Flows of up to 5 L per minute can be obtained by the extracorporeal centrifugal pump driven by a three-phase, brushless, DC servomotor.

The Impella system is a catheter-based impeller-driven axial flow pump which is placed percutaneously into the left ventricle usually via a femoral artery approach and can provide between 2.5 and 5.0 L per minute of flow, depending on which version of the device is used. When introduced via the femoral artery, the Impella VAD is passed around the aortic arch and sits across the aortic valve. Cannulation of the axillary artery can avoid manipulation of the arch in some circumstances and may permit ambulation. Once the Impella device is placed across the aortic valve, the microaxial pump located at the end of a 9-F catheter can pump up to 2.5 L per minute (Impella 2.5™, a percutaneous device) or 5.0 L per minute (Impella 5.0™, inserted by femoral cutdown). The pump uses an impeller at rotational speeds in excess of 30,000 rpm. Low-grade hemolysis is sometimes a consequence.

Devices for Long-Term Support

VADs designed for longer-term support are also divided into the pulsatile versus nonpulsatile VADs. Both subtypes have been used in multiple clinical scenarios with success. The search for the perfect device, however, remains elusive, and the management of the risks of sepsis, thromboembolism, and anticoagulant-related hemorrhage presents an ongoing challenge in the use of these devices in the long term. The intracorporeal systems have the advantage of enhanced patient mobility, with improved potential for rehabilitation. However, intracorporeal placement of devices made from foreign materials creates the potential for sepsis. Second generation axial flow devices and third generation centrifugal devices are smaller, cause less blood trauma, decrease the risk of device-related complications, and have become the VAD of choice in both the bridge to transplant and destination therapy groups, outside of the salvage setting.

Pulsatile Long-Term Ventricular Assist Devices

The pulsatile devices can be positioned paracorporeally (e.g., Thoratec PVAD) or intracorporeally (e.g., Heart Mate I XVE, or Thoratec IVAD).

Thoratec. The Thoratec VAD System (Thoratec Corp., Pleasanton, CA) is a paracorporeal or intracorporeal volume displacement pulsatile device. The pump either sits externally on the patient's anterior abdominal wall or is implanted subcutaneously or intra-abdominally. It is driven by a bedside pneumatic pump which compresses the distensible pump sac housed inside a solid polycarbonate shell (22). The pump delivers a maximal stroke volume of 65 mL and has adjustable suction to facilitate pump filling. The system houses two single tilting disk mechanical valves. Anticoagulation with a combination of aspirin and warfarin is required. The advantage of the Thoratec system is that the pump can be used either for LV or for RV support, and hence is often favored in situations where BiVAD support is required (Fig. 8.3).

HeartMate I XVE. The vented electric HeartMate I intracorporeal VAD has been approved for use in both the bridge to transplant and the destination therapy settings. There is considerable clinical experience with this device.

Continuous Flow Devices for Long-Term Support

The second generation axial flow VADs (e.g., HeartMate II) are electrically driven and powered by a single drive line which exits the patient. These VADs are all placed intracorporeally and are much smaller than previous designs. Intracorporeal placement of the pump itself reduces the external components which the patient must carry, making mobilization and rehabilitation of these patients much simpler. Power consumption is also lower. Given the often-extended waiting times for a donor heart in the bridge to transplant group and the potential to use these devices as destination therapy as an alternative to transplantation, the third generation devices represent the future of MCS. Furthermore, the design of these pumps, often without bearings and valves,

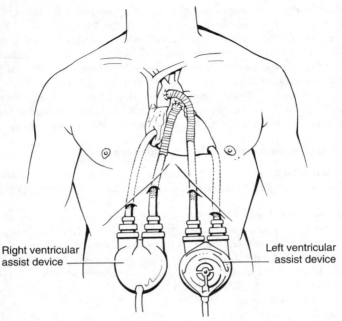

FIGURE 8.3 Cannulation scheme for Thoratec biventricular assistance. The left ventricular assist device withdraws blood from the left ventricular apex and returns it to the ascending aorta. The right ventricular assist device withdraws blood from the right atrium and returns it to the pulmonary artery.

minimizes both blood trauma and stasis within the device thus, reducing the potential for thromboembolism.

The long-term effect of a nonpulsatile circulation has not been clearly defined. Vascular remodeling has been documented with thinning of the aorta; however, end organ function appears not to be compromised (23). Reversal of heart failure–related end organ dysfunction has been clearly documented with the use of continuous flow devices, albeit with less echocardiographically measured LV unloading (24).

Ventricular Assist Device Physiology and Right Ventricular Function

In concept, VADs unload the assisted ventricle, draining blood either from the atrium or from the ventricular apex via the inflow cannula, and provide pressure to the returning column of blood via the outflow cannula to the ascending aorta or pulmonary artery, depending on the ventricle being supported. Management of a patient with an isolated left ventricular assist device (LVAD) requires optimizing the function of the right ventricle to ensure adequate filling of the left-sided VAD, which, in turn, will pump the blood to the systemic circulation. The insertion of an LVAD can precipitate or unmask underlying RV dysfunction. Significant RV dysfunction has been reported in up to 35% of patients receiving an isolated LVAD, and in 10% to 20% of patients, a right-sided device will also be required (25). Preoperative severe RV dysfunction, low RV stroke work index, elevated pulmonary vascular resistance, nonischemic etiology, and female gender all increase the risk of RV failure and the need for right-sided support.

It is also clear that the unloading of the left ventricle provided by the LVAD alters the function of the RV in a potentially deleterious manner. The alterations in the LV cause a reduction in RV contractility, an increase in compliance, and a decrease in RV afterload. The position and function of the ventricular septum are critical in this situation, and its tendency to shift left toward the LV during LVAD support can further change the shape of the RV and impair systolic function. In the normal heart there is no net effect on cardiac output. However, in clinical practice, where RV function is often subnormal, frank RV failure can be precipitated (26). This deleterious movement of the interventricular septum is easier to precipitate in the continuous flow VADs where the preload of the left ventricle is attenuated by continuous drainage. This highlights the need for careful titration of pump speed, best guided initially with transesophageal echocardiography in the operating room. Pump speed, the effective strength of suction placed on the blood in the LV cavity, controls the LV volume. Too little LV volume, and the RV attains a spherical appearance with the septum shifting toward the LV. This alteration in shape of the RV can severely impair its pumping ability, precipitating RV dysfunction.

Right ventricular function can be improved with manipulation of the patient's volume state, assessed by the central venous pressure (CVP), epicardial pacing, modulation of the pulmonary vascular resistance with ventilatory optimization, the use of specific pulmonary vasodilators such as nitric oxide and prostacyclin, and the use of inotropes such as milrinone, which has coincident dilating properties on the pulmonary vasculature. The right ventricle is also dependent on a critical perfusion pressure and diminished systemic pressures can precipitate RV failure.

The presence of a patent foramen ovale or atrial septal defect must be sought and corrected if present during deployment of an LVAD. An interatrial communication can lead to right-to-left shunting and systemic deoxygenation when the left atrial pressure is reduced, particularly in the presence of RV dysfunction with elevated RA pressures. In addition, the presence of more than mild aortic regurgitation must be corrected with either oversewing of the aortic valve or by aortic valve replacement.

Salvage VAD Use: Cardiogenic Shock,
Postcardiotomy Cardiogenic Shock

Despite improvements in medical and intensive care management, the outlook for patients with cardiogenic shock remains poor. In postcardiotomy cardiogenic shock, the decline in myocardial performance is often related to perioperative myocardial stunning, and recovery of ventricular function maybe anticipated; however, reported mortality in excess of 50% is common (20). Other etiologies of cardiogenic shock such as acute myocardial infarction or myocarditis carry similarly poor prognosis. The dual aim of therapy in these situations is to unload the injured ventricle to facilitate recovery and to provide sufficient end organ perfusion to prevent multiorgan failure. The patient who has undergone a technically complete operation but who cannot be weaned from CPB, despite use of an IABP, may be supported with a VAD (27,28).

Patient Selection. Preoperative assessment can identify patients at risk for profound postoperative ventricular dysfunction. Poor ventricular function is perhaps the strongest predictor of problems with weaning from CPB. If a patient has underlying left ventricular dysfunction in association with critical aortic stenosis or occlusive coronary artery disease in combination with viable myocardium, improved left ventricular function following either aortic valve replacement or coronary revascularization is anticipated (29). Should such a patient fail to be weaned from CPB, VAD support is a reasonable undertaking, with the expectation that myocardial recovery will occur. For patients with a low ejection fraction who have marginal potential for recovery of myocardial function following operative intervention, it is prudent to perform initial transplant evaluation. If such a patient requires VAD support upon completion of the operation, the end point changes from recovery of ventricular function to the bridge-to-transplant application.

Unfortunately, the inability to wean a patient from CPB is often unanticipated. Thus, the decision regarding the use of a VAD in this situation is made urgently in the operating room. Echocardiography or visual inspection will demonstrate poor left ventricular wall motion. In rapid sequence, the patient should be started on appropriate inotropic support, and an IABP should be placed. If the patient cannot be weaned from CPB despite these interventions, consideration should be given to the use of a VAD (30). Preoperative conditions that may negatively impact the potential for survival include renal failure, irreversible pulmonary hypertension, severe peripheral vascular disease, and advanced age. Operative events that may adversely impact the potential for patient recovery include a low flow state or prolonged hypotension, either of which might precipitate a neurological event or renal failure.

Device Selection and Implantation Technique. In the postcardiotomy cardiogenic shock scenario, centrifugal pumps either utilizing the bypass circuit cannulae or with device specific cannulae are used to allow weaning from bypass. In the nontransplant setting, patients who cannot be weaned from CPB usually suffer from predominant left-sided heart failure (see Table 8.1). Thus, left ventricular support is provided first. The usual configuration for short-term left heart support is VAD inflow from the patient's left ventricular apex with VAD outflow to the patient's ascending aorta (31,32). Left ventricular cannulation provides optimal ventricular drainage, and the use of concentric purse string sutures with pledgets to secure the cannula at the apex is highly hemostatic. An alternative for device inflow is to use left atrial cannulation. During pump start-up, caution must be exercised to avoid excessive negative pressure which can entrain air through needle holes, particularly when left atrial cannulation is used. Keeping the insertion site submerged, use of fibrin glue, and avoiding initial high flow rates can help minimize this risk.

For left atrial cannulation, the interatrial groove is developed, and the left atrial cannula is inserted via the right lateral wall of the left atrium. The outlet graft is anastomosed in an end-to-side fashion to the ascending aorta. If a centrifugal pump is used as an LVAD, a standard arterial CPB cannula can be employed for VAD outflow. For left-sided heart support utilizing a left atrial or left ventricular inflow cannula, the inflow and outflow cannulae exit the pericardium in the subcostal region. The cannulae are completely de-aired and connected to the VAD circuit.

Right-sided heart performance is optimized as discussed earlier using temporary pacing and selective inotrope infusion. Inhaled nitric oxide (10 to 20 parts per million) can help unload a failing right heart by reducing pulmonary vascular resistance (33). Left- and right-sided preload are monitored simultaneously using a combination of invasive pressure measurements and TEE. LVAD flow is initiated as CPB flow is decreased. The goal is a systemic systolic blood pressure in excess of 90 mm Hg with a cardiac index well above 2.0 L per minute per square meter. If the right heart is functioning satisfactorily, the CVP should remain below 10 to 15 mm Hg. If LVAD filling is satisfactory, the left atrial pressure will be below 10 mm Hg and the atrial septum should be in the midline on TEE.

Persistent right heart dysfunction despite the measures outlined above requires concomitant right ventricular assist device (RVAD) implantation (34). The usual configuration for RVAD implantation is right atrial inflow with pulmonary artery outflow. The Abiomed BVS 5000 or AB5000, Thoratec pumps, or any centrifugal pump can be configured for right-sided support. Inflow and outflow cannulae exit the chest via the left subcostal region. Fig. 8.4 shows RVAD and LVAD cannulation.

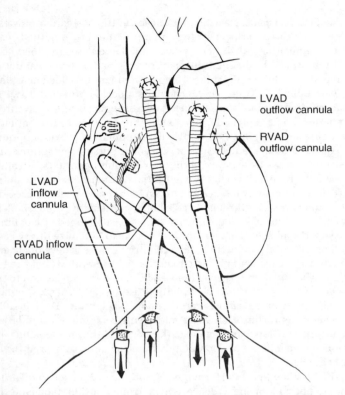

FIGURE 8.4 Cannulation scheme for biventricular assistance for postcardiotomy cardiogenic shock. Left ventricular assistance employs left atrial inflow and aortic outflow cannulae. Right ventricular assistance utilizes right atrial inflow and main pulmonary artery outflow cannulae. LVAD, left ventricular assist device; RVAD, right ventricular assist device.

Occasionally, a patient will develop isolated right ventricular failure most commonly following an inferoposterolateral infarct or secondary to acute right ventricular distention associated with a sizable pulmonary embolism. In this situation, the patient's left-sided heart will be decompressed and contracting vigorously. The right-sided heart will be distended and hypocontractile. The CVP will exceed 20 mm Hg, while pulmonary artery pressures will be low. If optimized ventilation, use of pulmonary vasodilators, and inotropic therapy do not result in improved left ventricular preload and right-sided heart decompression, RVAD implantation should follow. RVAD inflow is via the right atrium with return to the main pulmonary artery.

Following termination of CPB, protamine sulfate is slowly administered. Nonsurgical bleeding is the norm following an extended CPB time. Specific coagulation deficits are corrected with the administration of blood component therapy. Chest closure can be problematic due to the presence of VAD cannulae and coronary bypass conduits, but is attempted because reapproximation of the sternal edges and soft tissues reduces postoperative bleeding. If it is not possible to close the chest primarily, the sternum is stented open. As myocardial edema resolves over the ensuing days, delayed chest closure is often possible.

Postoperative Care

Management Issues with Ventricular Assist Devices. The primary postoperative consideration following LVAD implantation is to ensure adequate systemic perfusion. This relies on adequate function of the VAD and the ability of the right heart to deliver sufficient cardiac output to the device through the pulmonary vasculature. Assuming that the patient has an effective cardiac rhythm, the right heart is supported with inotropic agents, optimized pacing, and inhaled nitric oxide as described in "VAD physiology and RV function" beginning on page 316. The maintenance of adequate systemic pressures in this situation is essential. Failing these treatment modalities, an RVAD is used to replace the function of the native right ventricle.

The postcardiotomy cardiogenic shock patient is at high risk for postoperative hemorrhage. The etiology of this bleeding is multifactorial (35). Platelet dysfunction due to prolonged CPB and the IABP (if present) are prime causative factors. A reduction in serum clotting factors, excessive fibrinolysis, and the presence of multiple suture lines and cannula access sites also contribute. When this occurs, coagulation studies are obtained, and the coagulopathy is corrected with appropriate blood product and clotting factor administration. If the patient is considered to be a candidate for heart transplantation, leukodepleted blood products are used to help avoid antibody development. Blood products must be used judiciously, however, due to their potential effects on pulmonary vascular resistance and right heart function.

In the first 24 hours following VAD insertion, the patient is allowed to awaken for neurologic assessment. Early extubation helps avoid nosocomial pneumonia and improves RV function. Diuretic administration augments urinary output with the aim to remove the total body fluid overload that is often present following prolonged CPB. This is often in the form of a continuous furosemide infusion. Although the goal is to achieve a negative fluid balance, this is often difficult to do until the systemic inflammatory response has resolved, and the initial fluid management should be directed toward optimization of RV function and should be tailored to the CVP.

Within 12 to 24 hours of surgery, all noncritical tubes and lines are removed to avoid infectious complications. All of the extracorporeal blood pumps require systemic anticoagulation, but systemic anticoagulation is not begun until the patient's coagulation studies have returned to normal and mediastinal tube drainage has fallen below 50 mL per hour for 2 to 3 hours. Following this, heparin is administered with the goal of partial thromboplastin time 1.5 to 2.0 times control. The usual intensive care unit precautions are employed, including stress ulcer prophylaxis, aggressive nutritional support, and infection control.

Antibiotic Prophylaxis. Routine antibiotic prophylaxis is used and it is our practice to include vancomycin, a cephalosporin or levofloxacin, and fluconazole. As the initial phase of support elapses and stable circulatory support is achieved, less invasive monitoring will be needed. In this setting, antibiotic prophylaxis can be stopped to avoid emergence of resistant flora. This usually involves 3 to 5 days of coverage.

Weaning from Mechanical Circulatory Support. Following VAD implantation ventricular recovery usually requires 3 to 5 days of support. A combination of invasive pressure monitoring and serial echocardiographic assessment monitors the progress of cardiac function. The natural inclination is to rapidly wean the patient from the VAD for fear of a complication related to the presence of the device. Weaning attempts should be delayed, however, to allow time for ventricular recovery and to make sure that end organs have recovered from the acute insult of the initial operation.

For the LVAD-only patient, weaning should be performed slowly to avoid volume overloading of the left ventricle. Device flow is slowly reduced over a number of hours while monitoring the filling pressures and cardiac output without the use of additional inotropic drugs. If the left ventricle has recovered, these hemodynamic parameters will be maintained despite a mild to modest reduction in LVAD flow. If the reduced LVAD flow results in a significant elevation in left atrial or pulmonary artery pressures, LVAD flow should again be increased to decompress the left-sided heart, which facilitates left ventricular recovery. Complete unloading of the ventricle is not necessarily desirable in this recovery situation, and leaving the LV partially filled and ejecting is sufficient.

LVAD flow is reduced to a minimum of 1.5 to 2 L per minute, as dictated by each specific device, with flow maintained at that minimal rate for an extended period of time to ensure patient stability prior to device removal. We prefer that the patient be hemodynamically stable on a minimum of 2 L per minute of LVAD flow for at least 12 to 24 hours prior to device explantation. During this time, it is imperative that the patient's anticoagulation be therapeutic to avoid VAD thrombosis, and some devices may require additional anticoagulation during weaning at reduced flows.

If ventricular function is recovered, the patient is returned to the operating room for VAD removal. CPB is not usually required for explantation. If echocardiographic and visual inspection of the heart suggests that there is unequivocal recovery of ventricular function, the device is simply withdrawn. To be certain that the patient has recovered ventricular function, in the operating room we usually administer additional heparin and discontinue VAD support for 30 to 60 minutes prior to device explantation. By so doing, we ensure that the patient is hemodynamically stable without LVAD support. The left atrial cannula is then withdrawn; the outlet graft is transected adjacent to the aorta, and the stump of the graft is oversewn. Chest closure and patient care are conventional thereafter.

Advanced Heart Failure: Bridge to Recovery, Bridge to Cardiac Transplant, Destination Therapy

Patients with advanced congestive cardiac failure have a dismal prognosis, with a 20% 2-year survival (36). In these patients the only prospect of long-term survival is cardiac transplantation. Organ scarcity precludes immediate transplantation of most of these patients, and MCS with long-term VADs can be used to both rehabilitate these patients and prolong their lives while awaiting a donor allograft, effectively providing a bridge to transplantation (28).

Bridge to Recovery

Sustained ventricular unloading can allow the recovery of the heart sufficiently to allow explantation of the VAD. This occurs more commonly in patients with myocarditis and postpartum cardiomyopathy (37–39). Active areas of investigation include identifying patients who might benefit from interim circulatory support and the mechanism(s) by which recovery occurs (40). Bridge to recovery has been reported both with pulsatile and nonpulsatile devices (41). Of the patients in whom explantation of the device has occurred as a result of myocardial recovery, the majority remain transplant free at follow-up, with preserved LV and RV function and excellent functional class (42,43). For the majority of patients, however, who present with advanced heart failure, the implantation of a VAD is a means by which to rehabilitate the patients and prepare them for transplantation.

Indications for Ventricular Assist Device as Bridge to Transplant

Bridge to transplantation encompasses the full spectrum from the patient who presents in cardiogenic shock to the purely elective VAD inserted in the patient with elevated pulmonary vascular resistance, who is not currently a candidate for orthotopic transplantation. Furthermore, a separate subcategory of VAD insertion was created in 2002 when the Food and Drug Administration approved permanent use of an intracorporeal VAD in patients with end-stage heart failure who are not candidates for cardiac transplantation (36). In this instance, the VAD remains *in situ* for the remainder of the patient's life, so called "Destination Therapy."

The focus of patient care in the bridge-to-transplant patient is different from that in the postcardiotomy cardiogenic shock situation, as the heart is not expected to recover. Rather, the goal is to improve systemic perfusion and end organ function. Furthermore, the patient is rehabilitated, physically and nutritionally, in preparation for the subsequent heart transplant. Excellent pretransplant and posttransplant survival is possible.

Indications for Ventricular Assist Device Insertion as Bridge to Transplant

1. Cardiogenic shock resulting from decompensated heart failure.
2. Recurrent episodes of cardiac failure.
3. Progressive end organ dysfunction related to low cardiac output refractory to medical and inotropic support.
4. Elevated pulmonary vascular resistance precluding orthotopic transplant.
5. Uncontrollable, malignant ventricular arrhythmias

With some exceptions the patient being considered for VAD implantation must fulfill all cardiac transplant inclusion and exclusion criteria and be on the active transplant waiting list (44). In the past, VAD insertion was reserved for the approved cardiac transplant recipient who deteriorated hemodynamically and was hospitalized in an intensive care unit with invasive hemodynamic monitoring lines, maximized inotropic drugs, and often an IABP. However, as results with MCS in this patient population have improved, and the duration of waiting times prior to transplantation has increased, the use of VADs has expanded to encompass patients without IABP support, and even those not necessarily requiring intensive care therapy. Indications for VAD insertion have expanded and included recurrent heart failure, inotrope dependence, and increasing diuretic requirements with worsening renal function. The third generation axial flow pumps will allow a much more ambulatory existence for the VAD patient with lower complication rates. There is no doubt that the high morbidly and mortality seen using VADs in the critically ill patient can be vastly reduced if the patient in placed on support before reaching the extreme level of illness.

Management of the Patient with an Elevated Pulmonary Vascular Resistance

The development of pulmonary hypertension related to chronic heart failure has traditionally been a relative contraindication to orthotopic heart transplantation. Oversizing the donor allograft, heterotopic transplantation, or postoperative mechanical support were strategies used to deal with the RV dysfunction that resulted from placing an allograft into a recipient with pulmonary hypertension. Evidence has documented the reversal of pulmonary hypertension in this setting related to pulmonary vascular remodeling as a result of the unloading of the pulmonary circuit achieved with VAD insertion. Therefore, this subcategory of patients is unique, in that they are a bridge to become transplantable.

The reduction in PVR occurs over a period of weeks to months and is assessed by a combination of serial echocardiography and repeat right-sided heart catheterization. Adjunctive treatment with sildenafil and/or bosentan has been used to assist in the PVR reduction (45). Once sustained reduction in PVR below 4 Wood Units has been demonstrated, the patient can be listed for transplantation. The results of transplantation in patients in whom an LVAD has been used to achieve a sustained reduction in PVR are comparable to the results in the nonelevated PVR patient (46).

Patient Preparation

Optimization of the patient's hemodynamic, nutritional, and mental state prior to VAD insertion facilitates better outcomes. The patient should be infection-free. Systemic anticoagulation is discontinued if possible, or is converted to heparin infusion if continued thromboprophylaxis is required.

Pre- and intraoperative echocardiography is used to assess for left ventricular thrombus, aortic valve function, and the presence of a patent foramen ovale (47). Assessment is also made of RV function, as profound RV dysfunction with a high likelihood of BiVAD support may alter device selection.

The patient's abdomen is examined as previous intra-abdominal operations may provide technical hurdles for implantable LVAD insertion. A prior incision in the subcostal region may affect preperitoneal placement of an implantable blood pump. Patients who have received an implantable defibrillator in the distant past may have a generator in the left upper abdominal quadrant that may need to be removed or repositioned when the LVAD is implanted.

Optimization of hemodynamics, in particular aggressive diuresis or hemofiltration, can be used to unload the RV in preparation for LVAD insertion. These attempts to improve RV function are tailored to avoid the need for concomitant RVAD placement.

If a patient is a candidate for MCS as a bridge to cardiac transplantation, the operation is usually performed on an urgent, but not emergency, basis. All intravenous catheters and lines are moved to new sites before LVAD insertion to reduce the infection risk. The antibiotic regimen is specifically designed to provide prophylaxis against a broad spectrum of organisms associated with VADs.

Ventricular Assist Device Selection

The first decision in managing the bridge-to-transplant patient is device selection. A combination of the patient's size, clinical status, age, RV function, and likelihood of needing biventricular support determine device choice. Smaller patients have traditionally been implanted with a paracorporeal device, such as the Thoratec system. In patients who present in cardiogenic shock and mechanical support is a salvage procedure, using a paracorporeal Thoratec VAD is advantageous as it can be configured for either left- or right-sided heart support. However, this pneumatically powered blood pump lacks easy portability due to the presence of the external drive unit. Therefore, in the semielective or truly elective situation, electric implantable blood pumps, which by virtue of their size, are more portable have a clear advantage.

The patient in the elective setting who presents with profound or predominant right-sided failure remains a challenge. In this situation, the paracorporeal VAD remains our device of choice.

Operative Management

LVAD configuration for the bridge-to-transplant application usually involves placement of a cannula through the left ventricular apex for device inflow and a graft to the aorta for outflow. A standard sternotomy incision is employed (48). With intracorporeal devices, the pump pocket is fashioned prior to heparinization to achieve optimal hemostasis. CPB is initiated with an aortic perfusor and dual stage venous cannula unless a patent foramen ovale is present, in which case bicaval cannulation is necessary. The outlet graft-to-aortic anastomosis is usually performed prior to the initiation of CPB, and it is performed as low on the ascending aorta as possible to permit complete removal of the outlet graft at the time of cardiac transplantation. Cardioplegic arrest, vented ventricular fibrillation, or vented beating heart surgery can be used for left ventricular cannulation. The heart and VAD circuit are compulsively de-aired. The patient is weaned from CPB as LVAD flow is initiated. If the extracorporeal VAD is employed, the heart is approached through a standard median sternotomy, and the inflow and outflow cannulae traverse the skin in the left subcostal region. The remaining operative considerations are identical to those described above.

Left and right ventricular preload should be carefully monitored as left-sided heart support is initiated. As discussed, left ventricular decompression can unmask or even precipitate right ventricular failure, and if it occurs, it is managed as described previously. Transesophageal echocardiography is used to evaluate ventricular cannula position, the effectiveness of left ventricular decompression, septal position, and RV function. With left ventricular apex cannulation, the entire output of the left-sided heart should be via the VAD and native aortic valve should remain closed.

Chest closure details include placement of mediastinal and VAD pocket drains, positioning of the outlet graft to the right of the midline to avoid injury on reentry, and pericardial closure, using a prosthetic pericardial membrane, if necessary (49). These measures will facilitate reentry at the time of subsequent sternotomy for the transplantation operation.

Postoperative Care

Managing the bridge-to-transplant patient follows the same principles as outlined in the section "Management Issues with Ventricular Assist Devices" on page 321. In addition, the goal is to avoid development of a complication that would prevent subsequent cardiac transplantation. Initially, the VAD patient is removed from the cardiac transplant waiting list. The patient is activated on the transplant waiting list when recovery, wound healing, and relatively normal kidney, lung, and liver functions are achieved. This usually requires 6 to 10 weeks of recovery.

The patient is usually extubated, and the majority of tubes and lines are removed within 24 hours of VAD implantation. Perioperative antibiotics are continued for 5 days, during which time all invasive monitoring lines should have been withdrawn. Anticoagulation with intravenous unfractionated heparin is begun within the first 24 hours following VAD implantation once mediastinal drain tube losses have decreased to <50 mL per hour.

Enteral feedings are initiated with a small-diameter feeding tube. Patients are mobilized early, and aggressive cardiac rehabilitation initiated. Range-of-motion exercises are initiated within 12 to 24 hours. Ambulation begins as soon as invasive hemodynamic monitoring lines are withdrawn (50).

Patients who receive an implantable blood pump have drains placed in the blood pump pocket to avoid a pocket hematoma or seroma that might spontaneously drain through the driveline exit site, thus increasing the risk of driveline or pocket infection. Drainage from the driveline exit site also interferes with tissue in growth at the driveline skin exit site interface and may increase the potential for driveline bacterial colonization. In some centers, the pump pocket drains are not removed until therapeutic levels of oral anticoagulation have been achieved and heparin has been ceased.

The patient who is a candidate for home discharge and the family receive preoperative teaching regarding the concept of MCS (51). This may include a visit by a patient who is currently receiving VAD support. Thereafter, a staged training program is initiated. Following surgery, the patient learns to manage the power source and battery changes. The patient or family member performs driveline exit site care, and both are taught to deal with emergency troubleshooting and management of the VAD. At discharge, community members who might come in contact with the patient also receive specialized training. This list of community members might include local health care providers, community cardiac rehabilitation specialists, emergency medical services, as well as family members or friends. Patients at home on cardiac support devices are also placed on a priority status with their regional utility provider so that in the event of power outage, they will have priority for power restoration.

Anticoagulation for the Ventricular Assist Device Patient

The thrombogenicity of VADs makes the early institution of adequate anticoagulation essential to prevent both systemic thromboembolism and pump thrombosis. This must be balanced against the danger of mediastinal bleeding and tamponade. Postoperative care protocols generally allow the initial hours following implantation without anticoagulation so that initial surgical hemostasis can be achieved. When instituted, anticoagulation should be administered gradually to avoid overshoot in anticoagulation, which can reinstitute postoperative bleeding.

Patients receiving the HeartMate I device receive aspirin, whereas a combination of aspirin and warfarin is provided for all other patients. The therapeutic international normalized ratio is 2.5 to 3.5. While some centers have used thromboelastography to ensure that the patient is an aspirin responder and can provide an objective means by which to dose adjust antiplatelet therapy, we have not incorporated this into our practice.

Avoidance of infection is of paramount importance in the VAD patient who is to subsequently undergo cardiac transplantation with inherent immunosuppression (52). Standard endocarditis prophylaxis is employed when the patient visits the dentist or undergoes any procedure that carries a risk of bacteremia. Superficial driveline or cannula exit site colonization is usually treated with local wound care. If exit site colonization is associated with fever or an elevation in white blood count, empiric antistaphylococcal antibiotic therapy is commenced. The coverage continues for the duration of VAD support. Blood-borne sepsis can lead to VAD endocarditis that carries with it the risk of embolism. If endocarditis develops, consideration should be given to VAD replacement. In addition, sepsis increases the risk of thromboembolic complications, and extra care is needed in this setting to ensure that sufficient anticoagulant therapy is provided. VAD infection is not a contraindication to transplantation.

Heart transplant candidates with an implanted VAD undergo monthly measurement of panel-reactive antibody (PRA) titers (53). The purpose of this test is to identify preformed antibodies in the recipient's serum that may place the recipient at risk for hyperacute rejection or decreased long-term survival following cardiac transplantation (54). Recipients who are at increased risk for the formation of preformed antibodies include those who have had multiple previous blood transfusions or women who have been pregnant.

Ventricular Assist Device Explantation and Cardiac Transplantation

VAD explantation is an operation fraught with risk, particularly with regard to the potential for catastrophic hemorrhage. Notification of the impending transplant to the hospital blood bank is advised, in addition to the crossmatching of a minimum of 6 units of packed cells.

Timing of the cardiac transplant can be complex as these patients require a complex redo sternotomy that can require 2 or even 3 hours of dissection prior to implantation of the donor heart (55). Frequent communication between donor and recipient surgical teams is imperative. Standard antibiotic prophylaxis is employed. The patient is prepped and draped in a routine fashion, with the exception that cannula skin exit sites are excluded from the operative field to avoid mediastinal contamination.

The femoral regions are prepared, but routine peripheral cannulation is not employed. On sternal entry, the inlet side of the pump is not exposed until CPB is initiated to avoid the potential for air embolism. As CPB is initiated, VAD pumping is discontinued and the outlet graft clamped. The recipient cardiectomy and donor implant are performed in a fashion identical to that described in the "Cardiac Transplantation" section. Every effort is made to divide the aorta distal to the outlet graft-to-aortic anastomosis to eliminate the volume of foreign material retained in the mediastinum following cardiac transplant. Following the cardiac transplant and chest closure, the cannula, tubing, or driveline skin exit sites are exposed. These are debrided, irrigated, and closed primarily. Patient management is conventional thereafter.

CARDIAC TRANSPLANTATION

Although it is the established gold-standard therapy for end-stage heart failure, cardiac transplantation is still a therapy in evolution. The optimal immunosuppressive regimen, the optimal implant technique, the best method for myocardial preservation in the donor allograft, and more recently, the role if any of non–brain-dead donors are all subjects of active investigation. Rejection, opportunistic infections, donor allograft vasculopathy, and immunosuppression-related malignancy remain problems in the long-term management of these patients. Only when solutions to these problems have been found will we truly be able to say that cardiac transplantation is a mature therapy.

Cardiac Recipient Selection

Cardiac transplant recipient selection criteria are listed in Table 8.3. The patient must have sufficiently poor cardiac function to justify transplantation, with a comorbidity profile that excludes other major end organ diseases.

The typical candidate has New York Heart Association (NYHA) functional Class 3 or 4 heart failure and has an ejection fraction of <20%. A patient with NYHA Class 3 heart failure can be considered a candidate for transplantation if the measured exercise maximal oxygen consumption (VO_2 max) is <14 mL/kg per minute. Occasionally, a patient with intractable angina and non-bypassable occlusive coronary

TABLE 8.3   Cardiac Transplant Recipient Selection and Exclusion Criteria

Selection criteria
  NYHA Class 4 not amenable to surgical treatment
  Estimated 1-yr mortality >50%
  Chronologic age ≤65 yr
  No systemic illness (other than abnormalities related to heart failure)
  Normal pulmonary artery pressures or reversible pulmonary hypertension
  Emotional stability, with strong family support system

Exclusion criteria
  Fixed pulmonary hypertension
  Irreversible hepatic, renal, or pulmonary disease
  Active systemic or pulmonary infection
  Uncorrected systemic or cerebrovascular disease
  Active peptic ulcer disease
  Active history of substance abuse
  Active malignancy
  Diabetes mellitus with end-organ damage

NYHA, New York Heart Association.

artery disease or a patient with refractory life-threatening ventricular arrhythmias may be considered a candidate for cardiac transplantation despite freedom from NYHA functional Class 3 or 4 heart failure symptoms. Advanced age is a relative contraindication to cardiac transplantation. Although patients older than 65 to 70 years have successfully undergone transplantation, usual selection criteria limit this therapy to patients 65 years or younger (56). The majority of adults who undergo cardiac transplantation suffer from ischemic cardiomyopathy or idiopathic dilated cardiomyopathy, with most being between the ages of 35 and 64 years (57). Occasional older patients are placed on an "alternate waiting list" and may be offered only a donor heart that has been deemed unsuitable for use in patients on the standard waiting list (58).

A recent history of malignancy or other condition which precludes immunosuppression is a contraindication. Normal renal function is optimal, but an estimated GFR >30 mL per minute is acceptable. If GFR is less than 30 mL per minute, combined cardiac and renal transplantation should be considered.

Pulmonary Hypertension and Pulmonary Vascular Resistance

A careful assessment of pulmonary vascular resistance is required given the sensitivity of the donor heart to fail in the presence of pulmonary hypertension, particularly since methods of organ preservation are least effective at protecting the right ventricle. Right-sided heart catheterization is mandatory, and a PVR in excess of 4 Wood Units is a relative contraindication to orthotopic transplant. A PVR less than 4 Wood Units is acceptable for orthotopic transplant. Many centers prefer to measure the transpulmonary gradient (mean pulmonary artery pressure – pulmonary capillary wedge pressure), since at low cardiac output, pulmonary vascular resistance expressed as Wood Units is falsely elevated. A fixed transpulmonary gradient in excess of 15 mm Hg is a relative contraindication to transplantation. A fixed transpulmonary gradient in ≥20 mm Hg is an absolute contraindication to transplantation. Serial assessment of the high PVR patient with optimization of medical therapy is required prior to either including or excluding the patient from the transplant waiting list. We would consider these patients for VAD implantation as a bridge to transplant. Oversizing the donor allograft and the liberal use of perioperative RV MCS can be used as a strategy in borderline cases.

Operative reports from previous cardiac operations should be reviewed, especially in patients with congenital heart disease (59,60). Details of previous operations permit a better estimate of operative risk and may lead to modifications in the donor cardiectomy (61). If the patient has had previous coronary revascularization, knowledge of the presence and location of bypass grafts, and whether or not they are patent, facilitates risk assessment and operative planning.

Once a patient is deemed a suitable candidate for cardiac transplantation, the patient is placed on the cardiac transplant waiting list. The patient is listed with the United Network for Organ Sharing (UNOS) and is assigned a recipient status level. The status level determines the urgency with which the recipient is offered a donor heart. UNOS status levels are listed in Table 8.4 (62). The patient provides the listing center with a 24-hour telephone number and carries a pager to allow the transplant center to contact him or her immediately following a donor heart offer. Transplant waiting list times vary by recipient blood type and body weight, but can measure months to even 2 years (63,64). During that time, the patient is closely monitored and managed medically to preserve end-organ function. If end-organ dysfunction appears, consideration must be given to supporting the patient with a VAD. Any change in the patient's clinical condition would be reflected in the UNOS listing. Up to three quarters of patients are hospitalized or on life support at the time of cardiac transplant. Because of the shortage of donor hearts, up to one third of patients will die while awaiting cardiac transplantation.

Cardiac Donation

Cardiac Donor Selection Criteria

The majority of cardiac donors have suffered a traumatic injury or intracranial hemorrhage (Table 8.5) (65). When a patient fulfills brain death criteria, the regional Organ Procurement Organization (OPO) is

TABLE 8.4	UNOS Cardiac Transplant Recipient Status
Status 1A	The patient is admitted to the listing transplant center hospital and has at least one of the following:
	Mechanical circulatory support (VAD ≤30 d),[a] artificial heart, IABP
	Mechanical circulatory support >30 d, with device-related complication
	Mechanical ventilation
	High-dose inotropes, continuous hemodynamic monitoring
	Life expectancy <7 d
Status 1B	At least one of the following:
	VAD >30 d without complication
	Continuous i.v. infusion of inotropes
Status 2	All other actively listed patients
Status 7	Patient temporarily removed from the transplant waiting list

IABP, intra-aortic balloon pump; UNOS, United Network for Organ Sharing; VAD, ventricular assist device.
[a]VAD patients are permitted to accumulate 30 d of Status 1A time, following VAD implantation, regardless of whether or not they are hospitalized.

	Cardiac Donor Selection and Exclusion Criteria

Selection Criteria
Pronounced brain dead
Age < 46 yr (advanced age warrants further cardiac work-up)
No history of cardiac disease
Minimal vasopressor support
Normal hemodynamics
Normal echocardiographic wall motion
No untreated bacterial infection

Exclusion Criteria
Closed-chest injury resulting in myocardial contusion
Known history of cardiac disease (previous cardiac operation or history of ischemic or valvular heart disease)
Systemic infection including hepatitis B or C positivity
Unwitnessed cardiac arrest or prolonged cardiac resuscitation
HIV positivity or history of high-risk behavior
Systemic malignancy (primary brain tumor excluded)

HIV, human immunodeficiency virus.

notified of the presence of a potential organ donor. Informed consent for specific organ donation is obtained from the donor's nearest relative, and the OPO personnel assumes both medical and financial responsibility for the donor's care. OPO personnel access the UNOS transplant waiting list, and the heart is offered to a recipient based upon blood type, body weight, status, and time spent on the waiting list.

On receipt of a heart offer, the surgeon should request details concerning the donor's demise, including the cause of death, resuscitative efforts, if any, and events of note during the donor's hospitalization. The heart offer is directed to a specific recipient on the transplant waiting list. The blood types of both donor and recipient are confirmed, and the donor weight and height are requested to ensure that the size match between donor and recipient is appropriate. When a recipient is listed for transplantation, the cardiac transplant center is asked to select a minimum acceptable weight for a cardiac donor. Traditionally, the minimum acceptable weight for the cardiac donor is 80% of the recipient's body weight (66). However, matching by donor and recipient height is far more useful, since weight does not always reflect lean body mass, and proper height matching leads to improved matching of great vessel size. In general for dilated cardiomyopathy, using hearts that are slightly oversized is desirable. However, a donor who is 4 to 6 inches shorter than the recipient is usually safe for use. In patients with a smaller pericardial sac, such as those with restrictive myopathy or a VAD *in situ*, size matching is critical. We prefer to undersize such recipients to avoid transplanted heart tamponade.

If the potential donor has suffered from blunt chest injury, the electrocardiogram and cardiac enzymes are carefully reviewed. The electrocardiogram should be normal, although global ST-segment abnormalities and T-wave changes can occur in association with head trauma, unrelated to myocardial injury. The creatine phosphokinase determination is often difficult to interpret in the multiply injured patient due to skeletal muscle injury. Creatine phosphokinase isoenzymes or troponin allows identification of a myocardial source. The donor with a significant myocardial contusion is excluded from consideration for cardiac donation.

Potential cardiac donors undergo an echocardiogram to assess global ventricular function (67). Segmental wall motion abnormalities are located, valvular function is assessed, and valvular vegetations, if present, are identified. Echocardiography is useful to exclude structural heart disease; however, caution should be exercised is using transthoracic echo to evaluate LV function in this scenario. Regional wall motion abnormalities which resolve posttransplant are commonly seen, and their significance in an otherwise healthy donor is dubious.

Cardiac catheterization is used selectively in donors (68). Coronary angiography is strongly recommended in any donor >55 years of age. Coronary angiography is recommended in male donors 46 to 55 years of age and female donors 51 to 55 years of age. In males ≤45 years of age or females ≤50 years of age, angiography is recommended if the donor has ≥3 coronary disease risk factors. Angiography is strongly recommended or mandated for donors with a cocaine use history.

As part of the cardiac recipient screening process, a PRA screen is performed. If the PRA is >10% (and at some centers, if the PRA is anything other than 0%) a lymphocytotoxic cross-match is performed. For this, lymph node tissue from the prospective donor is mixed with the prospective recipient's serum. If the recipient serum contains preformed antibodies to the donor lymph node tissue, the test is positive and identifies the recipient as being at increased risk for hyperacute rejection if the donor heart is utilized. This usually precludes the use of this heart in this recipient.

Donor Management

Although the OPO is responsible for donor management, the transplant surgeon may be called upon to provide input (69,70). Appropriate management of the potential donor will serve to maximize the use of organs. Patients with a neurologic injury have often been fluid restricted. In addition, donors frequently suffer from diabetes insipidus. As a result, there is usually a volume deficit that must be corrected and will allow the weaning of inappropriate vasopressors.

Donors should have at the minimum a CVP and an arterial line for monitoring. Mean arterial blood pressure should exceed 60 mm Hg at a CVP of 5 to 10 mm Hg. If these criteria are met in the context of an ejection fraction ≥50% on echocardiography, it is safe to proceed. We advocate that all donors receive hormonal resuscitation comprising thyroid hormone, vasopressin, insulin, and corticosteroids. A review of the UNOS database shows that this hormonal replacement leads to increased utilization of all thoracic and abdominal organs and improved organ function. We also favor aggressive use of pulmonary artery catheters and apply the hemodynamic criteria codified at the Crystal City Consensus Conference to determine suitability (71).

Donor Cardiectomy

The heart is usually retrieved as part of a multiorgan harvest. Timing of donor cardiectomy is determined by the number of organs being retrieved, the transportation time between the donor and recipient hospitals, and the complexity of mediastinal dissection in the recipient. The issue of timing between donor and recipient operations is critical to minimize the donor heart ischemic time.

A midline incision is created from the suprasternal notch to the symphysis pubis. The heart is inspected to ensure that there are no signs of cardiac trauma. Chamber size and regional wall motion abnormalities can be identified by visual inspection or transesophageal echocardiography, if available. The surface of the heart should be gently palpated to identify occult coronary artery plaques, although care is taken in palpating the heart, as the donor heart tends to be prone to arrhythmias. Gross valvular lesions can be assessed with palpation.

The mediastinal dissection required for donor cardiectomy is minimal. The SVC and azygous vein are dissected free and encircled with a silk tie. The plane between aorta and pulmonary artery is opened. The pleuropericardial reflections are incised and lungs are inspected at this time if lung retrieval is required.

The abdominal team then completes the dissection prior to cardiac removal. When the chest and abdominal dissections are complete, the donor is fully heparinized. A cardioplegia needle is inserted into the ascending aorta (Fig. 8.5). The SVC and azygous veins are ligated and the inferior vena cava (IVC) is divided. Warm blood is evacuated from the chest to facilitate myocardial cooling. Alternatively, if the IVC is vented in the abdomen, the IVC is clamped above the diaphragm and divided above the clamp. This keeps warm blood out of the chest and minimizes the risk of injury to the hepatic veins. After venting the heart through the IVC, the aorta is cross-clamped and cold hyperkalemic cardioplegia administered into the aortic root (72). The left heart is

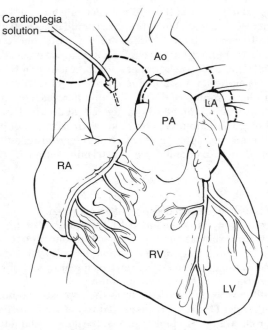

FIGURE 8.5 Schematic of donor cardiectomy. Cold cardioplegia is administered into the aortic root after an aortic cross-clamp is applied. The heart is vented by transecting the inferior vena cava and left inferior pulmonary vein. If there is a simultaneous lung dona-tion, the left-sided heart is vented by opening the left atrial appendage. Once the heart is arrested, the donor cardiectomy is completed by dividing the superior vena cava and remaining pulmonary veins and transecting the great vessels along the dotted lines shown in the figure. Ao, aorta; LA, left atrium; LV, left ventricle; PA, pulmonary artery; RA, right atrium; RV, right ventricle.

vented by cutting a pulmonary vein or in the case of concomitant lung retrieval, by cutting the left atrial appendage.

Although a variety of cardioplegic solutions have been employed, we find a simple, commercially available cardioplegia solution easiest to use in the variety of settings where organ donations occur (Plegisol™, Hospira). Ice-cold normal saline is applied to the surface of the heart as a topical coolant.

Following cardioplegia administration, the heart is excised. The supe-rior vena cava is divided well above the cavoatrial junction to avoid injur-ing the sinoatrial node, higher if the bicaval implant technique is used. The pulmonary veins are divided individually. The aorta is divided at the level of the innominate artery, and either the distal main pulmonary artery or the right and left main pulmonary arteries are divided. The donor cardiectomy is modified in the face of a simultaneous lung retrieval. If the lungs are being retrieved from the same donor, the donor cardiectomy can proceed in one of two ways. The donor heart can be removed first with the lungs to follow. Alternatively, the heart–lung bloc can be excised and moved to a back table where the three organs are separated (73). Regardless of technique employed, if the lungs are being retrieved, the pulmonary veins must accompany the lungs. The donor heart is briefly inspected for a patent foramen ovale, which if identified is closed. The valves are inspected to ensure that there is no evidence of occult endocarditis or valve abnormality. The heart is packaged in layered plastic bags filled with ice-cold saline solution, and the packaged heart is placed in an ice-filled cooler for transportation to the recipient hospital.

Cardiac Recipient Management

Cardiac Recipient Preparation

When the recipient hospital is contacted by the OPO with a cardiac offer, the heart is accepted for a specific patient on the cardiac transplant waiting list. If the PRA is elevated, a cross-match is performed using donor lymphocytes and recipient serum that is stored at the tissue-typing center and updated monthly. That recipient is immediately contacted and questioned with regard to the presence of any new conditions that might be a contraindication to transplantation such as an acute infection. The potential recipient is asked to take nothing further by mouth and to travel to the hospital immediately. On arrival, a history and physical examination are performed to confirm that the potential recipient remains a suitable candidate.

The recipient's anterior chest, abdomen, and both anterior thighs are clipped, and the patient subsequently showers with chlorhexidine. If the patient has been receiving warfarin, the prothrombin time may be corrected with vitamin K and fresh frozen plasma as indicated. Monitoring lines include a radial arterial line, one or two large-bore peripheral intravenous catheters, and a central venous catheter. We employ a pulmonary artery catheter routinely in all cardiac transplant recipients. This catheter is inserted via the left internal jugular vein, thereby preserving the right internal jugular vein for subsequent cardiac biopsies. It is important that all catheters and lines be inserted with meticulous sterile technique.

Preoperative immunosuppressive agents are administered according to the schedules described below. The patients receive gram-positive and gram-negative antibiotic coverage (vancomycin and levofloxacin). Perioperative antibiotic coverage continues for 48 hours following cardiac transplantation.

Timing of the Donor and Recipient Operations

Perhaps the most challenging portion of the cardiac transplant procedure is the timing of both the donor and the recipient cardiectomy. The
primary focus of this portion of the operation is to minimize the period
of time between application of the aortic cross-clamp in the donor and
removal of the aortic cross-clamp in the recipient. Myocardial preservation is always important, but this is particularly true in cardiac transplantation when the donor heart is sometimes undersized and is
expected to perform in a setting of pulmonary hypertension following a
period of prolonged ischemia. The donor heart should arrive as the
recipient cardiectomy is being completed. Close communication
between the cardiac and abdominal organ retrieval teams is paramount,
as abdominal organ retrieval time can vary dramatically depending
upon organs to be retrieved, as well as anatomic hurdles encountered
during the abdominal organ dissection.

Implant team considerations can have a profound impact upon the
speed with which the cardiac recipient is taken to the operating room.
It may take several hours for the patient simply to arrive at the hospital.
Preformed antibodies in the recipient's blood and the requisite lymphocytotoxic cross-match may require several additional hours prior to
determining that the potential recipient is suitable. In this instance, we
often bring a second backup recipient to the hospital to minimize any
potential delay should the lymphocytotoxic cross-match be positive in
the primary recipient. In addition, a patient who has had previous cardiac surgery or has a VAD *in situ* may require multiple hours of additional dissection before reaching the point in the operation when donor
heart implantation can occur.

The recipient is moved to the operating room well in advance of
the anticipated anesthetic induction time. We prefer that the recipient
not be anesthetized until the donor team has actually visualized the
donor heart and has communicated that it is functioning satisfactorily.
At that time, the recipient operation begins.

Recipient Operative Management

The beginning of anesthesia is dictated by the progress of the donor
operation. Because the recipient has advanced heart failure, anesthetic
induction and maintenance require careful monitoring and pharmacologic management. A narcotic-based anesthetic is employed to minimize myocardial depression. Volume administration is minimized, and
filling pressures are monitored with invasive hemodynamic monitoring
lines. The recipient cardiectomy is performed through a median sternotomy. CPB employs bicaval venous cannulation and aortic cannulation. If the recipient has had previous cardiac surgery or if a VAD is in

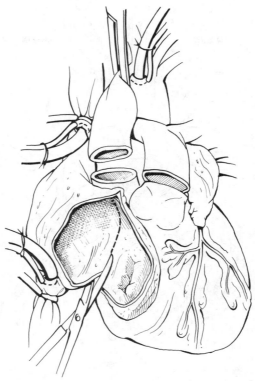

FIGURE 8.6 The recipient cardiectomy. The patient is placed on cardiopulmonary bypass using bicaval venous cannulation and aortic arterial cannulation. The heart is isolated from the blood path with caval snares and the aortic cross-clamp. The great vessels are divided at the level of the semilunar valves. The ventricles are removed by dividing the atria along the atrioventricular groove.

place, the femoral vessels may be accessed for arterial cannulation and inferior vena caval return, if necessary. If the patient is grossly fluid overloaded, we employ continuous ultrafiltration during CPB for volume removal. The patient is cooled to a core temperature of 28°C. The aorta is cross-clamped, and caval snares are applied to isolate the heart from the blood path. The recipient cardiectomy is accomplished by dividing the atria along the atrioventricular grooves (Fig. 8.6) (74). The great vessels are divided just distal to the semilunar valves. The recipient's left atrial appendage is excised to eliminate a potential source for intracardiac thrombus formation. The tips of the commissures are maintained on the pulmonary artery to facilitate orientation of the

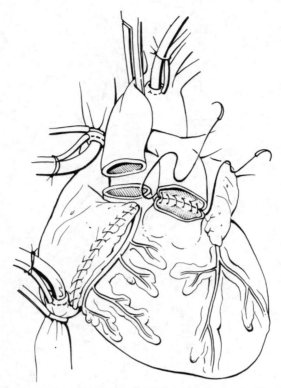

FIGURE 8.7 The cardiac implant is accomplished by anastomosing the donor atrial cuffs to their recipient counterparts. The great vessel anastomoses follow. Care is taken to avoid injuring the donor sinoatrial node.

pulmonary artery as the donor heart is implanted. This avoids pulmonary artery torsion, a potential cause of right-sided heart failure in the donor heart. Although the intrapericardial dissection is performed prior to the arrival of the donor heart, the recipient cardiectomy is not usually completed until the donor heart has safely arrived in the hospital.

During implantation, we give a dose of cold, blood cardioplegia via the aortic root at the start of the implant and between each anastomosis in addition to topical hypothermia. The donor implant is accomplished by anastomosing the left followed by the right atrial cuffs to the recipient counterparts (Fig. 8.7). The pulmonary artery anastomosis follows. Care is taken to trim the pulmonary artery to the appropriate length to avoid redundancy of this vessel that can result in kinking and

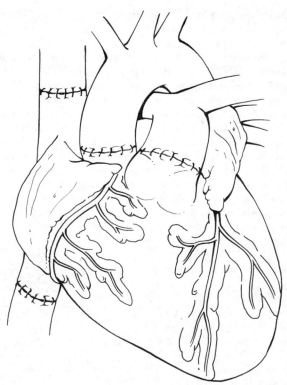

FIGURE 8.8 The bicaval cardiac implant utilizes the standard left atrial cuff anastomosis. However, the donor right atrium is not opened. The donor superior and inferior venae cavae are anastomosed directly to the recipient cavae.

increased afterload to the right-sided heart. Rewarming is completed as the aortic anastomosis is performed. Before completing the aortic anastomosis, the caval snares are removed, and the heart is permitted to fill with blood. The heart is de-aired and the aortic anastomosis completed.

We have converted from the standard biatrial implant technique to a bicaval implant technique (Fig. 8.8) (75,76). In the latter procedure, the recipient right atrium is excised in its entirety, and the recipient superior and inferior vena cavae are divided at the point at which they would normally have entered the recipient right atrium, leaving small cuffs of right atrial tissue attached to the cavae. The implant technique is modified such that a caval-to-caval anastomosis is performed on both the superior and the inferior vena cavae. This eliminates the redundant right atrium associated with the standard biatrial technique. Proponents of this procedure note improved right ventricular performance and reduction in the incidence of tricuspid regurgitation and perhaps a reduced incidence of atrial arrhythmias. Despite the anatomic elegance of the bicaval technique, the data are not conclusive that there are any clinically significant differences in long-term outcomes (77,78).

The patient usually converts to sinus rhythm upon release of the aortic cross-clamp. Because the donor heart is denervated, the recipient will require chronotropic support. Although we place temporary pacing wires on both the donor atrium and the ventricle, chronotropic support is usually achieved with isoproterenol (1 to 4 μg per minute i.v.). The goal is a heart rate of approximately 100 beats per minute, recognizing that younger hearts are much more responsive to this intravenous medication. If the donor heart does not respond to isoproterenol administration, temporary pacing can be employed. Atrial pacing or atrioventricular sequential pacing are the most physiologically effective pacing modes.

Right Ventricular Failure Posttransplant. Patients with chronic heart failure frequently have elevated pulmonary artery pressures and pulmonary vascular resistance. Analogous to the measures outlined earlier for managing RV function in the setting of LVAD implantation, the donor heart is particularly susceptible to right ventricular failure, as it is not accustomed to the increased afterload. In addition, size mismatch and the RV's enhanced susceptibility to injury during the procurement process and from prolonged ischemic times increase the risk of perioperative failure (79).

Management of right heart physiology is therefore critical in cardiac transplantation. Following release of the aortic cross-clamp, the CVP should be carefully monitored as CPB is discontinued. A CVP >15 mm Hg is a warning sign of impending trouble. Care should be used to avoid right-sided overload, particularly if blood products are needed to reverse coagulopathy. Isoproterenol is the drug of choice for support of right ventricular function as it increases the donor heart rate, has a positive inotropic effect, and reduces pulmonary vascular resistance. Right ventricular contractility is evaluated visually, and if impaired, milrinone, epinephrine, or dobutamine can be added to the drug regimen. Inhaled nitric oxide (10 to 20 parts per million) should be administered as a PVR-reducing agent irrespective of measured pulmonary pressures (80).

Profound RV failure requires mechanical support with an IABP, RVAD, or ECMO. An IABP may be sufficient if difficult to maintain systemic pressures are compromising RV function; however, profound RV failure requires more definitive therapy. The biventricular support provided by ECMO, despite the higher risks it presents with bleeding and thromboembolic complications, is potentially better at unloading the RV and facilitating recovery (81,82). If recovery of the right ventricle is achieved, excellent long-term outcomes can be anticipated, with survival equivalent to the patient who did not require perioperative support (83).

Many heart transplant recipients have received preoperative warfarin, and the warfarin effect may be reversed preoperatively, although time may not always allow for this and it may not be necessary (84). If the associated coagulopathy has not been corrected preoperatively, up to 8 U of fresh frozen plasma can be added to the CPB circuit during terminal rewarming. Excess water is removed with hemofiltration during CPB. Postoperatively, the patient will often require transfusion with either blood or blood products. This is particularly true in patients who have had a previous sternotomy or who have been supported with a VAD. Packed red blood cells and platelets are administered through a leukodepletion filter to avoid an antigen load. Clotting factor administration contributes to increased pulmonary vascular resistance (and, thus, right ventricular dysfunction). Intraoperative blood loss is minimized and transfusions given only as required.

Postoperative Management

Hemodynamics

In the absence of hyperacute rejection or a problem with donor heart preservation, the left ventricle usually contracts satisfactorily following cardiac transplant (85). Right ventricular dysfunction, however, can result in central venous hypertension and inadequate left ventricular preload. The CVP is carefully monitored, and right ventricular distention is avoided. Within 24 to 48 hours, the pulmonary vascular resistance usually falls, and medications used for right-sided heart support can be weaned. Tricuspid regurgitation, if present, usually improves as the pulmonary artery pressures fall. Chronotropic support with isoproterenol is often required for 4 to 7 days depending upon the patient's heart rate. Isoproterenol can be administered peripherally and does not require intensive care unit monitoring. Thus, this drug can be slowly withdrawn over a number of days using the heart rate as the end point. Early in the postoperative course, we attempt to maintain a heart rate above 90 beats per minute. Toward the end of the first postoperative week, we accept a heart rate above 70 to 80 beats per minute.

Infection

Patients undergoing heart transplantation receive perioperative antibiotic prophylaxis for both gram-positive and gram-negative organisms that is continued postoperatively until the mediastinal tubes and lines are removed, usually 48 hours following the heart transplant. Patient isolation and reverse precautions are not employed; however, traffic is minimized in the patient room. More important, all personnel who enter the patient room utilize good hand-washing technique.

Cytomegalovirus (CMV) and *Toxoplasmosis gondii* can be transmitted from a seropositive donor into a seronegative recipient. CMV, in particular, can produce a flulike syndrome with pneumonitis, enteritis, and hepatitis (86). Patients infected with CMV appear to be at increased risk for accelerated allograft coronary artery disease. Recipients who are seronegative preoperatively that receive a heart from a CMV-seropositive donor are treated with intravenous ganciclovir for 21 days, followed by oral ganciclovir for 3 months, followed by oral acyclovir for 1 year. CMV-seropositive recipients who receive a seropositive donor heart are treated prophylactically with intravenous ganciclovir until hospital discharge. This is followed by oral acyclovir. Seronegative recipients who receive a seronegative donor heart receive oral acyclovir starting immediately following extubation. CMV titers are checked every 6 months. If seroconversion occurs, oral ganciclovir is administered for 3 months, followed by oral acyclovir for 3 months. In all of these scenarios, low-dose oral acyclovir is continued for a minimum of 1 year following transplantation. Acyclovir is discontinued thereafter, provided the prednisone dose is <10 mg per day.

Seronegative recipients for *T. gondii* who receive a seropositive donor heart are prophylactically treated with pyrimethamine and folinic acid for 6 weeks (87). Oral candidiasis ("thrush") is prevalent in the immunosuppressed patient population. To avoid this infectious complication, the recipients receive nystatin oral suspension (100,000 U/mL, 5-mL p.o. swish and swallow after meals and at bedtime) for 4 to 6 weeks. Prophylaxis against *Pneumocystis carinii* consists of trimethoprim and sulfamethoxazole.

Immunosuppression

The drug protocols used for immune suppression therapy of cardiac transplant recipients vary from institution to institution and are constantly changing. The purpose of this discussion is to provide general patient care guidelines and examples of commonly used therapeutic regimens. Immunosuppression begins prior to the cardiac transplant (88–90). The backbone of immunosuppressive protocols is *triple-drug therapy*, utilizing a calcineurin inhibitor (cyclosporine or tacrolimus), mycophenolate mofetil, and steroids. We do not routinely use antilymphocyte preparations for "induction." However, we have a low threshold for using these cytolytic agents and delaying addition of a calcineurin inhibitor in patients with perioperative renal dysfunction. Our preference is to use rabbit antithymocyte globulin (Thymoglobulin™, Genzyme Corp.) and we adjust dosage to achieve an absolute CD3 count of 50 to 100.

An alternative immunosuppressive protocol commonly used in adult cardiac transplant recipients employs a monoclonal antibody specific for the activated T-cell interleukin-2 (IL-2) receptor (91). IL-2 receptor blockers are very safe but have less efficacy than antilymphocyte preparations. As with rabbit antithymocyte globulin, the IL-2 receptor blockers provide sufficient immunosuppression to delay the institution of calcineurin inhibitors (92).

Other Management Issues

If the cardiac transplant has been performed uneventfully and the implanted heart functions satisfactorily, the patient is weaned from mechanical ventilation and rapidly extubated. Chronic left ventricular dysfunction is frequently associated with preoperative pulmonary congestion. Postoperatively, the patient receives diuretic drug treatment to eliminate excess pulmonary extravascular lung water. To avoid a precipitous decline in preload, this diuresis is most effectively accomplished with a continuous furosemide infusion (adult dose 5 to 40 mg per hour i.v.) to maintain a urine output of 50 to 100 mL more than the total intravenous fluid intake each hour. Rapid extubation reduces the potential for hospital-acquired pneumonia. The incidence of infectious complications is further reduced by early withdrawal of percutaneous lines and tubes, including the urinary drainage catheter. Patients with chronic heart failure frequently suffer cardiac cachexia. Enteral nutritional via a feeding tube is instituted if the patient is unable to meet his or her caloric need in the first 48 hours following cardiac transplant. Cardiac transplant recipients, with the exclusion of those supported with a VAD, are usually deconditioned by their chronic heart failure. Therefore, physical therapy is begun in the intensive care unit following extubation (93).

Chronically ill heart failure patients who have a protracted hospitalization related to cardiac transplantation are at risk for the development of stress ulcers and thus are treated prophylactically with ranitidine or lansoprazole. Postoperative anemia is treated, in part, with iron sulfate (325 mg p.o.b.i.d., before meals), beginning on postoperative day 7, for 6 weeks. Aspirin (81 mg p.o. every day) is administered beginning on postoperative day 7. Patients who receive chronic steroid therapy are at risk for the development of osteoporosis (94). All patients receive calcium carbonate (500 mg p.o. t.i.d.) beginning on postoperative day 3 and a daily multivitamin that contains 400 IU of vitamin D beginning on day 7. Because patients who receive cyclosporine frequently develop hyperlipidemia, pravastatin (10 mg p.o. every day) is administered beginning on postoperative day 7 (95).

Long-Term Problems

Rejection

The risk of acute rejection is highest in the first 3 months following cardiac transplantation. Thereafter, the risk of rejection decreases but remains constant (96). Risk factors for rejection during the first year following cardiac transplantation include a recipient of younger age, a donor or recipient of female gender, CMV positivity, or a recipient who has had a significant prior infection. After 1 year following cardiac transplantation, the risk of recurrent rejection is more common in patients who have a CMV infection or who experienced multiple rejection episodes during the first posttransplant year. Cardiac rejection is often presaged by unexplained weight gain, unexplained arrhythmia, decrease in blood pressure, or increase in heart rate. Rejection surveillance is accomplished using endomyocardial biopsies. The first biopsy is performed 7 days following transplant and is followed by weekly or biweekly biopsies for the next 2 months. Thereafter, the biopsy schedule is individualized according to the occurrence of rejection. At the minimum, an endomyocardial biopsy is performed on an annual basis. The biopsy tissue is histologically graded according to the International Society for Heart & Lung Transplantation (ISHLT) criteria (Table 8.6) (97).

Patients who develop mild cellular rejection (ISHLT grade 1B, 2, or 3A) are treated with a prednisone pulse (50 mg p.o. b.i.d. for 5 days) followed by a taper in the dose back to the maintenance schedule. If there is hemodynamic instability, we would favor using cytolytic therapy with rabbit antithymocyte globulin, ATGAM, OKT3, or alemtuzumab. The patient is observed and undergoes a repeat biopsy in 7 to 14 days.

Moderate cellular rejection (ISHLT grade 3A, 3B, or 4) is treated in a manner dictated by the presence or absence of hemodynamic compromise. If the patient has no hemodynamic instability, pulse steroid

TABLE 8.6	International Society for Heart & Lung Transplantation Standardized Cardiac Biopsy Grading Scale
Grade	**Histologic Findings**
No rejection	–
1A	Focal (perivascular or interstitial) infiltrate without necrosis
1B	Diffuse but sparse infiltrate without necrosis; one focus only with aggressive infiltration and/or focal myocyte damage
3A	Multifocal aggressive infiltrates and/or myocyte damage
3B	Diffuse inflammatory process with necrosis; diffuse aggressive polymorphous infiltrate, ± edema, ± hemorrhage, ± vasculitis, with necrosis

coverage is provided using methylprednisolone followed by oral prednisone. If the patient demonstrates hemodynamic compromise as defined by the presence of relative hypotension (systolic blood pressure 20 mm Hg less than baseline), a new third heart sound, increase in jugular venous pressure, or a decrease in left ventricular systolic function as evidenced by echocardiography, the patient receives antithymocyte globulin, parenteral methylprednisolone, and then oral prednisone.

Infection

The patient experiences the greatest risk for infection in the immediate postoperative period and during periods of augmented immunosuppression used for the treatment of rejection (98). Infection is more common in older patients, those who have required mechanical ventilation or MCS prior to transplantation, and those for whom monoclonal antibody therapy was used for immunosuppression induction. Viral and bacterial infections predominate in this patient population. Any patient who demonstrates a fever or rise in white blood count should be aggressively examined, recognizing that a leukocytosis may accompany steroid treatment. The examination and management of a patient with suspected sepsis include wound and catheter site examination, urinalysis, sputum and blood cultures, and a chest radiograph. Should the patient develop a fever or evidence of peripheral thrombophlebitis, the intravenous catheter should be moved to a new site. In general, antibiotic therapy is reserved for treatment of a known infection.

Malignancy

Malignancies are the second most common cause of late death in patients who undergo a cardiac transplant, occurring in up to 15% of patients (99). The most common tumors are cutaneous neoplasms, non-Hodgkin's lymphoma, and lung cancer. Lymphoproliferative disorders occur more commonly in patients who received high-dose immunosuppressive therapy or induction therapy with OKT3. Lymphoproliferative malignancies, in particular B-cell lymphomas, are more common in recipients who were seronegative for the Epstein–Barr virus prior to transplant. When suspected, the cancers are diagnosed using standard techniques. Treatment is tumor specific and includes a reduction in the immunosuppressive dose.

Allograft Coronary Artery Disease

The etiology of allograft coronary artery disease is multifactorial (100,101). Because the donor heart is denervated, cardiac transplant recipients rarely present with angina. Shortness of breath, diaphoresis, nausea, edema, and a new cardiac murmur are suggestive of myocardial ischemia. Allograft coronary artery disease is the most common cause of late death following transplantation. Thus, vigilance must be maintained throughout the life of the transplant patient. Two months following cardiac transplantation, the patient undergoes right- and left-sided heart catheterization, including coronary angiography to provide a baseline evaluation with which subsequent coronary angiograms can be compared. Thereafter, patients undergo an annual assessment of left ventricular ejection fraction, echocardiogram, and cardiac catheterization to assess hemodynamics and coronary anatomy. If occlusive coronary artery disease or ventricular dysfunction develops, the frequency of follow-up is increased to every 6 months. Allograft coronary artery disease does not present as typical native coronary artery disease with segmental stenoses. Rather, the coronary arteries taper throughout their length, providing an angiographic appearance of a "pruned tree." These findings can sometimes be subtle, making it important to compare the current angiogram with the angiogram obtained previously. The only effective treatment for allograft coronary artery disease is repeat cardiac transplantation (102).

References

1. Ferguson JJ III, Cohen M, Freedman RJ Jr, et al. The current practice of intraaortic balloon counterpulsation: results from the Benchmark Registry. *JACC* 2001;381:456–462.
2. Duncan BW. Mechanical support for infants and children with cardiac disease. *Ann Thorac Surg* 2002;73:1670–1677.
3. Baskett RJF, Ghali WA, Maitland A, et al. The intraaortic balloon pump in cardiac surgery (review). *Ann Thorac Surg* 2002;74:1276–1287.
4. Dietl CA, Berkheimer MD, Woods EL, et al. Efficacy and cost-effectiveness of preoperative IABP in patients with ejection fraction of 0.25 or less. *Ann Thorac Surg* 1996;62:401–409.
5. Christenson JT, Simonet F, Badel P, et al. Optimal timing of preoperative intraaortic balloon pump support in high-risk coronary patients. *Ann Thorac Surg* 1999;68:934–939.
6. Kang N, Edwards M, Larbalestier R. Preoperative intraaortic balloon pumps in high-risk patients undergoing open heart surgery. *Ann Thorac Surg* 2001;72:54–57.
7. Burack JH, Uceda P, Cunningham JN. Transthoracic intraaortic balloon pump: a simplified technique. *Ann Thorac Surg* 1996;62:299–301.
8. Arafa OE, Pedersen TH, Svennevig JL, et al. Vascular complications of the intraaortic balloon pump in patients undergoing open heart operations: a 15-year experience. *Ann Thorac Surg* 1999;67:645–651.
9. De Robertis F, Birks EJ, Rogers P, et al. Clinical performance with the Levitronix Centrimag short-term ventricular assist device. *J Heart Lung Transplant* 2006;25:181–186.

10. Frazier OH, Rose EA, Oz MC, et al. Multicenter clinical evaluation of the HeartMate vented electric left ventricular assist system in patients awaiting heart transplantation. *J Thorac Cardiovasc Surg* 2001;122:1186–1195.

11. Holman WL, Kormos RL, Naftel DC, et al. Predictors of death and transplant in patients with a mechanical circulatory support device: a multi-institutional study. *J Heart Lung Transplant* 2009;28:44–50.

12. Farrar DJ, Hill JD, Pennington DG, et al. Preoperative and postoperative comparison of patients with univentricular and biventricular support with the Thoratec ventricular assist device as a bridge to cardiac transplantation. *J Thorac Cardiovasc Surg* 1997;113:202–209.

13. Zimpfer D, Zrunek P, Roethy W, et al. Left ventricular assist devices decrease fixed pulmonary hypertension in cardiac transplant candidates. *J Thorac Cardiovasc Surg* 2007;133:689–695.

14. Hoy FBY, Mueller DK, Geiss DM, et al. Bridge to recovery for postcardiotomy failure: is there still a role for centrifugal pumps? *Ann Thorac Surg* 2000; 70:1259–1263.

15. Curtis JJ, Walls JT, Wagner-Mann CC, et al. Centrifugal pumps: description of devices and surgical techniques. *Ann Thorac Surg* 1999;68:666–671.

16. Chung DA, Kizner L, Al-Deiri M, et al. Clinical utility of the Levitronix CentriMag™ in extracorporeal membrane oxygenation for severe cardiogenic shock. *J Heart Lung Transplant* 2007;26(suppl):S86–S87.

17. Bruschi G, Cannata A, Russo, et al. Single center experience with the Levitronix CentriMag™ circulatory support system as short-term cardiac assist in different clinical scenarios. *J Heart Lung Transplant* 2008;27(suppl):S154–155.

18. De Robertis F, Rogers P, Amrani M, et al. Bridge to decision using the Levitronix CentriMag™ short-term ventricular assist device. *J Heart Lung Transplant* 2008;27:474–478.

19. Sezai A, Minami K, El-Banayosy A, et al. Mechanical circulatory support with Abiomed BVS 5000 and BioMedicus BP-80 for postcardiotomy cardiogenic shock. *J Congest Heart Failure Circ Support* 2001;1:445–448.

20. Samuels LE, Holmes EC, Thomas MP, et al. Management of acute cardiac failure with mechanical assist: experience with the Abiomed BVS 5000. *Ann Thorac Surg* 2001;71:S67–S72.

21. Morgan JA, Stewart AS, Lee BJ, et al. Role of the Abiomed BVS 5000 device for short-term support and bridge to transplantation. *ASAIO J* 2004;50:360–363.

22. Farrar DJ. The Thoratec ventricular assist device: a paracorporeal pump for treating acute and chronic heart failure. *Semin Thorac Cardiovasc Surg* 2000;12:243–250.

23. Radovancevic B, Vrtovec B, de Kort E, et al. End-organ function in patients on long term circulatory support with continuous- or pulsatile-flow assist devices. *J Heart Lung Transplant* 2008;26:815–818.

24. Drews T, Jurmann M, Michael D, et al. Differences in pulsatile and non-pulsatile mechanical circulatory support in long-term use. *J Heart Lung Transplant* 2008;27:1096–1101.

25. Ochiai Y, McCarthy PM, Smedira NG, et al. Predictors of severe right ventricular dysfunction after implantable left ventricular assist device insertion: analysis of 245 patients. *Circulation* 2002;106 (Suppl 1):I198–202.

26. Santamore WP, Gray LA Jr. Left ventricular contributions to right ventricular systolic function during LVAD support. *Ann Thorac Surg* 1996;61:350–356.

27. Goldstein DJ, Oz MC. Mechanical support for postcardiotomy cardiogenic shock. *Semin Thorac Cardiovasc Surg* 2000;12:220–228.

28. Richenbacher WE. Ventricular assistance for postcardiotomy cardiogenic shock. In: Richenbacher WE, ed. *Mechanical Circulatory Support*. Austin, TX: Landes BioScience, 1999:78–105.
29. Mickleborough LL, Carson S, Tamariz M, et al. Results of revascularization in patients with severe left ventricular dysfunction. *J Thorac Cardiovasc Surg* 2000;119:550–557.
30. Samuels LE, Kaufman MS, Thomas MP, et al. Pharmacological criteria for ventricular assist device insertion following postcardiotomy shock: experience with the Abiomed BVS system. *J Cardiac Surg* 1999;14:288–293.
31. DiCorte CJ, Van Meter CH Jr. Abiomed RVAD and LVAD implantation. *Oper Tech Thorac Cardiovasc Surg* 1999;4:301–317.
32. Pae WE Jr, Lundblad O. Thoratec paracorporeal pneumatic ventricular assist device. *Oper Tech Thorac Cardiovasc Surg* 1999;4:352–368.
33. Argenziano M, Choudhri AF, Moazami N, et al. Randomized, double-blind trial of inhaled nitric oxide in LVAD recipients with pulmonary hypertension. *Ann Thorac Surg* 1998;65:340–345.
34. Fukamachi K, McCarthy PM, Smedira NG, et al. Preoperative risk factors for right ventricular failure after implantable left ventricular assist device insertion. *Ann Thorac Surg* 1999;68:2181–2184.
35. Pavie A, Szefner J, Leger P, et al. Preventing, minimizing, and managing postoperative bleeding. *Ann Thorac Surg* 1999;68:705–710.
36. Rose EA, Gelijns AC, Moskowitz AJ, et al. Long-term mechanical left ventricular assistance for end-stage heart failure. *N Engl J Med* 2001;345:1435–1443.
37. Chen JM, Spanier TB, Gonzalez JJ, et al. Improved survival in patients with acute myocarditis using external pulsatile mechanical ventricular assistance. *J Heart Lung Transplant* 1999;18:351–357.
38. Frazier OH, Benedict CR, Radovancevic B, et al. Improved left ventricular function after chronic left ventricular unloading. *Ann Thorac Surg* 1996;62:675–682.
39. Loebe M, Müller J, Hetzer R. Ventricular assistance for recovery of cardiac failure. *Curr Opin Cardiol* 1999;14:234–248.
40. Young JB. Healing the heart with ventricular assist device therapy: mechanisms of cardiac recovery. *Ann Thorac Surg* 2001;71:S210–S219.
41. Freilich M, Stub D, Esmore D, et al. Recovery from anthracycline cardiomyopathy after long-term support with a continuous flow left ventricular assist device. *J Heart Lung Transplant* 2009;28:101–103.
42. Farrar DJ, Holman WR, McBride LR, et al. Long-term follow-up of Thoratec ventricular assist device bridge-to-recovery patients successfully removed from support after recovery of ventricular function. *J Heart Lung Transplant* 2002;21:516–521.
43. Simon MA, Kormos RL, Murali S, et al. Myocardial recovery using ventricular assist devices: prevalence, clinical characteristics, and outcomes. *Circulation* 2005;112(suppl):132–136.
44. Williams MR, Oz MC. Indications and patient selection for mechanical ventricular assistance. *Ann Thorac Surg* 2001;71:S86–SS91.
45. Zakliczynski M, Maruszewski M, Pyka L, et al. Effectiveness and safety of treatment with sildenafil for secondary pulmonary hypertension in heart transplant candidates. *Transplant Proc* 2007;39:2856–2858.
46. Zimpfer D, Zrunek P, Sandner S, et al. Post-transplant survival after lowering fixed pulmonary hypertension using left ventricular assist devices. *Eur J Cardiothorac Surg* 2007;31:698–702.

47. Rao V, Slater JP, Edwards NM, et al. Surgical management of valvular disease in patients requiring left ventricular assist device support. *Ann Thorac Surg* 2001;71:1448–1453.

48. Slater JP, Williams M, Oz MC. Implantation techniques for the TCI HeartMate left ventricular assist systems. *Oper Tech Thorac Cardiovasc Surg* 1999;4: 330–344.

49. Vitali E, Russo C, Tiziano C, et al. Modified pericardial closure technique in patients with ventricular assist device. *Ann Thorac Surg* 2000;69:1278–1279.

50. Jaski BE, Lingle RJ, Kim J, et al. Comparison of functional capacity in patients with end-stage heart failure following implantation of a left ventricular assist device versus heart transplantation: results of the experience with left ventricular assist device with exercise trial. *J Heart Lung Transplant* 1999;18: 1031–1040.

51. Seemuth SC, Richenbacher WE. Education of the ventricular assist device patient's community services. *ASAIO J* 2001;47:596–601.

52. Gordon SM, Schmitt SK, Jacobs M, et al. Nosocomial bloodstream infections in patients with implantable left ventricular assist devices. *Ann Thorac Surg* 2001;72:725–730.

53. Tsau PH, Arabía FA, Toporoff B, et al. Positive panel reactive antibody titers in patients bridged to transplantation with a mechanical assist device. Risk factors and treatment. *ASAIO J* 1998;44:M634–M637.

54. Loh E, Bergin JD, Couper GS, et al. Role of panel-reactive antibody cross-reactivity in predicting survival after orthotopic heart transplantation. *J Heart Lung Transplant* 1994;13:194–201.

55. Oz MC, Levin HR, Rose EA. Technique for removal of left ventricular assist devices. *Ann Thorac Surg* 1994;58:257–258.

56. Blanche C, Blanche DA, Kearney B, et al. Heart transplantation in patients seventy years of age and older: a comparative analysis of outcome. *J Thorac Cardiovasc Surg* 2001;121:532–541.

57. Hosenpud JD, Bennett LE, Keck BM, et al. The Registry of the International Society for Heart and Lung Transplantation: eighteenth Official Report— 2001. *J Heart Lung Transplant* 2001;20:805–815.

58. Laks H, Scholl FG, Drinkwater DC, et al. The alternate recipient list for heart transplantation: does it work? *J Heart Lung Transplant* 1997;16:735–742.

59. Carrel T, Neth J, Mohacsi P, et al. Perioperative risk and long-term results of heart transplantation after previous cardiac operations. *Ann Thorac Surg* 1997;63:1133–1137.

61. Vouhé PR, Tamisier D, Le Bidois J, et al. Pediatric cardiac transplantation for congenital heart defects: surgical considerations and results. *Ann Thorac Surg* 1993;56:1239–1247.

62. Renlund DG, Taylor DO, Kfoury A, et al. New UNOS rules: historical background and implications for transplantation management. United Network for Organ Sharing. *J Heart Lung Transplant* 1999;18:1065–1070.

63. Chen JM, Weinberg AD, Rose EA, et al. Multivariate analysis of factors affecting waiting time to heart transplantation. *Ann Thorac Surg* 1996;61: 570–575.

64. Kauffman HM, McBride MA, Shield CF, et al. Determinants of waiting time for heart transplants in the United States. *J Heart Lung Transplant* 1999; 18:414–419.

65. Brock MV, Salazar JD, Cameron DE, et al. The changing profile of the cardiac donor. *J Heart Lung Transplant* 2001;20:1005–1009.

66. Morley D, Boigon M, Fesniak H, et al. Posttransplantation hemodynamics and exercise function are not affected by body-size matching of donor and recipient. *J Heart Lung Transplant* 1993;12:770–778.

67. Gilbert EM, Krueger SK, Murray JL. Echocardiographic evaluation of potential cardiac transplant donors. *J Thorac Cardiovasc Surg* 1988;95:1003–1007.

68. Hauptman PJ, O'Connor KJ, Wolf RE, et al. Angiography of potential cardiac donors. *JACC* 2001;37:1252–1258.

69. Wheeldon DR, Potter CDO, Oduro A, et al. Transforming the "unacceptable" donor: outcomes from the adoption of a standardized donor management technique. *J Heart Lung Transplant* 1995;14:734–742.

70. Holmquist M, Chabalewski F, Blount T, et al. A critical pathway: guiding care for organ donors. *Crit Care Nurse* 1999;19:84–98.

71. Zaroff JG, Rosengard BR, Armstrong WF, et al. Consensus conference report: maximizing use of organs recovered from the cadaver donor: cardiac recommendations. *Circulation* 2002;106:836–841.

72. Jahania MS, Sanchez JA, Narayan P, et al. Heart preservation for transplantation: principles and strategies. *Ann Thorac Surg* 1999;68:1983–1987.

73. Hinkamp TJ, Montoya A, Bakhos M, et al. Heart and lung grafts harvested en bloc: operative technique, utilization, and results. *Ann Thorac Surg* 1993;56:1381–1385.

74. Bolman RM III. Heart transplantation technique. *Oper Tech Thorac Cardiovasc Surg* 1999;4:98–113.

75. Brandt M, Harringer W, Hirt SW, et al. Influence of bicaval anastomoses on late occurrence of atrial arrhythmia after heart transplantation. *Ann Thorac Surg* 1997;64:70–72.

76. Aziz TM, Burgess MI, El-Gamel A, et al. Orthotopic cardiac transplantation technique: a survey of current practice. *Ann Thorac Surg* 1999;68:1242–1246.

77. Weiss ES, Nwakanma LU, Russell SB, et al. Outcomes in bicaval versus biatrial techniques in heart transplantation: an analysis of the UNOS database. *J Heart Lung Transplant* 2008;27:178–183.

78. Schnoor M, Schäfer T, Lühmann D, et al. Bicaval versus standard technique in orthotopic heart transplantation: a systematic review and meta-analysis. *J Thorac Cardiovasc Surg* 2007;134:1322–1331.

79. Bittner HB, Chen EP, Biswas SS, et al. Right ventricular dysfunction after cardiac transplantation: primarily related to status of donor heart. *Ann Thorac Surg* 1999;69:1605–1611.

80. Carrier M, Blaise G, Bélisle S, et al. Nitric oxide inhalation in the treatment of primary graft failure following heart transplantation. *J Heart Lung Transplant* 1999;18:664–667.

81. Taghavi S, Zuckermann A, Ankersmit J, et al. Extracorporeal membrane oxygenation is superior to right ventricular assist device for acute right ventricular failure after heart transplantation. *Ann Thorac Surg* 2004;78:1644–1649.

82. Arpesella G, Loforte A, Mikus E, et al. Extracorporeal membrane oxygenation for primary allograft failure. *Transplant Proc* 2008;40:3596–3597.

83. Marasco SF, Esmore DS, Negri J, et al. Early institution of mechanical support improves outcomes in primary cardiac allograft failure. *J Heart Lung Transplant* 2005;24:2037–2042.

84. Morris CD, Vega JD, Levy JH, et al. Warfarin therapy does not increase bleeding in patients undergoing heart transplantation. *Ann Thorac Surg* 2001;72:714–718.

85. Jahania MS, Mullett TW, Sanchez JA, et al. Acute allograft failure in thoracic organ transplantation. *J Cardiac Surg* 2000;15:122–128.
86. Rubin RH. Prevention and treatment of cytomegalovirus disease in heart transplant patients. *J Heart Lung Transplant* 2000;19:731–735.
87. Holliman RE, Johnson JD, Adams S, et al. Toxoplasmosis and heart transplantation. *J Heart Transplant* 1991;10:608–610.
88. McGoon MD, Frantz RP. Techniques of immunosuppression after cardiac transplantation. *Mayo Clin Proc* 1992;67:586–595.
89. Taylor DO, Olsen SL, Renlund DG. State of the art immunosuppressive regimens: routine and rescue. *Coronary Artery Dis* 1992;3:806–816.
90. Almenar L, Rueda J, Osa A, et al. Incidence of side effects of immunosuppressants commonly used in heart transplantation. *Transplant Proc* 1999;31:2519–2521.
91. John R, Rajasinghe HA, Chen JM, et al. Long-term outcomes after cardiac transplantation: an experience based on different eras of immunosuppressive therapy. *Ann Thorac Surg* 2001;72:440–449.
92. Beniaminovitz A, Itescu S, Lietz K, et al. Prevention of rejection in cardiac transplantation by blockade of the interleukin-2 receptor with a monoclonal antibody. *N Engl J Med* 2000;342:613–619.
93. Braith RW, Edwards DG. Exercise following heart transplantation. *Sports Med* 2000;30:171–192.
94. Cremer J, Strüber M, Wagenbreth I, et al. Progression of steroid-associated osteoporosis after heart transplantation. *Ann Thorac Surg* 1999;67:130–133.
95. Fellström B. Impact and management of hyperlipidemia posttransplantation. *Transplantation* 2000;70:SS51–SS57.
96. Kubo SH, Naftel DC, Mills RM Jr, et al. Risk factors for late recurrent rejection after heart transplantation: a multiinstitutional, multivariable analysis. *J Heart Lung Transplant* 1995;14:409–418.
97. Billingham ME, Cary NRB, Hammond ME, et al. A working formulation for the standardization of nomenclature in the diagnosis of heart and lung rejection. *J Heart Lung Transplant* 1992;11:1116–1124.
98. Fishman JA, Rubin RH. Infection in organ-transplant recipients. *N Engl J Med* 1998;338:1741–1751.
99. Kwok BW, Hunt SA. Neoplasia after heart transplantation. *Cardiol Rev* 2000;8:256–259.
100. Weis M, von Scheidt W. Coronary artery disease in the transplanted heart. *Annu Rev Med* 2000;51:81–100.
101. McGiffin DC, Savunen T, Kirklin JK, et al. Cardiac transplant coronary artery disease. A multivariable analysis of pretransplantation risk factors for disease development and morbid events. *J Thorac Cardiovasc Surg* 1995;109:1081–1089.
102. Srivastava R, Keck BM, Bennett LE, et al. The results of cardiac retransplantation: an analysis of the Joint International Society for Heart and Lung Transplantation/United Network for Organ Sharing Thoracic Registry. *Transplantation* 2000;70:606–612.

Note: Page numbers followed by f refer to figures and those followed by t refer to tables.

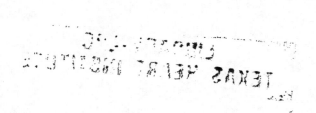